D0842840

Cost-Effectiveness in Health and Medicine

Cost-Effectiveness in Health and Medicine

Edited by

MARTHE R. GOLD
U.S. Public Health Service

JOANNA E. SIEGEL
U.S. Public Health Service

LOUISE B. RUSSELL
Rutgers University

MILTON C. WEINSTEIN
Harvard University

New York   Oxford
OXFORD UNIVERSITY PRESS
1996

Oxford University Press

Oxford   New York
Athens   Auckland   Bangkok   Bombay
Calcutta   Cape Town   Dar es Salaam   Delhi
Florence   Hong Kong   Istanbul   Karachi
Kuala Lumpur   Madras   Madrid   Melbourne
Mexico City   Nairobi   Paris   Singapore
Taipei   Tokyo   Toronto

and associated companies in
Berlin   Ibadan

Published by Oxford University Press, Inc.,
198 Madison Avenue, New York, New York 10016

Oxford is a registered trademark of Oxford University Press

Library of Congress Cataloging-in-Publication Data
Cost-effectiveness in health and medicine /
edited by Marthe R. Gold . . . [et al.].
p. cm.   Includes index.
ISBN 0-19-510824-8
1. Medical care—Cost effectiveness—Research—Methodology.
I. Gold, Marthe R.
[DNLM: 1 Cost-Benefit Analysis.
2. Health Care Costs.
W 74   C8415 1996]   RA410.5.C688   1996
338.4'33621—dc20   DNLM/DLC for Library of Congress   96-4753

9 8 7 6 5

Printed in the United States of America
on acid-free paper

Foreword

Two realities provide compelling context to health policy decisions in a world preparing for the twenty-first century: The availability of health-related interventions now in the marketplace exceeds by a considerable margin our societal ability to afford them; and current decision rules are inadequate to guide choices toward those interventions that are likely to yield the most benefit for the population. In the abstract, these are not new developments. People have long sought cures for ailments using a variety of methods, settings, and caregivers. The assortment of approaches has been fed by uncertainties about the nature and treatment of illness. Although on an individual basis cost may have had significant implications for which therapies people chose, aggregate spending on health care has been of little concern historically.

But things have changed, with respect both to the reliability and to the costs of available interventions. Until relatively recently, the notion of efficacy was frequently left to anecdote, at least as much a function of the salesmanship of the purveyor as of any salutary effect of the therapy. Medical science has rapidly progressed in this century to the point that many interventions succeed at a predictable level of reliability. High blood pressure can be controlled, coronary arteries can be cleared, colon cancers can be removed, degenerated joints can be replaced, severed limbs can be reattached, kidneys can be transplanted. These are genuine advances that offer real improvements for the individuals concerned.

They come with a price. In the United States, each coronary bypass procedure costs nearly $50,000; a kidney transplant is $70,000. And these prices do not count the cost of diagnosis. The major expansions over the last generation in health care technology, and its costs, have come on the diagnostic side, with rapid growth in the costs of laboratory tests and imaging procedures.

The nature of the purchase and payment mechanisms has served as a prod to the growth of the health care industry. The traffic in commodities in the marketplace generally operates according to the normal laws of supply and demand. People come to some understanding of what they need and want, and budget accordingly. But, unlike food, clothing, shelter, or other consumable goods and services, health care needs are for the most part neither predictable nor discretionary.

Hence, insurance has been widely applied as a social instrument to distribute the burden of payment more evenly across time for individuals, and more equitably across sectors of the population. This has given the service provider primary responsibility for the number and types of services purchased. Both professional and economic incentives have worked to the expansion of those services, to the point that between 1965 and 1995, the share of the U.S. gross domestic product devoted to health care grew from 5% to 15%; more than $1 trillion dollars was spent in 1995.

Investments of this magnitude prompt questions as to the nature of the returns. Those questions take on greater urgency in the face of what appears to be a widening gap between investments in treating diseases and investments in preventing those diseases from occurring in the first place.

Medical care has been surprisingly limited in its ability to alter the national health profile. Available estimates generally indicate that medical care has been accountable for only about 10% to 15% of the declines in premature deaths that have occurred in this century—the remainder attributable to factors that have helped prevent illness and injury from occurring. This suggests that the promise implicit in many technological interventions may exceed their ability to deliver genuine health gains, at least on a population-wide basis. However, they certainly consume resources. Ninety-nine percent of health expenditures in the United States goes to individually targeted medical care, leaving little for public health and prevention programs that bring benefit to the entire population.

Despite mounting evidence that preventive measures can effectively reduce morbidity and mortality due to many conditions, including heart disease, stroke, diabetes, injuries, many cancers, and pneumonia, prevention has found itself at a competitive disadvantage for time and for money. Attention falls naturally to acute concerns, as opposed to those that can be put off for the moment. In general, the tendency of those allocating resources has been to consider preventive services and population-based interventions as non-essential and to require evidence of their potential to generate cost savings, prior to considerations of providing funding for them. This approach diverts attention from a fundamental policy question: What are the most efficient methods of creating health for Americans?

From the perspective of a societal aim of maximizing the years of healthy life gained for its population in return for a given level of investment, it makes little sense to use one set of standards to assess preventive interventions and a different set to assess therapeutic interventions. Rather, approaches are needed that rely upon more informed and more comparable data—approaches that provide all candidate interventions a level playing field and that carefully investigate which investments will yield the greatest payoff for the health of the nation. The issue cannot only be whether an intervention accomplishes what it sets out to do. It must also be how efficiently it works and how it compares to other potential interventions in improving society's health status.

The challenges of predicting returns on investments are difficult in any field. In most sectors of commerce a reliable predictive model requires an accurate notion of the cost of production of goods or services, the level of demand, how the demand will fluctuate with price, and how the price will fluctuate with competition. But health care investments are qualitatively different from other goods and services. The stakeholders are not merely investors purchasing stocks. They are individuals seeking good health prospects, employers seeking a productive work force, taxpayers seeking equitable access for vulnerable populations to needed services. The anticipated returns are therefore assessed in different ways and in different time frames. Rather than profit margins registered at quarterly intervals, the returns take form in terms of actual or anticipated health status at various points on a time horizon that may extend out many years. Even the investment side of the equation may look different, as costs incurred may include factors other than money spent on an intervention—for example, time required for the intervention, or an undesired side effect that carries its own costs.

The analytic complications that have resulted because of efforts to address these differences have introduced a high degree of variability into the conduct of analyses designed to estimate returns on investments in health. For example, screening for breast cancer has been variously estimated to save money, and to cost amounts ranging from $3,000 up to $80,000 per year of life gained. These discrepancies stem from different approaches taken in creating economic analyses.

The lack of a common set of techniques in cost-effectiveness analysis has restrained the applicability of these studies in a policy context. As it sought an affordable means to ensure health insurance coverage of all its' citizens, the state of Oregon attempted to use cost-effectiveness as a tool to decide how to prioritize services for coverage. This bold effort to implement a policy that required explicit examination of what services Oregonians would and would not be willing to pay for fell victim to both political and methodologic factors. We are still in the early stages of exploring what our society will sanction with respect to the explicit rationing of health care services, but the Oregon experiment was criticized as much for its lack of methodologic rigor as it was for the difficult ethical questions it raised. The data upon which to create a ranking of interventions based on their relative cost-effectiveness were simply unavailable, and the methods employed were inadequate to the task.

This book, a report of a U.S. Public Health Service–appointed expert panel, makes an important contribution toward improving the methods of cost-effectiveness analysis. The overarching goal for this work has been to move the field forward so that over the next decade, state and federal decision makers will have access to robust information with respect to the true cost per health effect gained for the continuum of health-related interventions—be they preventive, palliative, curative, or rehabilitative.

The Panel on Cost Effectiveness in Health and Medicine was charged with assessing the state of the science in cost-effectiveness analysis; with identifying methodologic inconsistencies and fragilities in the technique; with fostering consensus, where possible, with respect to standardizing the conduct of studies; and with proposing steps that can be taken to address remaining issues and uncertainties in the methodology. The authors of this report have recognized that in order for cost-effectiveness studies to be useful they must be made comparable to one another through agreement on a common set of standards.

The panel has addressed this need for standardization by outlining an explicit set of recommendations for use in a *Reference Case analysis*. A Reference Case analysis will provide important reassurance to decision makers in government and in industry—reassurance that the results of different cost-effectiveness analyses can be meaningfully compared to one another.

To arrive at the recommendations for a Reference Case analysis, the panel members showed an uncommon openness to accommodating the many intellectual traditions that converge in cost-effectiveness methodology, bridging the perspectives of economics, decision analysis, outcome measurement, clinical medicine, and ethics. Often the authors were required to return to their parent disciplines in order to examine underlying theory so that seemingly irreconcilable differences could in fact be reconciled. The panel's efforts to forge consensus have resulted in an important document that is certain to move the field forward.

A final point bears making here. Improvements in the quality and comparability of cost-effectiveness analyses do not in themselves provide the answer to how, as a society, we should allocate resources in pursuit of health. As the panel takes care to point out, cost-effectiveness analyses provide information which can help locate the tradeoffs associated with different decisions, but these studies do not in themselves make decisions. Stronger methodology assures only that our information is more reliable. The difficult decisions as to how we use this information lie ahead.

J. Michael McGinnis, M.D.
Assistant Surgeon General (ret.)
Scholar-in-residence, National Academy of Sciences

Acknowledgments

This book and the project from which it arose have benefitted from the interest and contributions of many people. Michael McGinnis, who directed the Office of Disease Prevention and Health Promotion from 1978–1995, provided vision and support for this work. Steve Teutsch, of the Centers for Disease Control and Prevention prodded us at every turn toward public health and pragmatism. Martin Brown of the National Cancer Institute, and Larry Braslow and Laurie Burke of the Food and Drug Administration, through their active participation in panel discussions and their careful review of manuscripts, provided important insights with respect to methodology, as well as to political process. Alison Kelly and Anne Haddix of the Centers for Disease Control and Prevention and Aaron Stinnett of Harvard University devoted tremendous effort to implementing the panel's recommendations in the analyses they prepared for this book, a task made more difficult by the shifting sands beneath the final Reference Case recommendations. Peter Franks of the University of Rochester, Ted Ganiats and Robert Kaplan of the University of California, San Diego, and Alan Williams, of the University of York, gave guidance in the development of values for health states for use in the worked examples. Bernie O'Brien of McMaster University graciously shared his work-in-progress on uncertainty during an early meeting of the panel. Joan Rivera, Director of the HARMET project (The Harmonisation by Consensus of the Methodology for Economic Evaluation of Health Technologies in the European Union), provided careful review of a major portion of the manuscript. Mollie McEvoy and Dale Kasab contributed diligent coordination and recording of panel meetings.

Many others, from academia and from government, contributed thoughtful review of earlier drafts of the manuscript and the recommendations. In many instances, their insights resulted in the reopening of discussion, the redrafting of language, and, ultimately, the recrafting of recommendations. Their names appear below.

Finally, the tireless research, coordination, and editorial eye provided by Kristine McCoy were critical to the production of this volume.

Our thanks to all.

Federal Reviewers

Katy Benjamin, S.M., M.S.W., *Agency for Health Care Policy and Research*, Ed Brann, M.D., M.P.H., *Centers for Disease Control and Prevention,* Larry Braslow, Ph.D., *Food and Drug Administration,* Martin Brown, Ph.D., *National Institutes of Health,* Laurie Burke, M.P.H., *Food and Drug Administration,* William S. Cartwright, Ph.D., *Substance Abuse and Mental Health Services Administration,* Paul Farnham, Ph.D., *Centers for Disease Control and Prevention,* Robin D. Gorsky, Ph.D. (deceased), *Centers for Disease Control and Prevention,* Anne Haddix, Ph.D., *Centers for Disease Control and Prevention,* William Harlan, M.D., *National Institutes of Health,* Tom Hodgson, Ph.D., *Centers for Disease Control and Prevention,* Mary Jansen, Ph.D., *Substance Abuse and Mental Services Administration,* Arnold Potosky, Ph.D., M.H.S., *National Institutes of Health,* Elaine Power, M.P.P., (formerly at) *Office of Technology Assessment, U.S. Congress,* Dixie E. Snider, Jr., M.D., M.P.H., *Centers for Disease Control and Prevention,* Steve Teutsch, M.D., M.P.H., *Centers for Disease Control and Prevention,* and Judith Wagner, Ph.D., (formerly at) *Office of Technology Assessment, U.S. Congress.*

Outside Reviewers

Donald Berwick, M.D., M.P.P., *Institute for Healthcare Improvement,* Scott B. Cantor, Ph.D., *University of Texas,* Allan S. Detsky, M.D., Ph.D., F.R.C.P.C., *University of Toronto, Canada,* Michael Drummond, D.Phil., *University of York, Great Britain,* Floyd J. Fowler, Jr., Ph.D., *University of Massachusetts,* Daniel M. Fox, Ph.D., *Milbank Memorial Fund,* Peter Franks, M.D., *University of Rochester,* Deborah Freund, Ph.D., M.P.H., *Indiana University,* John Graham, Ph.D., *Harvard School of Public Health,* James Hammitt, Ph.D., *Harvard School of Public Health,* Robert M. Kaplan, Ph.D., *University of California (San Diego),* Emmett Keeler, Ph.D., *RAND Corporation,* Robert Lawrence, M.D., *Johns Hopkins School of Hygiene and Public Health,* Hilary Llewellyn-Thomas, Ph.D., *University of Toronto, Canada,* Kathleen N. Lohr, Ph.D., *Institute of Medicine, Washington, D.C.,* John Mullahy, Ph.D., *Trinity College (CT),* Robert Nease, Jr., Ph.D., *Washington University,* Duncan Neuhauser, Ph.D., *Case Western Reserve University,* Erik Nord, Ph.D., *National Institute of Public Health, Oslo, Norway,* Bernard O'Brien, Ph.D., *McMaster University, Canada,* Stephen Pauker, M.D., *New England Medical Center,* Joan Rovira, Ph.D., *University of Barcelona, Spain,* Frans Rutten, Ph.D., *Erasmus University, The Netherlands,* Kevin Schulman, M.D., *Georgetown University Medical Center,* Donald S. Shepard, Ph.D., *Brandeis University,* Harri Sintonen, Ph.D., *University of Kuopio, Finland,* Jane E. Sisk, Ph.D., *Columbia University School of Public Health,* Tammy Tengs, Sc.D., *Duke University,* Anna Tosteson, Sc.D., *Dartmouth Medical School,* Alan Williams, Ph.D., *University of York, Great Britain,* Nancy Wolff, Ph.D., *Rutgers University,* and Steven H. Woolf, M.D., M.P.H., *Medical College of Virginia.*

Contents

List of Contributors

Panel Members

NORMAN DANIELS, Ph.D.
Tufts University

DENNIS G. FRYBACK, Ph.D.
University of Wisconsin, Madison

ALAN M. GARBER, M.D., Ph.D.
Department of Veterans Affairs and
    Stanford University

DAVID C. HADORN, M.D., M.A.
Ministry of Health
New Zealand

MARK S. KAMLET, Ph.D.
Carnegie Mellon University

JOSEPH LIPSCOMB, Ph.D.
Duke University

BRYAN R. LUCE, Ph.D.
MEDTAP International

JEANNE S. MANDELBLATT,
    M.D., M.P.H.
Georgetown University

WILLARD G. MANNING, Jr.,
    Ph.D.
University of Minnesota

DONALD L. PATRICK, Ph.D.
University of Washington

Panel Co-Chair

LOUISE B. RUSSELL, Ph.D.
Rutgers University

GEORGE W. TORRANCE, Ph.D.
McMaster University

Panel Co-Chair

MILTON C. WEINSTEIN, Ph.D.
Harvard University

PHS Staff

MARTHE R. GOLD, M.D., M.P.H.*

KRISTINE I. McCOY, M.P.H.

JOANNA E. SIEGEL, Sc.D.*

* This work was conducted while Drs. Gold and Siegel were on leave respectively from the University of Rochester and Harvard University.

Introduction

This book summarizes the discussions and recommendations of the Panel on Cost-Effectiveness in Health and Medicine, a group of 13 non-government scientists and scholars with expertise in cost-effectiveness analysis (CEA). Convened by the U.S. Public Health Service in 1993, the panel was charged with assessing the current state-of-the-science of the field and with providing recommendations for conduct of studies in order to improve their quality and encourage their comparability. The panel's creation was motivated by (1) the keen interest of the Public Health Service (PHS) in using CEAs to enhance perspectives for health-related decisions and by (2) its accompanying discomfort with the variability of the range of techniques used in these analyses. The burgeoning of this form of economic analysis creates an opportunity to rationalize health policy, but only if the technique and its applications are well understood and implemented.

Over the past decade, as pressures to control health care spending have accelerated, the term ''cost-effective'' has come increasingly into common parlance. Its usage by groups as disparate as the Congress, the business community, managed-care organizations, the pharmaceutical industry, and the press is insufficiently precise, however, to provide guidance to the many who might use the information generated by a cost-effectiveness analysis in improving the quality and efficiency of the health care system.

Imprecision comes, in part, from the manner in which CEA methodology has arisen over the past three decades. Developers of the field and analysts who apply its methods come from a number of academic disciplines, including economics, medicine, operations research, medical sociology, psychology, public health, and ethics. Each brings a particular set of concepts and a unique language that have been melded in the building of the technique. In addition, the related method of cost-benefit analysis (CBA) shares enough common features with CEA so that the intertwining of these methodologies has found its way into many analyses, leading to difficulties in conceptualizing the separate tasks.

The imprecision attached to the term ''cost-effective'' stems also from the variety of masters the concept serves. Purchasers of health care use the term to convey a careful assessment of the relative value of different health care services; producers of health care technologies and programs use the idea to support marketing claims; advocates for particular illnesses or constituencies use the term to garner resource investments. All of these parties are agreeing to the notion of value for money that is connoted by the term, and this notion does allow for common conceptual ground to be found. However, notions of what is cost-effective held by the pharmaceutical industry, by managed-care organizations, or by other participants in the health care system may well be at variance with each other, or with what is thought of as cost-effective by society at large.

The central purpose of CEA is to compare the relative value of different interventions in creating better health and/or longer life. The results of such evaluations are typically summarized in a cost-effectiveness ratio, where the denominator reflects the gain in health from a candidate intervention (measured, for example, in terms of years of life gained, premature births averted, sight years gained) and the numerator reflects the cost of obtaining that health gain. A cost-effectiveness analysis provides information that can help decision makers sort through alternatives and decide which ones best serve their programmatic and financial needs. Decision makers may be federal, state, or local. They may be in the private sector or the public sector. They may control dollars or they may run programs. CEA provides a framework within which decision makers may pose a range of questions.

Information from the CEA Framework

Cost-effectiveness analyses furnish information that can be useful in a variety of settings. For example, a managed-care organization might wish to know the cost per low-birthweight birth averted as a consequence of a prenatal outreach program. Or it might wish to take the question further and ask the cost of this program per year of life saved for its enrolled population. Or, recognizing that programs that avert premature births may not primarily save lives but rather avert disability over the lifetime of an individual, it might want to know the cost of this intervention for each quality-adjusted life year (QALY) gained. This latter question is addressed by a particular type of CEA, sometimes termed ''cost utility analysis,'' where adjustments for the value assigned to health-related quality of life are built into the calculation.

As another example, a pharmaceutical manufacturer might wish to use CEA in pricing and marketing a new cholesterol-lowering drug. It might ask the question, How much does our medication cost per year of life gained compared to a similar product manufactured by a different company? Or, if clinical trials show clinically insignificant changes in cholesterol level between the two products but significantly decreased side effects associated with the new drug, a drug purchaser or payer might wish then to calculate the cost per QALY gained in using the new drug. An industry investigator might decide to extend the considerations of the analysis and explore the cost per year of life or QALY gained when comparing pharmaceutical treatment with surgical treatment for coronary artery disease.

Or, an analysis for a state health department might wish to explore different strategies for control of blood lead levels in the population. It might choose to assess the cost-effectiveness of screening all children, compared to screening only those thought to be

at particular risk for elevated lead levels by reason of housing or environmental sur-
roundings. The study might frame the question in a larger context by asking what the
cost per case of high blood lead level averted would be using an educational intervention
to reduce household dust and peeling paint, rather than any kind of clinical intervention.
Or the analysis might draw its boundaries even wider by comparing the cost per QALY
gained of either of these blood lead level treatment programs to the cost per QALY
gained of a program that improves the nutrition of school-age children.

The conduct of particular studies may be constrained by lack of required information
on the effectiveness of the interventions being compared, their impact on health-related
quality of life, and their costs—but the answers to all of the questions posed above—
can, in theory, be determined by using the methods of cost-effectiveness analysis. In
cases where primary or secondary data are unavailable or inconclusive (e.g., a therapy
has been shown to have an effect in one population, but the CEA is being conducted
on a different population for whom the benefit may differ) CEAs must rely on explicitly
described assumptions and models that can be examined for credibility.

In addition to addressing each of the above cases in isolation, it is useful to be able
to make comparisons across health interventions. Ultimately, health care resources are
finite and comparisons of cost-effectiveness across health interventions can provide
important information about how health care resources might be allocated in the most
effective and efficient manner. Ideally, one would wish to be able to array all CEAs on
a "league table," where cost per health effect gained using one intervention is assessed
side by side with the cost per health effect gained using others. Comparisons of this
sort would allow decision makers to understand the relative efficiencies of different
health investments. Closer appraisal of effective interventions that are costly per health
effect gained can suggest approaches for improving their efficiency or alternative strategies for maximizing health for the resources invested. Although cost-effectiveness is
but one element of public decisions about health care, gaining a clearer quantitative
understanding of this important element cannot help but improve decision processes.

A number of problems currently interfere with the broadest use of CEAs in informing
larger health care resource allocation decisions. These difficulties are detailed throughout this book, but we note two at the outset because of their overarching importance.

First, the perspective taken by an individual CEA will determine the final ratio of
cost per health effect. When managed-care organizations or the Health Care Financing
Administration (HCFA) use their own perspective in a CEA, they consider the costs
they will experience in producing or arranging for medical care for subscribers and
beneficiaries. The costs that a patient bears, such as help required at home as a consequence of early hospital discharge, or medication that allows outpatient management
of an illness, are not relevant to that perspective. Although the costs are real, they are
borne elsewhere. On the effect side, it is not relevant to a managed-care organization
or to the government (as a payor for health care services) how rapidly, or indeed if, an
enrollee can return to work, although it may make a great deal of difference to the
insured, their employers, or even another government agency from whose coffers the

disability payments must come. At present, not only are differing perspectives used, but many CEAs do not articulate a perspective, or do not follow the implications of that perspective fully in their analyses.

Second, the measure of outcome used in an analysis determines whether the analysis can be considered alongside other CEAs conducted on different interventions. For example, while from the perspective of a state health department it may be useful to calculate the cost per case of acquired immune-deficiency syndrome (AIDS) prevented by one program when compared to another AIDS prevention program, that analysis would not furnish useful information regarding the relative value of a program that calculated its benefit in cost per case of high blood pressure controlled. Current measures of effect vary from highly specific information particular to specific conditions (e.g., millimeters of mercury decrease in blood pressure) to the broader, but still non-comparable, outcomes, years of life and quality-adjusted life years gained.

Differences in perspective or measures of effect do not pose a problem when studies are used to address the specific issues that motivated them, but they do prevent the broader comparisons across studies that could help inform larger issues of resource allocation for health care. Thus an important potential for cost-effectiveness studies has yet to be realized.

It is important to note, however, the limitations of even the most exactingly created cost-effectiveness analyses. Resource allocation decisions can never be shaped by the mechanical ranking of cost-effectiveness ratios. Ratios provide information about one type of ''value,'' health benefit per dollar spent. But other values of society, including considerations of distributive justice and fairness (e.g., giving priority at times to the sickest of individuals) require that CEA be viewed as an informer of decision making rather than a decision maker per se.

The Reference Case

In seeking to improve comparability of CEAs designed to inform decision making more broadly, while allowing analysts the flexibility to design studies that answer issues specific to a particular problem or industry, the panel proposes the use of a Reference Case. The Reference Case is a standard set of methodologic practices that an analyst would seek to follow in a cost-effectiveness study. These suggested practices are outlined in recommendations as they arise from the discussions within the individual chapters. A summary of the recommendations, together with the rationales that support them is found in Appendix A. For example, recommendations for the perspective and the health effect measure for use in a Reference Case analysis flow from discussions contained respectively in chapters on roles and limitations of CEA (Chapter 1) and on valuing and measuring outcomes (Chapter 4).

Although an investigator might well choose to include other cases in a study with assumptions and methods that differ from those in the Reference Case (in order to best serve the purpose of the analysis), the Reference Case would serve as a point of comparison across studies. The results for the Reference Case in any two studies could then be compared with confidence that the comparison is an appropriate one. The larger the number of CEAs that include a Reference Case, the larger the number of meaningful comparisons. Thus each study contributes to a pool of information about the broad allocation of resources as well as to the specific questions it was designed to address.

The inclusion of a Reference Case in an analysis should not be construed as a requirement for performing a valid CEA. Nor does adherence to Reference Case recommendations mean that a study fulfills the needs of its primary audience. CEA is a technique that can legitimately serve many needs. There will be some situations in which the primary purpose of an analysis is a confined comparison of simple alternatives, so a Reference Case will then be of only secondary interest. At the other end of the continuum, an analyst may seek to compare interventions that cross sectors, for example, into environment and food safety, and CEA may not in fact be the appropriate form of economic analysis. To try to include a Reference Case in these circumstances might lead the analysis too far from its primary purpose. In a number of situations, however, the analyst may want to contribute to the larger body of information on cost-effectiveness of health care programs, or, indeed, that may be the primary purpose of the analysis. Since comparability with other studies is critical for this purpose, the analyst will want to include a Reference Case.

In crafting the recommendations for a Reference Case, the panel sometimes disagreed about the best advice to give. When the disagreement involved a major aspect of the analysis, and guidance from theory or the current state of work in the field did not point clearly to a single answer, the relevant recommendation narrows choices and offers options. For some analyses, the requirements of the study audience may dictate that analysts pursue only one of these options. In other cases, the panel decided to settle on a single recommendation, but the recommendation is not regarded as "right" in an absolute sense. Instead, the panel agreed that comparability was sufficiently important that a consensus recommendation was needed. In addition to defining a Reference Case, the panel offers a number of recommendations to help build the CEA methodology. These recommendations outline a research agenda intended to advance the field and lead, over time, to continued refinements in the Reference Case.

Audience, Boundaries, and Content of the Report

This text is directed primarily at those who conduct, or who direct the conduct, of CEAs. It is not a "how-to-do it" manual; rather it provides an overview of the state of the field and a discussion of the component methods used in CEA in a manner that should be accessible to persons with some familiarity with CEA. Because these analyses have many different technical aspects built from extensive theoretical and operational literatures of their comprising disciplines, a number of issues cannot be dealt with in depth. Instead, references are given so that the reader may pursue details elsewhere.

This book should also prove useful to those who wish to evaluate CEAs critically. While parts of the chapters provide in-depth discussion of technical areas, the recommendations are designed to be accessible to people who wish simply to be sophisticated consumers of these studies. We anticipate that it should therefore be of use to managed care organizations, insurers, health departments, and state and federal policy makers.

We bound the considerations within this document to the application of CEA methods to interventions that occur within the medical care and public health sectors, including medical technologies, pharmaceuticals, and clinical and population-based prevention. This is, we acknowledge, an arbitrary bounding of both interventions and economic analysis techniques. Certainly there are many strategies occurring in a variety of arenas ranging from environment to agriculture to education that make highly significant and efficient contributions to health. There are also other methods available for evaluating economic impact. Two major factors, one philosophical and the other pragmatic, motivate this drawing of the line at CEAs conducted in the health sector.

First, the health sector has traditionally favored economic analyses that assess cost per unit of health effect, resisting the use of the closely associated technique of cost-benefit analysis (CBA), where both costs and effects of programs and interventions are valued in dollars. A number of ethical difficulties ranging from the macro issue of what constitutes fairness in allocation of resources, to more micro issues, such as the effect of valuing the time people spend pursuing medical treatment according to their wages, are already embedded in CEA. CBA adds an additional difficulty in that it presumes to put a dollar figure on the value of human life and uses controversial methods to do so. The panel has shared the dominant bias of the health sector—that monetizing the price of life in these ways introduces ethical concerns that are avoided by CEA, albeit at some sacrifice of generalizability.

Second, as the stalwart reader will discover, this volume discusses a host of technical issues that a long history of scientific inquiry has not yet settled. Cost-benefit analysis's primary valuation method is *willingness to pay* (WTP), an approach whose difficulty lies in its intrinsic favoring of the programs and diseases of the affluent over those of the poor. Until more widely accepted ways to compensate for the inherent discrepancies in health purchases that differential wealth will confer become available, the technical problems of basing a Reference Case economic analysis on CBA remain formidable. This is a field of active research, however, and subsequent developments here may influence the future viability of CBA for analyses in the health field.

Because CBA is the dominant form of economic evaluation used to assess health-producing interventions in other sectors, we acknowledge that certain opportunities to compare the efficiency of competing interventions in the production of health are lost by our emphasis on CEA. This is particularly true in public health, where many of the interventions share at least as much common ground with other sectors as they do with

clinical medicine. We have tried, therefore, to make bridges within this document between the techniques of CEA and CBA: The need to cross sectors when considering
best value in the production of health will only increase in the future.

This book presents the results of the panel's deliberations. The panel met 11 times
over a 2½-year period. Once the agenda was determined, Panel members and staff
drafted papers on the major topics and controversies in different aspects of cost-effectiveness analysis. Each paper presented the salient issues for that topic and suggested
specific recommendations that were debated by panel members in successive meetings
until some form of consensus was reached, and in a few cases, until it became clear
that consensus could not be reached. In areas where consensus was particularly difficult,
or was in fact elusive, text was revised in order to lay out the arguments on each side
of the discussion. Methodologists from relevant PHS and HCFA activities served as
liaisons to this process throughout and together with the academic community have
reviewed and helped shape this work.

The book consists of nine chapters addressing, in turn: the roles and limitations of
CEA; its theoretical foundations; how to frame an analysis; identifying and valuing the
outcomes of programs; estimating effectiveness; estimating costs: discounting future
effects and costs; evaluating the uncertainty of study results; and reporting results. A
final section presents two "worked examples" in which we perform, in essence, a
reality check on what we have recommended. We hope that this volume will prove as
useful and stimulating to its audience as the discussions from which it was formed were
to its drafters.

The Editors

Cost-Effectiveness
in Health
and Medicine

1

Cost-Effectiveness Analysis as a Guide to Resource Allocation in Health: Roles and Limitations

L.B. RUSSELL, J.E. SIEGEL, N. DANIELS,
M.R. GOLD, B.R. LUCE and J.S. MANDELBLATT

Cost-effectiveness analysis (CEA) is a method used to evaluate the outcomes and costs of interventions designed to improve health. It has been used to compare costs and years of life gained for such interventions as screening for breast cancer (Eddy, 1989), bypass surgery for coronary artery disease (Weinstein and Stason, 1982), and vaccination against pneumococcal pneumonia (Willems et al., 1980). The results of an analysis are usually summarized in a series of cost-effectiveness ratios that show the cost of achieving one unit of health outcome—for example, the cost per year of life gained—for different kinds of patients and variations of the intervention (Table 1.1).

By providing estimates of outcomes and costs, CEA shows the tradeoffs involved in choosing among interventions or variants of an intervention. Put another way, it helps define and illuminate the "opportunity cost" of each choice: the health benefits lost because the next-best alternative was not selected. It thus gives decision makers in diverse settings—physicians' offices, health maintenance organizations (HMOs), or state or federal programs—important data for making informed judgments about interventions.

When the same measure of health outcome, such as years of life gained or cases of a particular disease prevented, is used for all interventions, they can be ranked on the basis of their cost-effectiveness ratios. Those with the lowest cost per year or per case are the most efficient ways of improving health; the ratios show which interventions produce the most years of life, or prevent the most cases of disease, for a given expen-

Table 1.1 Cost-Effectiveness Analysis: An Example

Cost-effectiveness analysis (CEA) involves estimating the net, or incremental, costs and effects of an intervention—its costs and health outcomes compared with some alternative, which might be the care that would be given if the intervention were not used at all, or a different intensity of the intervention, such as less frequent screening. The cost-effectiveness ratio that compares two alternatives is calculated as the difference in costs between the alternatives (net costs) divided by the difference in health outcomes (net effectiveness).

A study of screening for cervical cancer illustrates the main features of CEA. The study compared outcomes and costs associated with different schedules of screening (Eddy, 1990). We return to consider this analysis in greater detail later in the chapter.

The measure of health outcomes is years of life gained (increase in life expectancy). The estimates were developed from a model of the natural history of cervical cancer and the screening process based primarily on data from a study of 1.5 million women screened over many years in eight countries (IARC, 1986). The estimates took into account the accuracy of the test, the fact that not all cervical dysplasia progresses to cancer, and the effectiveness of treatment when cervical cancer is detected at various stages.

Costs were estimated from a variety of sources, including Medicare claims files. They include the costs of regular screening with the Papanicolaou smear, follow-up physician visits for abnormal tests, and treatment for dysplasia or cancer when it occurs.

Screening starts at age 20 and ends at 75. The discount rate, used to allow comparison of screening schedules which have outcomes and costs occurring in different years, is 5%.

The table presents some of the estimated increases in life expectancy (LE) and costs, expressed in days and dollars per woman. In the first column, screening at intervals of 4 years is compared with no screening. Almost 94 days of life are gained by screening (9.54 days after discounting) at a cost of $264; thus the cost-effectiveness ratio is $10,101 ($264 divided by 9.54 days yields the cost per day of life, which is then multiplied by 365 days to get the cost per year).

The second column shows the gain in days of life and the additional cost if screening takes place more frequently, every 3 years instead of every 4. The final column compares screening every 3 years with a schedule that begins instead with three annual tests, dropping back to screening at 3-year intervals only if all three initial tests are normal.

| | Screening Frequency | | |
	4 Years/No Screening	*3 Years/4 Years*	*3 Years After 3 Normal Annual Tests/3 Without Annual Testing*
LE increase in days	93.8	1.6	0.3
LE increase in days, discounted	9.54	0.18	0.06
Cost increase in dollars, discounted	264.00	91.00	112.00
Cost per life year	10,101.00	184,528.00	681,336.00

diture. Additional factors are almost always involved in selecting the final set of interventions, but CEA provides a useful guide to achieving a central objective, better health.

This chapter considers the uses of CEA and its limitations as an aid in the allocation of resources, broadly defined. The first section of the chapter asks which perspective is appropriate for CEA studies intended for this purpose. We conclude that the societal perspective is best, spell out some of the implications for identifying and valuing the health outcomes and costs included in an analysis, and consider the sort of information that CEAs conducted from the societal perspective can and cannot supply. Given this background, we discuss how CEA can be used as an aid to decision making. We then contrast CEA with other methods of evaluating choices in the allocation of health resources. Two examples show that CEA can suggest very different decisions from those reached by other methods. A discussion of the current and potential uses of CEA follows. We summarize our conclusions in the form of recommendations.

What Is the Appropriate Perspective?

When choices about the broad allocation of health resources are considered, who is affected? On whose behalf are decisions made? The answers to these questions define the perspective of the analysis, which, in turn, plays a crucial role in determining the relevant health outcomes and resources and how they should be measured and valued.

The broad nature of the problem suggests that the perspective should be equally broad. An analysis needs to consider not only those who gain health but those who pay for it. Relevant health outcomes include unwanted side effects, which can even occur in people who are not the intended recipients of the intervention, as well as longer life and improvements in health. Resource costs—which consist of all resources used, whether or not money changes hands for those resources—would be included regardless of who incurs them.

Programs to increase the folic acid intake of pregnant women in order to reduce the incidence of neural tube defects in their infants demonstrate the value of taking a broad view. One approach to delivering folic acid is to add the nutrient to cereal grains. This approach would allow women to improve their diets with no extra effort on their part, and is especially helpful for those who may not have adequate access to medical care and thus to other means of supplementation. The cost is borne by everyone who pays for products made with cereal grains. But fortification poses a risk, mostly for older people, because it masks pernicious anemia, which, undetected, can cause neurological problems. This adverse effect on the elderly should be counted as well as the gains for infants. A CEA intended to contribute to information about the broad allocation of health resources would need to evaluate all these health outcomes and costs, which would lead to consideration of the entire national population, not just pregnant women, as might appear to be the case at first.

What is described in this example is the societal perspective. When a CEA is conducted from the societal perspective, the analyst considers everyone affected by the intervention and counts all significant health outcomes and costs that flow from it, regardless of who experiences the outcomes or costs. Depending on where and how the intervention is applied, those affected could be confined to a small geographic area or subpopulation or could encompass the entire national population. The measure of health needs to be comprehensive and to include longer life, better function, and unwanted side effects. Costs include not only medical and other resources, but also the time of patients and unpaid caregivers.

By contrast, CEA done from other perspectives can reasonably omit some outcomes and costs if they are not of interest to the decision maker. For example, a CEA done for an employer might consider only outcomes and costs that affect the employer directly, such as the intervention's effect on workers' productivity or on medical bills reimbursed through the employee health plan; costs paid by employees might be excluded. Or an analysis done for a public program might consider only the health outcomes experienced by the program's beneficiaries and the costs paid by the program, not outcomes or costs experienced by others.

Implicit in the societal perspective is the recognition that societal resources are limited and that health should not be exempted from these limits. The societal perspective incorporates the value that many other social investments—in education, environmental quality, law enforcement, and the like—have merit. Thus no single activity, including health, should have such dominance that it always displaces other activities. Whether limits on health budgets are explicit or tacit, the societal perspective implies that resources devoted to health care should be invested wisely. Cost-effectiveness analysis offers a method for evaluating the choices made within these limits, attempting to account for all parties affected by the decisions.

This value—that health should be subject, at least to some degree, to the resource limits that constrain society—does not sit easily with everyone because it implies that CEA based on the societal perspective may sometimes recommend a course of action that is at odds with the wishes of individuals. Decisions about programs and coverage based in part on cost-effectiveness might mean, for example, that coverage would be denied for bypass surgery for individuals who are so old or in such poor health that the operation would add little to their life expectancies. Instead the insurer, public program, or HMO might choose to pay for exercise programs for the elderly because the resources would do more to improve health when used that way. But the individuals denied bypasses, and their doctors, might still value those benefits and want them.

What arguments can be advanced for choosing the societal perspective over others, when at times it may give less weight to the outcomes and costs of certain groups than they would like? One way to see the desirability of the societal perspective—of giving fair weight to all individuals and to all activities—is to imagine for a moment that we are looking at the world before we are born, or at least before we encounter any serious health problems, and to ask what kind of world we would like it to be. In that "ex ante'' position we would not yet know what health problems we were destined to develop—only that there was some chance that we might develop any of them. From that perspective, we would not want any health problem to be entirely neglected— after all, it might be ours some day. Nor would we want investments other than health to be neglected since we would live in the world created by that neglect.

This device—thinking about the world before we are born—has been used by many philosophers, operating from different philosphical perspectives, to argue for just ways of making decisions (Harsanyi, 1953, 1955; Rawls, 1971; Daniels, 1985, 1988; Menzel, 1992; Dworkin, 1981; Eddy, 1991). It is compatible with the common view that decisions are most likely to be fair if they are made by people who do not stand to gain or lose from them and with the related idea that decisions can be made in the public interest.

Viewing the situation from that perspective, we might reasonably prefer a system in which decisions about health interventions reflected the seriousness of the problem and the ability of the intervention to do something about it, without reference to the specific individuals with the problem or to particular budgets or special interests. In short, we would want a system that adopted the societal perspective. Some people would not get everything they want. But neither would anyone categorically be excluded.

If individual CEA studies are to serve this larger goal, they must be comparable. As noted in the Introduction, the mechanism proposed by the panel to promote comparability is a Reference Case, defined by the recommendations in this chapter and those that follow. A common perspective is the foundation for comparability. We recommend the societal perspective as the appropriate perspective for the Reference Case.

The societal perspective does not represent the situation from the viewpoint of particular agents in society, but it is the only perspective that never counts as a gain what is really someone else's loss. If an intervention adopted by an employer reduces the employer's costs for health insurance but increases costs for Medicare, the societal perspective includes both changes. Beyond the philosophical arguments in its favor, there is value in beginning with a perspective that includes all costs and effects because it provides a background against which to assess results from other perspectives. Analysts may, of course, include other perspectives in the same analysis.

Defining Outcomes and Costs from the Societal Perspective

The societal perspective has implications for which outcomes and costs should be measured and how they should be measured in a CEA. But in real-world situations the societal perspective, that is, a comprehensive viewpoint that tries to give proper weight to most or all of the significant aspects of a decision, can involve considerations than are not reflected, and in some cases cannot be, in the measures of outcome or cost used in CEAs. In this section we illustrate the problem with some examples.

In CEA done from the societal perspective, health outcomes are often represented by years of life gained. This is an important outcome for many interventions, but hardly the only one. When they work, health interventions do more than extend life: They relieve suffering, improve functioning, provide information, and convey care and compassion. Many effective interventions— acetominophen for headache, for example— have no effect on the length of life. They may also cause unintended and undesirable side effects. Ideally the measure of outcomes used in CEA should be defined more broadly to include these other outcomes.

Research conducted over the last 25 years has produced summary measures of health that reflect the quality as well as the quantity of life and increasingly CEAs have used these measures to estimate the quality-adjusted years of life (QALYs) gained from an intervention (Boyle et al., 1983; Oldridge et al., 1993; Patrick and Erickson, 1993; Spilker, 1990; Weinstein and Stason, 1976). The development of QALYs as an outcome measure has made it possible to encompass the diverse effects of a single intervention and to compare interventions with quite different kinds of outcomes, thus greatly expanding the applicability and usefulness of CEA. In Chapter 4, we discuss the use of health-related quality-of-life measures in the Reference Case and describe alternative approaches.

If these more comprehensive measures of health captured everything that mattered, then, with their use, CEA could identify the interventions that would contribute the most to societal goals. But even QALYs do not fully reflect what decision makers would like to accomplish in the public interest. To calculate the total health effect of an intervention, analysts sum all quality-adjusted life years. This simple addition implies that QALYs are of equal value no matter who gains them or when they occur during the life span. Both intuition and research suggest that this is not the case and that deviations from this assumption are substantial and important (Harris, 1987; Daniels, 1993). As a case in point, surveys of the general public (including the elderly) have revealed a strong consensus on the part of the general public, including the elderly, to the effect that the young should be favored over the old (Williams, 1988; Lewis and Charney, 1989).

The assumption that all QALYs are of equal value implies, for example, that it makes no difference whether extra years of healthy life go to people in good health or to people in poor health—perhaps people with a serious disability. Yet decision makers might give preference to those in poor health out of a sense that their need is greater. As another example, a therapy that saved the lives of a few people, allowing them to live many more years in good health, might produce the same number of quality-adjusted life years as treating mild arthritis in many people. Yet much of the general public would place a higher value on the intervention that helped fewer individuals because it made such a large difference for them. This ''aggregation problem'' occurs because the numerical sums are equal but we do not in fact value them equally.

These are difficult issues of equity and distributive justice that get to the core of what we care about as a society. In principle, QALYs received by different people at different times could be weighted before they were added together to reflect the values society places on different circumstances. But societal values are not understood fully enough, or perhaps not even fully enough formed, to make it possible to define such weights (Daniels, 1993). In practice, then, we do not know what the weights should be and are not likely to solve the problem anytime soon.

Equity issues arise on the cost side of the cost-effectiveness ratio as well. The valuation of time provides an example. CEA studies frequently do not include the time of patients and unpaid caregivers among the resource costs of a medical intervention. It is difficult to measure, but the societal perspective requires that it be included whenever it is significant. The societal perspective also requires that all resources be valued at their "opportunity cost." The best approximation of the opportunity cost of time for working-age adults is the wage they are, or could be, making in paid work. Chapter 6 gives analysts a choice, recommending that time be valued either at the average wage for persons of that age and sex or at the average wage for all workers.

But wage estimates that differ depending on characteristics such as gender and race raise troubling issues of fairness. Women are paid less than men. The lower wages of women mean that, other things equal, the same intervention will appear more cost-effective for them than for men because their time is valued at a lower rate. Yet most people would probably think it unfair to provide more of the intervention to women, or to provide it only to them—the health of men and women is equally valuable. Thus decision makers might choose to ignore differences in cost-effectiveness ratios that arise because of the difference in wages between men and women, or analysts might choose to substitute the wage for all workers.

Other important public values simply cannot be incorporated into CEA in any useful way. This problem arises in part because health interventions affect things other than health. For example, society's views on individuals' rights can affect the desirability of some health interventions: the right to privacy has made mandatory human immunodeficiency virus (HIV) testing unacceptable outside of special situations such as the military, even though life-lengthening treatments are available for individuals diagnosed early. Thus the measures of health outcomes used in CEAs must remain an incomplete representation of societal goals and values. Where nonhealth benefits or costs are relatively minor, CEA of health outcomes and costs may be sufficient to inform decisions. When nonhealth benefits are substantial, it may be helpful to use the method of cost-benefit analysis, or to supplement the CEA with legal, ethical, or other kinds of analyses.

CEA as an Aid to Decision Making

The textbook exposition of CEA explains that once cost-effectiveness ratios are computed from the societal perspective and placed in rank order, a decision maker can select the intervention with the lowest cost per QALY and continue down the list selecting interventions, until the available funds are exhausted. The resulting set of interventions are those that produce the largest possible number of QALYs for the expenditure. In textbook terms, the decision maker has selected the interventions that maximize health, represented by QALYs, within the constraint set by available resources.

For the kinds of reasons discussed in the last section, decisions in the real world are more complicated. Cost-effectiveness analysis provides valuable information about tradeoffs in the broad allocation of health resources, but other factors need to be considered as well—concepts of fairness and justice that are not fully captured in the sums of QALYs or in the way costs are valued, benefits and costs outside the health sector, and practical questions of feasibility. Thus, although it is possible to use CEA in a mechanical way, it is often not appropriate to do so. CEA is not a complete decision making process. The information it provides is, however, crucial to good decisions.

CEA can serve much the same function as the tables in an article in *Consumer Reports* (the well-known publication that evaluates consumer products). For example, typical tables show the benefits and costs of different models of cars, on various dimensions: repair records, crash tests, handling and style, fuel economy, space, and price. Summary indexes such as reliability or repair cost may be included as well. The final decision, however, is the reader's and differs from one reader to the next. Readers apply their own values to the information and decide which car to buy. And not all will choose the model recommended as ''The Best Buy'' because not all will share the values reflected in that recommendation.

In this role, CEA makes a simple, but crucial, contribution to decision problems by providing estimates of the magnitudes of costs and health outcomes. Accurate information is essential and can, by itself, lead to very different decisions, especially since many interventions are complex in their application and common beliefs about the magnitudes of costs and outcomes can be seriously mistaken. As appropriate for the problem, CEA can show the costs and health benefits of different frequencies and amounts of each intervention, when applied to different subgroups in the population, under circumstances that reflect different costs and service delivery systems. In addition, CEA's structured process of evaluating the strength of the evidence, stating assumptions explicitly, and working out their implications for cost-effectiveness can be as helpful as the final estimates in understanding alternatives.

The potential value of these estimates is exemplified by the common belief that preventive interventions save more money than they cost. According to the common belief, costs need not be considered, since they are outweighed by savings, and preventive interventions should be provided to all people for whom they are effective. Yet CEA shows that, depending on how they are applied, some effective forms of prevention can be very expensive. For example, screening for cervical cancer is effective in preventing deaths from the condition, but screening annually rather than every 2 years has been estimated to cost all payers more than $1 million per year of life gained because the health gain from annual screening, compared with biennial screening, is so small (Eddy, 1990). Simply knowing that costs are very large for a small benefit could influence decisions about screening frequency.

Ranking interventions by their cost-effectiveness ratios is a step beyond the *Consumer Reports*–style presentation of information on costs and effects. Rankings of ratios for a variety of interventions, sometimes termed "league tables," show how the interventions compare in terms of their cost per unit of health outcome, usually years of life in published studies (Drummond et al., 1993). Properly calculated cost-effectiveness ratios help the user interpret the data on costs and effects correctly and show, in simple, summary fashion, which interventions do the most to promote health.

Direct comparison of cost-effectiveness ratios can be useful across the spectrum of decisions to varying degrees: more useful when interventions and populations receiving them are less diverse and less useful when diversity is greater. At one end of the spectrum, cost-effectiveness ratios can be used to rank alternative interventions for the same group of people—say, treatments for people with end-stage renal failure or with severe hypertension. In these circumstances—a range of interventions which could be applied to a single condition in the same group of people, preferably a group that is similar in its other characteristics as well—it will often be possible to define health goals in terms that everyone can agree on and that are well represented by QALYs. If some facets of the effects and costs must be omitted, they may affect all patients in much the same manner, so omitting them does not bias the decision. Thus the cost-effectiveness ratios can provide strong guidance to the best choices.

For decisions that involve greater diversity in interventions and the people to whom they apply, cost-effectiveness ratios continue to provide essential information, but that information must, to a greater degree, be evaluated in light of circumstances and values that cannot be included in the analysis. Individuals in the population will differ widely in their health and disability before the intervention, or in age, wealth, or other characteristics, raising questions about how society values gains for the more and less healthy, for young and old, for rich and poor, and so on. The assumption that all QALYs are of equal value is less likely to be reasonable in this context. Similarly, differences in the values assigned to the time of different groups may raise questions of fairness. The issue of defining benefit packages—which of all the services available in the health care system to provide to the population in an HMO, a community, or the nation, and under what circumstances—lies at this end of the spectrum.

To serve well in any of these situations, the components of cost-effectiveness analysis and the cost-effectiveness ratios must follow generally accepted principles so that they are correct within studies and comparable across studies and interventions. Comparability among analyses is the foundation of CEA's usefulness as an aid to decision making. Because CEA methods have varied widely among studies in the past, authors comparing CEAs performed to date must be especially careful to check that the ratios presented are in fact comparable. The definition of the Reference Case in this volume is, as noted in the Introduction, intended to make such comparisons easier and more informative in the future.

Finally, even with QALYs and standardized methods, cost-effectiveness ratios cannot yet offer useful comparisons across all health interventions. This is the case when an intervention has important health outcomes that are not incorporated in existing QALY systems. For example, CEA can be used to evaluate interventions for treating schizophrenia and interventions for treating heart disease. But the health outcomes are so different that it is difficult to capture them in the same measurement system, and direct comparisons of the QALYs created by the two kinds of interventions may not yet be possible. In choices of this kind, CEA still provides useful information, but a greater part of the decision-making process occurs outside of the analysis.

Other Methods for Making Decisions in Health

In general decision makers have used methods other than CEA to evaluate choices about health interventions, methods based on notions of "medical necessity," on "standards of evidence," on whether an intervention is "experimental," or other criteria. These criteria are commonly perceived to be technical statements—objective and free of value judgments—and are supposed to exclude consideration of cost. In practice, however, they usually involve important value judgments and costs often play a part without explicit acknowledgment. Moreover, decision makers still face the distributive issues that arise with CEA

Consider "medical necessity." Judgments about medical necessity, which can determine whether an insurer covers a procedure or a provider offers it, are interpreted as stating that particular medical problems cannot be addressed except by particular interventions. While they appear to be technical statements, they often disguise three important types of value judgment. The first is a judgment about the goals of medicine. If we ask, for example, whether growth hormone treatment is "medically necessary" for children who are not growth hormone deficient but are simply in the bottom 1% of the population in projected adult height, we are asking about the goals of medicine. Is medicine aimed at the treatment of disease and dysfunction or is the elimination of other sources of unhappiness and disadvantage an equally legitimate aim?

A second type of value judgment often implicit in statements of medical necessity is based on prior decisions about the social division of responsibility. A home health service may respond effectively to the medical condition of a frail, elderly person, making the difference between independence and institutionalization. Yet a payer may decide that the service is not "medically necessary" on the unstated ground that it is up to family or a social support agency, not the health care system, to offer the assistance, even when it is clear that the service will not be provided through these other sources. Thus, the decision may be in part a decision about costs and who should bear them.

Medical-necessity judgments also turn on beliefs about the limits of our obligations, for example, about when we have done enough to try to rescue a seriously ill patient. Should an HMO's medical director authorize a bone marrow transplant for a case of advanced cancer because the oncologist insists it is medically necessary—it is the patient's last hope? The director is well aware that authorizing the procedure may mean not staffing a program that provides other medically necessary benefits.

Other criteria thought to be technical often involve similar value judgments, including hidden judgments about costs and their relation to benefits. An insurer may be reluctant to decide that a new technology is no longer "experimental" if its expected benefits are modest and its costs high. Evidence about effectiveness is not so clear and objective that it cannot be made to flex in response to such assessments. When the evaluation of outcomes and costs is not based on the systematic considerations that govern CEA, the result is likely to be less consistent and less informed judgments about what is experimental and what is proven effective.

Since we face the same distributive issues when using these methods but lack information about costs, we make a difficult decision more difficult. How we address distributive problems is affected by costs. We must know what we are giving up by treating the more seriously ill—the opportunity cost—before we can evaluate whether we have gone beyond the limits of our obligations to help those who are sickest. Neither medical necessity nor expected medical benefit nor CEA gives us a decision procedure for resolving these distributive problems, but CEA offers more complete information relevant to our decision.

Results of CEA and Other Methods Compared

If other decision-making methods generated similar recommendations, there would be little reason to advocate the use of CEA. The examples summarized in this section demonstrate that the conclusions supported by CEA can be very different from those based on other methods. Thus the choice among methods is of real importance. Guidelines promulgated by professional societies are used as examples of decisions based on other methods and are contrasted with the results of CEAs for the same intervention. We discuss two examples: screening for cervical cancer and treatment of high blood cholesterol.

We draw here on CEAs that were done well but that nonetheless do not meet all the requirements for the Reference Case (Russell, 1994). For example, all of them use years of life gained rather than QALYs as the measure of health and none count among the costs of the intervention the time that patients spend receiving it. All of them use a discount rate of 5%, which makes them comparable with each other on this point but differs from the rate of 3% recommended for the Reference Case. (See Chapter 7).

Cervical Cancer

Professional recommendations for cervical cancer screening have undergone several revisions in recent decades. Initially, Papanicolaou (Pap) smears were recommended annually for all women (ACOG, 1980). It was suggested that screening begin at age 18, and there was no upper age limit.

In 1980, the American Cancer Society (ACS) recommended that women aged 20–65 could be screened less often than annually if two consecutive annual tests were negative. And in 1988, after some disagreement with these ACS guidelines, more than ten professional organizations, led by the National Cancer Institute, the American College of Obstetricians and Gynecologists, and the American Cancer Society, issued a joint recommendation that screening start no later than age 18 and occur less frequently than annually at the discretion of the physician, but only after three consecutive annual smears were negative (e.g., Fink, 1988). No alternative frequency was suggested and many physicians continue to advise annual screening.

The ACS based its 1980 recommendation on a cost-effectiveness analysis of different screening schedules. We describe here an updated version of the analysis published later by the same author, which produced similar results (Eddy, 1990; some results from this study are shown in Table 1.1). The analysis estimated the costs and life years saved by screening at intervals of 1, 2, 3, and 4 years; by beginning screening at ages from 17 to 29; and by ending screening at age 65 or at later ages.

Compared with no screening, screening every 4 years—the longest interval shown—was estimated to cost about $10,000 for each year of life saved in 1985 dollars (Table 1.2, first row). To choose among screening frequencies, however, the decision maker needs to know how different frequencies compare with each other. Thus the study calculated the *additional* cost required to save an *additional* year of life by screening more often—every 3 years rather than every 4, say, or annually rather than every 2.

Table 1.2 Cost per Year of Life Saved for Different Frequencies of Screening[a] (in 1985 Dollars)

	Screening Every			
	4 Years	*3 Years*	*2 Years*	*1 Year*
Compared with no screening	10,101	—	—	—
Compared with screening at the next longer interval[b]	—	184,500	262,800	1,100,000
Worst-case scenario[c]				
Compared with no screening	—	15,500	—	—
Compared with screening at the next longer interval	—	—	167,900	503,700

Source: Eddy, 1990.

a. Future life years and costs are discounted at 5% per year. Costs are for 1985. All assumptions are based on data for an average woman who is asymptomatic when she begins screening at age 20 and who is screened to age 74 or 75.

b. For example, the number for a screening interval of 3 years, $184,500, shows the *additional* cost for each *additional* year of life saved due to screening every 3 years instead of every 4, and so on.

c. The worst-case scenario assumes that incidence is three times the U.S. rate of the mid-1980s and has increased among younger women in recent years, that 20% of cancers are of the fast-growing type rather than 5%, and that the rate of missed cancers is 15% higher than actual experience in centralized screening programs in Canada and Europe.

The study showed that increasing frequency is an expensive way to extend lives (Table 1.2, second row). Compared with screening every 4 years, screening every 3 is estimated to cost an additional $185,000 for each life year saved. Shortening the screening interval from 3 years to 2 brings additional life years at a cost of almost $263,000 each. And compared with screening every 2 years, annual screening costs more than $1 million for each additional life year saved. The analysis also showed that varying the age to begin screening from 17 to 29 years, or ending screening at age 65 for women who had been screened regularly up to that age, made little difference to health outcomes. As well, requiring three negative annual smears before allowing less-frequent screening was very costly and produced, on average, only hours of additional life expectancy. These results reflect the fact that cervical cancer can take years to develop and most cases are detected early enough by screening at intervals of several years; more frequent screening yields only a few more cases.

By contrast, screening women who have not been screened on any regular schedule brings substantial health benefits. The same analysis showed that screening women who have never been screened saves about 60 days of life per woman compared with the 3 days saved by screening women once a year rather than every 3 years. A study of screening for low-income elderly women who had not been screened in recent memory found that it not only extended lives; it reduced medical expenditures (Mandelblatt and Fahs, 1988). These findings are relevant to the one-quarter of all women in the United States who, according to a national survey done in 1987, had not had a Pap smear in the last 3 years (Harlan et al., 1991).

If the cost of screening annually is not much more than that of screening every 2 or 3 years, the choice of screening schedule makes little difference. The available estimates suggest that the cost is substantial, even though they include only the costs of the initial test itself, not the costs of follow-up tests or the (net) costs of treatment. Eddy estimated that screening every woman in the United States every year would cost about $6 billion (Kolata, 1988) compared with $2 billion for screening every 3 years.

Thus less frequent screening would free up substantial resources with relatively little loss of health benefits. A decision maker reviewing the broad allocation of health resources might well decide that some of the money spent on annual screening would be better, and more fairly, spent elsewhere—for example, to recruit and screen women who have not been previously screened.

Treatment of High Blood Cholesterol

In 1985, in response to the first evidence from a randomized controlled trial that reducing cholesterol reduces the risk of death from heart disease (Lipid Research Clinics Program, 1984), the National Institutes of Health created the National Cholesterol Education Program (NCEP). Three years later the NCEP published guidelines for the management of high blood cholesterol which recommended that all adults have their cholesterol checked at least every 5 years and that those with high levels (240 mg/dl or higher), or borderline-high levels (200–239 mg/dl) plus other risk factors, be tested further. It was suggested that those whose low-density lipoproteins (LDL) levels were also high should be treated by changes in diet or with cholesterol-lowering drugs (NCEP, 1988). It has been estimated that more than one-third of the adult population requires dietary change and/or drugs when judged by these criteria (Sempos et al., 1989).

Cost-effectiveness analyses done in the wake of the 1988 guidelines focused on the management of high blood cholesterol once detected. Both lovastatin, a frequently prescribed drug, and dietary counseling were shown to vary widely in cost-effectiveness depending on age and other risk factors for heart disease.

One study examined the use of lovastatin for people initially free of heart disease and for those who had already suffered a heart attack (Goldman et al., 1991). The authors found that, for healthy people, saving a year of life is much more costly among those with cholesterol as their only risk factor than it is for those with several risk factors, even when cholesterol is very high; the cost ranged up to $330,000 for men aged 35–44 with no other risk factors and up to $1.5 million for women in the same category (Table 1.3, top half). The cost was considerably lower for people with other risk factors, reflecting the widely accepted assumption that risk factors interact to make the adverse effects of any one greater when others are present. Lovastatin treatment

Table 1.3 Cost per Year of Life Saved by Lovastatin[a] (in 1989 dollars)

Healthy, Blood Cholesterol ≥ 300	Cost per Year of Life[b]	
	Low-Risk Patient	High-Risk Patient
Women 35–44	$1,500,000	$195,000
Women 55–64	130,000	34,000
Men 35–44	330,000	24,000
Men 55–64	58,000	15,000
Heart Disease, Blood Cholesterol ≥ 250	*All Patients*	
Women 35–44	4,500	
Women 55–64	8,100	
Men 35–44	—[c]	
Men 55–64	1,600	

Source: Goldman et al., 1991.

a. Dose is 20 mg of lovastatin daily. Costs include physician visits and tests required to monitor people taking lovastatin. Costs and health gains are discounted at 5% per year.

b. A low-risk person is a nonsmoker with diastolic blood pressure below 95 who is not more than 10% overweight. A high-risk person is a smoker with a diastolic pressure of 105 or higher who is 30% or more overweight.

c. Lovastatin estimated to save lives and money.

was still more costly per life year gained for people with levels in the range 250–299 (data not shown).

By contrast, the study found that it is potentially very cost-effective to treat people with elevated cholesterol who have had heart attacks (Table 1.3, bottom half). Costs per life year gained are relatively low and for some, such as men aged 35–44, drug treatment might save money as well as extend life.

Another study found similar results for a program of intensive diet therapy modeled after the one in the Multiple Risk Factor Intervention Trial (MRFIT) (Taylor et al., 1990). For example, diet therapy costs more than $500,000 per year of life for 20-year-old men with an initial cholesterol of 240 mg/dl and no other risk factors (Table 1.4, top line). For men with several risk factors, the cost per life year gained is much lower.

These results suggest that management of high cholesterol in people without heart disease is often very costly per life year saved. Since they show that treatment of people whose blood cholesterol levels are not far above 240 mg/dl can be extremely costly, they suggest that the same would be true for people with levels in the borderline-high range, although the studies did not analyze this group. Taken together, cost-effectiveness results suggest that resources might better be concentrated on those with very high cholesterol levels and/or other risk factors for heart disease (and on those in whom heart disease is already present). Revised guidelines, published by NCEP in 1993 (NCEP, 1994), were somewhat more modest in their aims, in response to studies like these as well to the ongoing debate over whether reducing cholesterol lengthens life in those without heart disease.

If NCEP's 1988 guidelines were followed to the letter, it would cost, depending on the effectiveness of diet in reducing blood cholesterol levels, $20 billion to $27 billion

Table 1.4 Cost per Year of Life Saved by Diet[a] (in 1986 Dollars)

Age	Blood Cholesterol	Cost per Year of Life for a:[b]	
		Low-Risk Man	High-Risk Man
20	240	$510,000	$99,000
	300	300,000	56,000
40	240	180,000	21,000
	300	94,000	11,000
60	240	280,000	23,000
	300	160,000	13,000

Source: Taylor et al., 1990.

a. Diet is assumed to reduce initial blood cholesterol levels by 6.7 percent, the average reduction in the MRFIT trial. Costs and health gains are discounted at 5% per year.

b. A low-risk man is a nonsmoker with systolic blood pressure lower than all but 10% and high-density lipoprotein (HDL) cholesterol equal to or higher than 90% of men of the same age. A high-risk man is a smoker with systolic blood pressure equal to or higher than 90% and HDL cholesterol lower than all but 10% of men of the same age.

to provide lovastatin at doses of 20 mg per day, and $47 billion to $67 billion to provide a higher, more effective, dose of 80 mg per day (Garber and Wagner, 1991). Again, as in the case of cervical cancer, the savings from a more selective strategy would be substantial, freeing resources to be applied elsewhere. The CEA results suggest that more selective treatment strategies could be designed that would lose little in health benefits.

Current and Potential Uses of CEA

In recent years, the number of CEAs of health and medical interventions has grown steadily (Elixhauser, 1993). Well over 100 studies per year are published in general medical, medical specialty, public health, and policy journals. CEAs are conducted and funded by agencies of the federal government, industry, insurers, consulting firms, and universities.

The strongest current focus of interest is in the area of pharmaceuticals, where a number of factors have converged to generate interest in CEA. Cost-effectiveness analysis in this area is supported by the relative availability of data on effectiveness, since effectiveness studies are required for the approval of pharmaceuticals. In the United States, higher market-entry prices for innovative drugs coupled with tighter budgets throughout the health care system appear to be inducing a demand for studies. Formulary committees in hospitals, HMOs, and Medicaid agencies require information on the value drugs offer before agreeing to purchase them (Luce and Brown, 1995). Pharmaceutical firms compete with one another to demonstrate that products are cost-effective. As a result, they are funding studies at a high rate, either in-house or through consulting firms or academic institutions.

Outside the US, the demand by pharmaceutical firms for CEAs of their products is driven by government requirements or price regulation. Australia requires pharmaceutical companies to submit CEAs in order to be reimbursed on the national formulary (Henry, 1992). Canada is instituting a similar regulation (Ontario Ministry of Health, 1994; CCOHTA, 1994). While these two countries explicitly require CEA, European governments are implicitly promoting CEA by requiring drug companies to demonstrate during price negotiations that a medication is of sufficient value to justify its price (Drummond, 1992).

For other health care services and technologies, CEA is believed to have played a key role in some policies, although its influence is not well documented. For instance, Congress is thought to have based its decision to make the pneumoccocal vaccine the first preventive service covered by Medicare on a CEA conducted by the Congressional Office of Technology Assessment (OTA, 1979). Blue Cross/Blue Shield of California is said to have adopted cancer screening policies based on a series of CEAs done by David Eddy (1980).

There is little indication, however, that CEA contributes systematically to resource allocation decisions in United States medicine. On the contrary, both HMOs and insurers deny considering cost when they make coverage decisions (Luce and Brown, 1995). Presumably, their reluctance to use CEA—at least formally—stems from a reluctance to risk the perception that they explicitly limit care due to cost.

Although it is difficult to identify an existing formal role for CEA, interest in the method suggests that CEA is able to influence policy makers' views in informal ways. CEAs are often cited as evidence of the value (or lack of value) of a particular program, technology, or type of intervention in order to promote (or discourage) its use. For example, federal agencies and consumer advocates have publicized cost-effectiveness results for prevention strategies (CDC, 1993; Institute for Women's Policy Research, 1994). These publications assemble the range of available information on cost-benefit and cost-effectiveness of prevention with the purpose of informing decision makers and the public. CEA is most convincing in this role when an intervention has a very low cost per unit of health outcome, or a very high cost, relative to medical technologies generally.

Few have taken issue with the dissemination of this type of cost-effectiveness information—whether these efforts were motivated by interest group or government politics or by public interest concerns. However, cost-effectiveness claims by commercial interests, such as pharmaceutical companies and medical device manufacturers, have generated greater concern. Clearly, it is possible for producers of medical technologies to use studies selectively to demonstrate the cost-effectiveness of their own products for specific conditions. Professional organizations and individual practitioners, similarly, can conduct or sponsor CEAs in areas where they have a professional, financial, or ideological stake, obtaining results that justify the recommendations they support. The lack of guidelines for conducting cost-effectiveness analyses and of standards by which to judge their quality have contributed to the potential for bias.

Efforts to assure the quality of cost-effectiveness analyses have begun on several fronts. Seeking to uphold its requirements for "adequate and well-controlled studies" (21 CFR Part 314.126), the Food and Drug Administration (FDA) currently applies strict standards to claims of cost-effectiveness by pharmaceutical companies. In general, the type of claim reviewed by the FDA compares a given drug to a competitor. The FDA requires that the evidence of effectiveness used in CEAs be obtained from rigorous studies that directly compare the drugs in question.

On another front, *The New England Journal of Medicine* has developed a policy for the review of cost-effectiveness analyses intended to preclude financial conflicts of interest that might affect the choice of methods or data used in an analysis (Kassirer and Angell, 1994). The journal reported that it would not consider CEAs for publication if an author has a financial relationship with a sponsoring company—a stronger restriction than the disclosure requirements it applies to other forms of original research.

To develop voluntary ethical guidelines for the sponsorship and conduct of CEA, faculty at the Leonard Davis Institute organized the Task Force on Principles for Economic Analysis of Health Care Technology. This committee, sponsored by pharmaceutical companies, consisted of academics and representatives from industry and the federal government and issued guidelines for the pharmaceutical industry (Task Force on Principles for Economic Analysis of Health Care Technology, 1995). Efforts to standardize CEA methodology address concerns about bias by reducing discretion in the choice of methodology and by providing a benchmark for judging the quality of analyses.

With improvements in the standardization of CEA methods, policy makers will be able to move toward a more systematic use of CEA. One set of potential applications involves reimbursement decisions for new procedures and treatments. A drug or procedure could be required to meet standards of cost-effectiveness before it could be reimbursed. This gatekeeping function would parallel the international efforts to use cost-effectiveness in the development of drug formularies.

Cost-effectiveness analysis could also be used in the development of medical and public health practice guidelines. Guidelines are currently developed on the basis of effectiveness; when costs are examined, they play a secondary role. For example, the guidelines panels sponsored by the Agency for Health Care Policy and Research (AHCPR) have considered the cost of implementing a proposed guideline, but to date no formal cost-effectiveness analyses have been factored into guideline development (OTA, 1994). The recommendations of the U.S. Preventive Services Task Force for clinical preventive services are based primarily on evidence of effectiveness. While the task force acknowledges that clinical decisions may be made on other grounds, and that these grounds may include cost, it does not consider cost-effectiveness formally (USPSTF, 1989). The introduction of CEA into guidelines processes would allow expert panels to weigh the cost implications of various protocols along with differences in effectiveness, side effects, and other risks.

The development of benefit packages for government and private insurance coverage is a potential use of CEA, but a controversial one. In Oregon, pioneering efforts to prioritize medical benefits for the Medicaid program initially attempted to use a cost-effectiveness formulation (Klevit et al., 1991). The results contained counterintuitive rankings (e.g., suggesting a higher priority for dental caps than for appendectomy) and were widely criticized. (See Hadorn, 1991; Brown, 1991; Fox and Leichter, 1991; Tengs et al., 1996, for descriptions of the process and reviews of the reactions Oregon received.) Although the Oregon Health Services Commission attributed problems in the rankings to inadequate data, it ultimately backed away from cost-effectiveness as a decision criterion.

Much of the controversy over this kind of application concerns whether medical services should be limited explicitly in any way. If policy makers opt for explicit, as opposed to implicit, means of allocating resources, CEA will provide critical information about the value of alternative investments in health.

Conclusion

The perspective of a CEA—the study's point of view—determines which health outcomes and costs are relevant and plays a part as well in how they should be valued. In this chapter, we considered the appropriate perspective for CEAs used to inform the broad allocation of health resources and concluded that the societal perspective best serves that purpose. Some implications of the societal perspective were discussed in the chapter and more are brought out in the chapters that follow.

Although CEA done from the societal perspective is comprehensive, counting the health effects and costs experienced by all those who are significantly affected by the intervention, it does not reflect everything of importance to decision makers. The chapter discussed in particular some of the distributive values that are not yet reflected in the methods used in CEA. Because of this, we envision CEA as a crucial aid to decision making, but not as a complete decision-making procedure.

Screening for cervical cancer and treatment of high blood cholesterol, the two examples discussed in the chapter, demonstrate that CEA suggests resource allocations very different from the allocations that flow from recommendations based on other methods of decision making. These analyses suggest changes from current policy in order to direct health care resources where they would do the most to extend life and improve its quality. Although other factors may sometimes offset cost-effectiveness considerations, we urge decision makers to take good CEAs into account when they are available. The policy debate would also be served, in many cases, if the decisive tradeoffs between health and other goals were more explicitly identified.

The use of the CEA approach for making decisions about the broad allocation of resources requires comparisons of health outcomes and costs across a wide range of interventions. To facilitate these comparisons it is important to standardize CEAs so that comparisons are valid. Differences in reported health outcomes, costs, and cost-effectiveness ratios should reflect, as much as practicably possible, true differences in the consequences of the interventions and not be artifacts introduced by unnecessary differences in method.

The main task of the Panel on Cost-Effectiveness in Health and Medicine has been to develop standards for the conduct of CEAs for decisions in the public interest. The Introduction of this book introduced the notion of the Reference Case, which is defined in the rest of the book. We summarize the contribution of this chapter in the following recommendations.

Recommendations

    1. CEAs intended to contribute to discussion of the broad allocation of health resources should include the Reference Case.

    2. The Reference Case is based on the societal perspective.

3. CEAS are an aid to decision making, not a complete procedure for making decisions, because they cannot incorporate all the values relevant to the decisions.

4. The use of CEA in decision making should be studied in a collaborative effort by decision makers and analysts to improve its usefulness.

References

American Cancer Society (ACS). 1980. *Guidelines for the cancer-related health checkup: Recommendations and rationale.* New York: ACS.

American College of Obstetricians and Gynecologists (ACOG). 1980. *Periodic screening for women: Statement of policy.* Washington, DC: ACOG.

Boyle, M.H., G.W. Torrance, J.C. Sinclair, and S.P. Horwood. 1983. Economic evaluation of neonatal intensive care of very-low-birth-weight infants. *N Engl J Med* 308:1330–37.

Brown, L.D. 1991. The national politics of Oregon's rationing plan. *Health Aff* 10:29–51.

Canadian Coordinating Office of Health Technology Assessment (CCOHTA). 1994. *Guidelines for economic evaluation of pharmaceuticals: Canada.* Ottawa: CCOHTA.

Centers for Disease Control and Prevention (CDC). 1993. *An ounce of prevention: What are the returns?* Atlanta: CDC.

Daniels, N. 1993. Rationing fairly: Programmatic considerations. *Bioethics* 7:223–33.

Daniels, N. 1988. *Am I my parent's keeper? An essay on justice between the young and the old.* New York: Oxford University Press.

Daniels, N. 1985. *Just health care.* Cambridge, MA: Harvard University Press.

Drummond, M. 1992. Cost-effectiveness guidelines for reimbursement of pharmaceuticals: Is economic evaluation ready for its enhanced status? *Health Econ* 1:85–92.

Drummond, M., G. Torrance, and J. Mason. 1993. Cost-effectiveness league tables: More harm than good? *Social Sciences in Medicine* 37:33–40.

Dworkin, R. 1981. What is equity? Part 2: Equality of resources. *Philosophy and Public Affairs* 10:283–345.

Eddy, D.M. 1991. The individual vs. society: Resolving the conflict. *JAMA* 265:2399–2406.

Eddy, D.M. 1990. Screening for cervical cancer. *Ann Intern Med* 113:214–26.

Eddy, D.M. 1989. Screening for breast cancer. *Ann Intern Med* 111:389–99.

Eddy, D.M. 1980. *Screening for cancer: Theory, analysis, and design.* Englewood Cliffs, NJ: Prentice-Hall.

Elixhauser, A., ed. 1993. Health care cost-benefit and cost-effectiveness analysis (CBA/CEA) from 1979 to 1990: A bibliography. Appendix C. *Med Care* 31:JS139–JS141.

Fink, D.J. 1988. Change in ACS check-up guidelines for the detection of cervical cancer. *CA Cancer J Clin* 38:127–28.

Fox, D.M., and H.M. Leichter. 1991. Rationing care in Oregon: The new accountability. *Health Aff* 10(2):8–27.

Garber, A.M., and J.L. Wagner. 1991. Practice guidelines and cholesterol policy. *Health Aff* 10(2):52–66.

Goldman, L., M.C. Weinstein, P.A. Goldman, and L.W. Williams. 1991. Cost-effectiveness of HMG-CoA reductase inhibition for primary and secondary prevention of coronary heart disease. *JAMA* 265:1145–51.

Hadorn, D. 1991. Setting health care priorities in Oregon: Cost-effectiveness meets the rule of rescue. *JAMA* 265:2218–25.

Harlan, L.C., A.B. Bernstein, and L.G. Kessler. 1991. Cervical cancer screening: Who is not screened and why? *Am J Public Health* 81:885–91.

Harris, J. 1987. QALYfying the value of life. *J Med Ethics* 13:117–23.

Harsanyi, J.C. 1953. Cardinal utility in welfare economics and in the theory of risk-taking. *J Political Economy* 61:434–35.

Harsanyi, J.C. 1955. Cardinal welfare, individualistic ethics, and interpersonal comparisons of utility. *J Political Economy* 63:309–21.

Henry, D. 1992. Economic analysis an an aid to subsidisation decisions: The development of Australia's guidelines for pharmaceuticals. *PharmacoEconomics* 1:54–67.

IARC Working Group on Evaluation of Cervical Cancer Screening Programmes. 1986. Screening for squamous cervical cancer: Duration of low risk after negative results of cytology and its implications for screening policies. *BMJ* 293:659–64.

Institute for Women's Policy Research. 1994. *Preventive health services: Benefits and cost-effectiveness.* Washington, DC: Institute for Women's Policy Research.

Kassirer, J.P., and M. Angell. 1994. The journal's policy on cost-effectiveness analysis. *N Engl J Med* 331:669–70.

Klevit, H.D., A.C. Bates, T. Castanares, E.P. Kirk, P.R. Sipes-Metzler, and R.Wopat. 1991. Prioritization of health care services: A progress report by the Oregon Health Services Commission. *Arch Intern Med* 151:912–16.

Kolata, G. Medical groups reach compromise on frequency of giving Pap tests. *New York Times* January 7, 1988, B13.

Lewis, P.A., and M. Charney. 1989. Which of two individuals do you treat when only their ages are different and you can't treat both? *J Med Ethics* 15:28–32.

Lipid Research Clinics Program, 1984. Lipid research clinics coronary primary prevention trial results, II: The relationship of reduction in incidence of coronary heart disease to cholesterol lowering. *JAMA* 251:365–74.

Luce, B.R., and R. Brown. 1995. The use of technology assessment by hospitals, health maintenance organizations, and third party payers in the United States. *Int J Technol Assess Health Care* 11:79–92.

Mandelblatt, J.S., and M.C. Fahs. 1988. Cost-effectiveness of cervical cancer screening for low-income elderly women. *JAMA* 261:2409–13.

Menzel, P.T. 1992. *Strong medicine.* New York: Oxford University Press.

National Cholesterol Education Program (NCEP). 1988. *High blood cholesterol in adults: Report of the expert panel on detection, evaluation, and treatment.* Bethesda, MD: National Institutes of Health, Department of Health and Human Services.

National Cholesterol Education Program (NCEP). 1994. The second report of the Expert Panel on Detection, Evaluation, and Treatment of High Blood Cholesterol in Adults. *Circulation* 89:1329–1445.

Office of Technology Assessment (OTA), U.S. Congress. 1994. *Identifying health technologies that work: Searching for evidence.* OTA-H-608. Washington, DC: U.S. GPO.

Office of Technology Assessment (OTA), U.S. Congress. 1979. *Review of selected federal vaccine and immunization policies based on case studies of pneumococcal vaccine.* Washington, DC: U.S. GPO.

Oldridge, N., W. Furlong, D. Feeny, G. Torrance, G. Guyatt, J. Crowe, and N. Jones. 1993. Economic evaluation of cardiac rehabilitation soon after acute myocardial infarction. *Am J Cardiol* 72:154–61.

Ontario Ministry of Health. 1994. Ontario guidelines for economic analysis of pharmaceutical products.

Patrick, D.L., and P. Erickson. 1993. *Health status and health policy: Quality of life in health care evaluation and resource allocation*. New York: Oxford University Press.

Rawls, J., 1971. *A theory of justice*. Cambridge, MA: Harvard University Press.

Russell, L.B. 1994. *Educated guesses: Making policy about medical screening tests*. Berkeley, CA: University of California Press and Milbank Memorial Fund.

Sempos, C., R. Fulwood, C. Haines, M. Carroll, R. Anda, D.F. Williamson, P. Remington, and J. Cleeman. 1989. Prevalence of high blood cholesterol levels among adults in the United States. *JAMA* 262:45–52.

Spilker, B. 1990. *Quality of life assessment in clinical trials*. New York: Raven Press.

Task Force on Principles for Economic Analysis of Health Care Technology. 1995. Economic analysis of health care technology: A report on principles. *Ann Intern Med* 123:60–69.

Taylor, W.C., T.M. Pass, D.S. Shepard, and A.L. Komaroff. 1990. Cost effectiveness of cholesterol reduction for the primary prevention of coronary heart disease in men. In *Preventing disease: Beyond the rhetoric*, ed. R.B. Goldbloom and R.S. Lawrence, 437–41. New York: Springer-Verlag.

Tengs, T.O., G. Myer, J.E. Siegel, J.S. Pliskin, J.D. Graham, and M.C. Weinstein. 1996. Oregon's Medicaid ranking and cost-effectiveness: Is there any relationship? *Med Decis Making* 16:99–107.

U.S. Preventive Services Task Force (USPSTF). 1989. *Guide to clinical preventive services: An assessment of the effectivness of 169 interventions*. Baltimore: Williams and Wilkins.

Weinstein, M.C., and W.B. Stason. 1982. Cost-effectiveness of coronary artery bypass surgery. *Circulation* 66:III-56–III-66.

Weinstein, M.C., and W.B. Stason. 1976. *Hypertension: A policy perspective*. Cambridge, MA: Harvard University Press.

Willems, J.S., C.R. Sanders, M.A. Riddiough, and J.C. Bell. 1980. Cost-effectiveness of vaccination against pneumococcal pneumonia. *N Engl J Med* 303:553–59.

Williams, A. 1988. Economics and the rational use of medical technology. In *The economics of medical technology*, ed. F.F.H. Rutten and S.J. Reiser. Berlin: Springer Verlag.

2

Theoretical Foundations of Cost-Effectiveness Analysis

A.M. GARBER, M.C. WEINSTEIN, G.W. TORRANCE, and M.S. KAMLET

Cost-effectiveness analysis (CEA) informs resource allocation decisions in health and medicine: How well it does so depends on the comparability and consistency of analyses of diverse interventions. But even a cursory examination of the literature reveals that investigators have made different assumptions about such issues as which costs and effects should be included in the analysis, which rate (if any) should be used to discount health effects that occur in the future, and the ways in which the cost of people's time should be incorporated. In the absence of uniform methods and perspectives—or of time-consuming efforts to reconstruct analyses that have used disparate methods—the results of different analyses cannot be compared.

If cost-effectiveness studies adhered to a fixed set of methodological standards, such problems might disappear. But why should one set of standards be adopted in preference to others? One way to answer this question is to seek consistency with a theoretical foundation that is broadly acceptable and informative. Such a theoretical construct, if followed through to its logical consequences, would have specific implications for the structure of CEA. An examination of the theoretical foundations of CEA will potentially resolve controversies and assist in the development of standards. This chapter describes possible theoretical foundations of CEA and their implications for the performance and interpretation of analyses.

Historically, there is no single theoretical foundation for CEA. Its roots can be traced to a variety of sources, prominent among them such fields as decision analysis and operations research. Many tools of CEA, such as the optimization techniques required for its application and the instruments developed to measure health-related quality of life, reflect the contributions of researchers of diverse backgrounds. Indeed, it might be said that CEA developed as an applied engineering technique for allocating resources.

Only recently (see, for example, Garber and Phelps, 1995) have economists sought to graft CEA to theoretical roots in welfare economics.

What kind of theory can serve as a foundation for CEA? Consider firstwhat one may mean by a theory. A theory can be defined as a coherent group of general propositions or principles (*Random House Dictionary of the English Language*, College Edition, 1968). A theory of decision making can be (1) *descriptive* if its objective is to explain phenomena or (2) *normative* if its objective is to define a standard of correctness or a norm. To the extent that CEA is designed to be a practical tool for achieving societal goals, we believe that such a theory must be normative. We do not claim that CEA adequately *describes* the behavior of health care decision makers; if it did, it would not be needed. Hence, the following discussion focuses on normative theory underlying CEA.

Perhaps no theoretical foundation can answer all of the questions that arise in setting policies for the allocation of health care. In this chapter we emphasize welfare economics as a theoretical foundation for CEA. We do so because welfare economics represents a comprehensive framework that provides answers to more methodologic questions that arise in decisions from the ''societal perspective'' than do any alternatives. We acknowledge, however, that CEA can be based on first principles outside of welfare economics and, therefore, that not *all* of the principles of welfare economics are essential to the practice of CEA.

The particular advantage of the welfare-theoretic framework, however—and the basis for our reliance on this theoretical foundation—is that it can inform specific issues in the application of CEA from the ''societal perspective.'' Welfare economics provides guidance on such elements of CEA as how *society* should value resource costs and choose a discount rate for evaluation. This is not true, for example, for optimization techniques—themselves based on theoretical principles from applied mathematics. Optimization techniques are essential to any application of CEA, but they address the question of which approach is best *if* one adopts a particular decision-making perspective in which the constrained resources and the decision maker's objectives are explicit. They cannot directly answer questions that require reference to a fundamental set of values.

Despite its appeal as a comprehensive framework, the values implicit in welfare economics are not shared by all decision makers, even those working from the societal perspective. Hence, on some matters it may be preferable to depart from the recommendations of welfare economics to accommodate alternative formulations of social goals regarding health and health care. We return to alternative, ''extra-welfarist'' perspectives later in the chapter.

What Is Cost-Effectiveness Analysis?

Cost-effectiveness analysis is a method designed to assess the comparative impacts of expenditures on different health interventions. As Weinstein and Stason (1977) state, it is based on the premise that "for any given level of resources available, society . . . wishes to maximize the total aggregate health benefits conferred." For example, we might wish to know whether spending a certain amount of money on a public campaign to stop smoking will have greater or lesser effect on health than spending the same amount on colorectal screening. Cost-effectiveness analysis can also be used in decision making by groups or individuals, but we focus here on resource allocations at the societal level.

The Cost-Effectiveness Ratio

The central measure used in CEA is the cost-effectiveness ratio. Implicit in the cost-effectiveness ratio is a comparison between alternatives. One alternative is the intervention under study, while the other is a suitably chosen alternative—"usual care," another intervention, or no intervention. The cost-effectiveness ratio for comparing the two alternatives is the difference in their costs divided by the difference in their effectiveness, or C/E.

The C/E ratio is essentially the incremental price of obtaining a unit health effect (such as dollars per year, or per quality-adjusted year, of life expectancy) from a given health intervention when compared with an alternative. When the intervention under study is both more effective and less costly than the alternative, it is said to *dominate* the alternative; in this situation there is no need to calculate a cost-effectiveness ratio. In the circumstances under which C/E analysis is typically performed, though, the intervention is both more costly and more effective than the alternative. Interventions that have a relatively low C/E ratio are "good buys" and would have high priority for resources. In the contemporary climate of cost-consciousness, C/E analysis can also inform decisions in which a new intervention is less costly but somewhat less effective than existing alternatives. In either case, the value of a unit of the health effect is the greatest "price," or incremental C/E ratio, that we would pay for an intervention relative to its less costly alternative.

A decision rule based on adopting all interventions with C/E ratios less than or equal to a particular value will be optimal in the following two respects: (1) the resulting set of interventions will maximize the aggregate health effect achievable by the resources used, and (2) the resulting aggregate health effect will have been achieved at the lowest possible cost. There are other ways to use cost-effectiveness ratios as well. For example, they can be used to provide information to consumers about the relative values of alternative health interventions. As discussed in Chapter 1, there may be contexts in which optimization strictly according to cost-effectiveness ratios may not be ethically acceptable owing to concerns about distributive fairness, but in which knowledge of the ratios may be informative nonetheless.

Cost-Effectiveness Analysis and Cost-Benefit Analysis

Cost-benefit analysis (CBA) is similar to cost-effectiveness analysis in many respects but has a closer and better-established connection with welfare economics. The usual cost-benefit criterion from program evaluation in CBA, that the benefits of a program exceed its costs, leads to decisions that meet the requirements for an "optimal" solution under the welfare-economic framework.

Because of CBA's explicit grounding in welfare-economic principles, it is natural to ask why one would use cost-effectiveness rather than cost-benefit analysis if one wants to build from a welfare-economic foundation. Our interest in cost-effectiveness analysis derives largely from its broad acceptance within the health care field, in contrast to the skepticism that often greets cost-benefit analyses in that arena.

It is the distinguishing feature of CBA that offends some sensibilities: In CBA, the benefit of the health intervention is expressed in dollar terms rather than in terms of a nonmonetary effectiveness measure (Kamlet, 1992). The monetary measurement is obtained by estimating individuals' willingness to pay for life-saving or health-improving interventions, a measure that inherently favors the wealthy over the poor.[1] It is thus the dependence of CBA on the monetary valuation of health benefit and the method for obtaining this estimate that have motivated the reliance on CEA in the field of health and medicine.

The valuation requirement for CBA is both its greatest disadvantage and its greatest strength. It presents a difficult measurement challenge, requiring the dollar valuation of all health outcomes of importance, including changes in pain, suffering, functional status, and mortality. The valuation exercise is so daunting that few analyses attempt it. But because CBA values health in dollars rather than in units of health outcomes, it entails no distinctions between cost and effect, input or outcome. Perhaps more importantly, its scope of application is broader than that of CEA. CEA can only compare interventions whose benefits are measured in the same units of effectiveness. Thus CEA cannot be used to inform decisions about how much we should spend on housing, food, or education in relation to health care. At least in principle, CBA can handle such disparate comparisons.

For those who are uncomfortable about attaching dollar valuations to health outcomes such as life expectancy, CEA offers much of the same information. Often the two techniques will lead to similar or identical decisions concerning the allocation of health resources, so the distinction may be more important for the sake of appearance than for its practical consequences (Phelps and Mushlin, 1991).

A Metric of Health Effect: Quality-Adjusted Life Years

It may appear that CEA cannot even be used to compare interventions whose effects on health are qualitatively different, such as prevention of coronary artery disease and treatment of arthritis. However, such a comparison is possible if the measure of effectiveness is general enough to capture all of the important health dimensions of the effects of the interventions. Using the quality-adjusted life year (QALY) as the unit of effectiveness approaches this ideal within the framework of CEA, thus expanding considerably the range of application of CEA. The QALY is a measure of health outcome which assigns to each period of time a weight, ranging from 0 to 1, corresponding to the quality of life during that period, where a weight of 1 corresponds to perfect health and a weight of 0 corresponds to a health state judged equivalent to death. The number of quality-adjusted life years, then, represents the number of healthy years of life that are valued equivalently to the actual health outcome. Chapter 4 gives a more detailed description of the theory and methods of quality-adjusted life years in CEA. The following discussion assumes that health effects are measured in QALY units.

Theoretical Foundations for Valuing Individual and Social Well-Being

If the fundamental purpose of CEA is to serve as an instrument to improve well-being by improving health, the overriding question is: Under what circumstances do decisions made on the basis of CEA lead to better distributions of resources? If such circumstances are artificial or uncommon, the technique is unlikely to be broadly useful. But if the circumstances pertain approximately in the settings in which it might be applied, CEA can have great value. Even when reality and the conditions of the theoretical model fundamentally differ, an exploration of the theoretical framework can reveal how and why CEA might need to be modified to remain a valid guide to decisions under such conditions.

By describing CEA as a tool for improving general welfare, we place it squarely within the context of welfare economics. Welfare economics is concerned with the means by which we can assess the desirability—from the societal point of view—of alternative allocations of resources. The central problem of welfare economics has been described by Arrow (1963) as "achieving a social maximum derived from individual desires." Welfare economics is based on the assumptions (1) that individuals maximize a well-defined *preference function* (in other words, their "utility" or sense of well-being depends on, among other things, material consumption, and the utility or preference function follows certain conditions of rationality and logical consistency), and (2) that the overall welfare of society is a function of these individual preferences. Much of the literature of welfare economics is concerned with developing criteria to determine whether a program improves the welfare of the affected population.

To make that determination, then, it is necessary to first measure well-being at the individual level and then aggregate individual well-being to measure welfare at the societal level.

Individual Utility Maximization

The starting point of economic theory, including welfare economics, is the behavior of individuals and the implications of individual economic behavior for interactions of groups of people in markets. Individuals are assumed to have well-defined preferences. These preferences are represented by individuals' utility functions, which relate their well-being to their levels of consumption of a number of goods and services.

The simplest economic models pertain to a world of complete certainty. Prices are known, there are no random events, and all information is freely available to everyone. These conditions bear little relation to the usual circumstances of health and medical care. Disease and its treatment have at their core substantial uncertainty. Kenneth Arrow's classic essay (1963) on the welfare economics of medical care claims that many of the distinguishing characteristics of health services delivery are direct consequences of uncertainty: the uncertainty inherent in the risk of disease and the uncertainty attending treatment—because our knowledge of its impact is imperfect.

Because both health status and the effects of health care involve pervasive uncertainty, the principal approach used in modeling preferences in cost-effectiveness analysis, as well as in other applications of health economics, has been expected utility theory. It has proven to be an extremely useful, if imperfect, descriptive framework with which to analyze individual behavior under uncertainty. When risk and uncertainty are significant factors, it has been used even more successfully to prescriptively guide decisions. According to expected utility theory, alternative actions are characterized by a set of possible outcomes and a set of probabilities corresponding to each outcome. Quantitative representations of preference, or utilities, are assigned to each possible outcome (e.g., health state) that may occur. To choose the best action, the probability of each outcome is multiplied by the utility of that outcome; these products are then summed across all possible outcomes in order to derive the expected value of utility. The numerical quantities used as utilities, then, reflect both ordinal rankings of outcomes and strength of preference for these outcomes when they are embedded in uncertain gambles. Expected utility theory is presented in many textbooks of economics (Hirshleifer and Riley, 1992), and it is at the heart of the prescriptive methodology of decision analysis (Raiffa, 1968; Holloway, 1979; Weinstein et al., 1980; Sox et al., 1988).

Valuing Individual Health Effects

Expected utility theory supplies a theoretical foundation for the quantification of effectiveness in cost-effectiveness analysis conducted at the individual level. Many analysts agree that the measure of effectiveness should reflect individual preferences under uncertainty: Specifically, the measure of health benefit to an individual should reflect the gain in expected utility for the individual. Quality-adjusted life years (QALYs) are one such measure.

The theoretical foundations of expected utility theory may be applied to answer the question: Under what circumstances can health-related utility be represented in terms of quality-adjusted life years? Pliskin et al. (1980), as modified by Johannesson et al. (1994), have shown that QALYs can be used to represent utility only if (1) individuals are willing to trade off years of life in a given health state for fewer years at an ideal health state at a constant rate, irrespective of the number of years spent in the state (the constant proportional tradeoff assumption), and if (2) individuals are indifferent among various survival curves that have the same life expectancy (they are risk neutral).[2] These assumptions may not hold in practice, but QALYs may still offer a close enough approximation to health-related utility to justify their use in cost-effectiveness analysis, especially when one views CEA as an input to, rather than a procedure for, decision making.[3]

Having defined individual health-related utility in terms of quality-adjusted life expectancy, the question of how to aggregate changes in health-related utility across individuals remains. We turn next to the issues at the level of a group or population.

The Role of Health in Determining Social Welfare

Health is an important component of individual utility, but not the sole consideration. Consumption of other goods and services, such as food, shelter, clothing, and recreation, also contributes to overall well-being. Different people may be willing to exchange other sources of utility for health at different rates. For example, a wealthy individual might be willing to reduce other consumption of nonhealth goods more sharply in order to improve health than would a poor person, who cannot afford to give up as much. One issue from the point of view of social welfare is whether to accept individual preferences for health vis-à-vis other commodities or whether to base social policy on the assumption that the goal of health policy is to maximize health.

To illustrate the distinction between these two approaches to social policy, consider a society consisting of rich people and poor people in which opportunities to provide health services to both groups are available. Suppose that society has allocated health care resources in order to maximize the aggregate number of quality-adjusted life years across the population. Now it may be that the poor people would gladly give up some of their health care (say, 100 QALYs' worth) in exchange for cash (which they can use to buy other valued items), and the rich people would gladly give up an equivalent amount of cash in order to get more health care (say, 90 QALYs' worth). Welfare economics would recognize this situation as an opportunity for a trade which could make both rich and poor people better off, according to their own preferences. Such a trade would, however, result in less aggregate health for the society as a whole. Moreover, it would leave the poor people in worse health than the rich, although they would consider themselves better off than under the initial state of affairs. Is this trade socially desirable? Neoclassical welfare economics says yes, because everyone perceives themselves as better off. However, an "extra-welfarist" perspective (Williams, 1993) might regard this trade as unacceptable because society values health as a "merit good," that is, a good which people should have regardless of their willingness to pay for it. According to the latter view, since the posttrade society has 10 fewer QALYs' worth of health than the pretrade society, society is worse off. This illustrates a fundamental difference in values between the implications of defining the output of health care in terms of its contribution to overall well-being and instead, defining it in terms of its contribution to health itself. In either case, individual preferences determine the magnitude of health improvements, but society's approach to aggregating these would be very different.

Welfare Economics as a Theoretical Foundation for CEA

In welfare economics, a *social utility function* is defined as some aggregate of individual utilities; economists view the maximization of the social utility function as the ultimate goal of any resource allocation scheme. One approach, which is frequently and incorrectly equated with the welfare-economic approach generally, is *strict utilitarianism*. The specific form of the social welfare function under strict utilitarianism is the sum of the utilities of the individuals who comprise society. But the usual reason to address social welfare in this framework is to propose or at least explore other forms of aggregation; typical measures allow for the possibility that different people should receive different weights in the social accounting. For example, greater weight might be given to the welfare of persons who are either in poor health or impoverished.

A substantial literature, spanning economics, philosophy, and political science, addresses the possible specifications of the social welfare function and the ways that such a distributive scheme might be elicited from the views of members of society. The literature suggests that there is no consensus on the specific form the social utility function should take; it appears to be impossible to select a specific weighting scheme from any universally accepted set of first principles (Sen, 1995). Consequently, much of the economic literature concerned with improvements in well-being avoids choosing weights to be attached to the utilities of different individuals. Instead it seeks less-demanding assumptions under which it is possible to make firm statements about the relative desirability of alternative resource allocations.

If there is no consensus about how individual utilities should be combined to form a social utility function, can anything useful be said about the effect of any reallocation of resources on social welfare? The concept of *Pareto optimality*, which is the benchmark used in nearly all mainstream microeconomics, has proven to be a simple but powerful guide to testing for whether a resource reallocation might improve social welfare. A resource distribution is considered to be Pareto-optimal when any change in the distribution must make someone worse off, even if others are better off. This implies, of course, that if an allocation is not Pareto-optimal, it is possible to reallocate so as to improve at least one person's welfare without making anyone worse off. A strict criterion for deciding whether a reallocation of resources represents an improvement in welfare is closely related to this concept. If the reallocation makes at least one person better off, and no one worse off, it is said to represent a *Pareto improvement*. Thus, when the effects of a change in policy or prices on individual utilities are known, but the specific social welfare function is not, the Pareto criterion can be used to test whether social welfare is improved.

A reallocation that makes some people better off and none worse off seems unexceptionable, but unfortunately it is rarely attainable. Few public programs produce only winners; typically, funds must be raised by taxes or another mechanism that imposes costs on some people that exceed the benefits they can expect to receive. In fact, packages of programs are often constructed to enable every voter to gain in at least some dimension, while perhaps sacrificing in others—or at least to appear to offer gains to everyone—but such efforts rarely achieve unqualified success. Thus, although this criterion is extremely useful in economic theory for determining the optimality of alternative schemes for pricing, taxation, and so on, it has limited applicability in testing the consequences of real-world policy options.

A less-restrictive standard, variously called *potential Pareto improvement*, the *Kaldor-Hicks criterion*, or the *compensation test*, has been proposed to evaluate situations in which there are both gainers and losers from a reallocation. Under the compensation test a program is considered to be welfare-enhancing if the gainers are willing to pay enough for their gains in order to compensate the losers. The rationale behind this standard is that *if* there were a mechanism for such payment to occur, the program would result in an actual Pareto improvement. Cost-benefit analysis is directly based on the potential Pareto-improvement criterion. It can be shown that if a program is undertaken whose (properly measured) benefits exceed their costs, a potential Pareto improvement will occur.[4]

Central to the compensation test for potential Pareto improvement is the proposition that the appropriate measures of value are the amounts of money that individuals are willing to pay for goods and services. The compensation test is tantamount to the following thought experiment. When a program is being considered, imagine passing a hat to each member of society. Individuals who would gain from the program must put into the hat the maximum amount of money that they are willing to pay for the program. Individuals who would lose, including taxpayers who would pay a share of the cost without receiving any benefit, take from the hat the amount of money that would be just enough to compensate them for their losses or tax payments. (For this reason, willingness to pay is also called ''compensating variation'' in welfare economics.) If there is more money in the hat at the end than there was at the beginning, then the program represents a potential Pareto improvement.

The drawback of this approach, of course, is that the reallocation from gainers to losers may not occur. Then the desirability of a program from the societal perspective cannot be determined without reference to the distribution of welfare, and a well-defined way of combining the welfare of different people into a social welfare function must again be invoked.

The welfare-economic framework facilitates derivation of the cost-effectiveness approach from fundamental principles, and in particular clarifies the conditions under which decisions based on C/E ratios are equivalent to tests of the Kaldor-Hicks criterion. Garber and Phelps (1995) describe a set of assumptions under which rankings derived from cost-effectiveness ratios provide the optimal expenditure of health resources. One such assumption is that individual utility in any period of life is the product of two factors: the utility attached to health-related quality of life in that period (i.e., a quality weight) and the utility attached to the individual's material consumption in that period. Under this assumption, Garber and Phelps show that individuals will optimally set priorities for health care expenditures by selecting those with cost/QALY ratios less than some threshold.

In essence, this approach rests on the assumption that QALYs are a valid representation of individual utilities for health outcomes. Because of the flexibility afforded by the adjustments for health-related quality of life, in many instances this will be reasonable; although the QALY formulation appears restrictive, it represents a close approximation for a much broader set of plausible utility functions than those that can be described in precise terms as QALYs (Garber and Phelps, 1995). Sometimes, however, QALYs will not be adequate; for example, an individual with a terminal illness may place very high value on living until a particular milestone (a child's wedding, a holiday, a reunion with a relative or friend), and care less about length of life after the event. The approximation to health-related utility that QALYs offer will be inexact. However, such phenomena may be unimportant when CEA is applied at the *population* level.

Maximizing QALYs as Social Policy

As an alternative to defining social utility as an aggregate of individual utilities, special status may be given to health in the social accounting. According to this view, health per se is viewed as the output of the health care sector, and the social objective is to maximize health subject to resource constraints (Culyer, 1991; Williams, 1993).[5]

The connection with individual expected utility theory is not that individual utilities provide any normative basis for aggregation, since clearly they do not, but that individual utilities allow for the possibility of creating a social utility function based on explicitly stated societal preferences, as determined, for example, by a decision-making body or official. For example, it might be asserted, as an ethical principle, that the marginal social utility of 1 year of quality-adjusted life expectancy is equal for all individuals. This assumption would lead to the use of aggregate QALYs as the quantity to be maximized in health resource allocation.

One approach to justifying a procedure for aggregating utilities (i.e., QALYs) appeals to a hypothetical choice situation, or "contract," among citizens who we assume are impartial because they operate behind a "veil of ignorance" (see Harsanyi, 1953, 1955). Imagine individual citizens in a state prior to their birth, uncertain of which of many prospects, including possible health scenarios, await them. Then rational individuals, seeking to make themselves as well-off as possible but blinded to the specifics of their futures, would opt for societal decision rules based on maximizing aggregate (or average) utility across the "population" of possible lives; they would choose a pure utilitarian distribution.[6] This conceptual basis for maximizing aggregate health-related utility has been described also as a "Constitutional Convention" by Kamlet (1992). If (1) deliberators behind such a veil of ignorance would choose to maximize expected utility across possible life scenarios, and (2) we assume that individual preferences for health outcomes are expressed by quality-adjusted life years, then we are led to a societal effectiveness measure equal to the sum of quality-adjusted life years gained.

Others have challenged the claim that rational citizens behind such a veil of ignorance would choose to maximize expected utility in this way. Rawls (1971)—who in any case rejects social utility as an appropriate measure of well-being for purposes of justice, appealing instead to "primary social goods"—argues that agents deliberating upon their life prospects behind a veil of ignorance should adopt as their principle of rational choice a "maximin" rule, that is, a rule which seeks to maximize the well-being of the worst-off member of society. Rawls refuses to assume that life prospects are equally probable in the absence of any information when the stakes are so high. Other contractarian theorists (Scanlon, 1982) have also argued that our moral concerns about the "separateness of persons," including the fact that the losses of some people are not compensated for by the gains of others, preclude accepting the "gamble" involved in choosing a utilitarian distribution or its specific implication here, namely, a measure of social effectiveness equal to the sum of QALYs.

It is possible to accommodate some of these worries about distributive effects, since we might aggregate individual utilities in ways other than the simple sum of QALYs. In extreme form, this could lead to a distributional principle based on maximizing the utility of the worst-off individual (the maximin rule). However, the maximin aggregation rule attaches no weight to improvements in the utility of the better-off or even average members of society. In the health context, the question is whether, behind the veil of ignorance, people would rather have increases in quality-adjusted life expectancy if their initial endowment of quality-adjusted life years turns out to be low, or if they would choose to receive the same gains in quality-adjusted life expectancy under all life scenarios. As an alternative, *changes* in QALYs could be weighted more heavily for members of society whose initial level of health is poorer (Nord, 1992). The problem is to justify any weighting scheme in a principled or morally acceptable way.

Implications of Alternative Foundations for Distributional Equity

It should be noted that, in the formulation of cost-effectiveness analysis founded upon the compensation test, the optimal cost-effectiveness threshold differs across individuals (Garber and Phelps, 1995). Wealthier individuals would spend a larger amount per QALY than poorer individuals, reflecting their greater willingness to sacrifice material consumption for increased quality of life and probability of survival. The resulting potential Pareto improvement can be converted to an actual Pareto improvement by requiring the wealthy, who would receive health interventions according to a more generous criterion, to compensate their poorer counterparts with a portion of their wealth. But because there is no guarantee that this redistribution will occur, the resulting distribution of health benefits may be unacceptable.

Would an allocation rule based on assigning equal value to all QALYs result in a more equitable distribution of welfare than an allocation rule based on the Kaldor-Hicks criterion? One cannot say. It depends on whether the transfers of wealth from rich to poor, as compensation for a greater willingness to invest in their health care, outweigh the inequities in the provision of health care based on allowing the C/E cutoff to vary by income.

Even the assumption that all QALYs are valued equally may lead to some ethically unsettling distributional implications. Applying this principle rigorously in CEAs would lead to calculations of societal benefit that give less weight to saving the lives of persons with life expectancies that are reduced because of age, race, or socioeconomic status. Similarly, the extension of lives of persons with chronic disabilities would count for fewer QALYs gained than the extension of healthy lives. From behind the veil of ignorance, perhaps this practice can be justified ethically, but some observers may find unacceptable the ethical implications of counting all QALYs equally. We return to this issue in Chapter 4.

Theoretical Foundations for Valuing Costs in CEA

The welfare-theoretic foundation of CEA facilitates resolution of numerous methodologic issues relating to the valuation of costs. Of particular importance for CEA, it provides guidance about how to assign monetary costs to the resources that are used or freed up by health care services.

The real cost to society of a resource consumed or freed up as part of a health intervention (or as a result of it) is the value of that resouce in its next best use to society. Because resources are more scarce than the needs for which they can be used, doing more of a given health service—employing more doctors or nurses, utilizing more space and equipment for hospital beds, using more chemical or biological products—means forgoing something else of value. In an ideal analysis from the societal perspective, therefore, resources should be valued at an amount equal to their best alternative use—their opportunity cost.

Economic theory shows that if the economy exhibits certain characteristics, then the prices prevailing in the marketplace fully reflect the values for resources in alternative uses. That is, the price of a good or service equals the resource cost of producing the last unit produced, and the resource cost of the marginal unit produced equals the value of its inputs used elsewhere. A common and tractable method useful in calculating the societal opportunity cost of a health intervention in a cost-effectiveness analysis thus locates and assigns a price to each of the resources consumed or saved by the intervention. Market prices are multiplied by incremental quantities of consumer goods or inputs to health care to calculate incremental costs.

The practice of substituting market prices for value in cost-effectiveness analyses may be less than ideal for two reasons. First, the theoretical equivalence between market prices and the value of the resources consumed does not hold in many circumstances. It assumes (1) the existence of perfectly competitive[7] markets for all goods and services, (2) the absence of externalities and public goods, and (3) the absence of distorting incentives (e.g., due to insurance, subsidies, or taxes). It is generally agreed that these conditions do not hold generally in the health sector. Second, the use of market prices does not account for changes in price that may occur as a result of the implementation of an intervention. A cost-effectiveness analysis performed before widespread use of a treatment, based on existing prices, might not reflect the true marginal cost of the treatment if substantially more (or less) of that treatment were consumed.[8] For example, if a national program began to cover the costs of bone marrow transplantation, demand would likely increase, causing a price increase due to limited short-term supply. A long-run price decrease might also occur as a result of improvements in the technology over time through a learning curve.

If observed market or transaction prices are inadequate as measures of value, the analyst may need to adjust current market prices or investigate alternatives, as discussed in Chapter 6. However, the principle of using opportunity costs provides a guide for determining the value of resources consumed and for use of market prices.

Applications of Theory to Methodologic Controversies

If the goal is to define and adopt a uniform set of practices to be followed by all cost-effectiveness analyses (see Drummond et al., 1993), then an appeal to theoretical foundations may seem unnecessary. For example, investigators might reach an agreement to ignore time costs in computing cost-effectiveness ratios. There might be strong reasons to favor such an approach, not the least among them the practical difficulty of measuring and valuing time costs. But the consensus is more likely to endure and earn wide acceptance when the logic supporting it is clear and persuasive. We now discuss how economic theory can provide a logical foundation for use in analysis. We will look at the consequences of adopting different approaches to three controversial issues in cost-effectiveness analysis—handling time costs, incorporating health care costs that occur during years of added life, and discounting future costs and health effects.

Time Costs

A complete analysis of the costs and benefits of an intervention should include all costs, including those that are due to time lost during illness or while in treatment. The need to incorporate time costs is widely accepted, yet many details about which time costs should be included in cost-effectiveness analyses and how they should be included are unresolved. Published analyses include three categories of time costs: (1) costs related to the treatment in question that involve the time of patients, their families, or others not considered to be formal health care providers; (2) costs associated with lost or impaired ability to work or to enjoy leisure activities due to morbidity; and (3) lost economic productivity due to death. Although some authors regard each of these categories as "indirect costs" of health care, we will refer to them as "time costs." An exception is the time spent by uncompensated caregivers, which will be considered to be included among the health care services costs.

Useful guidelines for handling of all three categories of costs emerge directly from the principle that time costs should be counted but not double-counted (either included as a [health] consequence or a change in monetary cost, but not both). The need to incorporate time costs follows from the motivation for performing cost-effectiveness analysis—to use limited resources as effectively as possible. Because time, like money, is a limited resource that can be put to other (valuable) uses, time should be incorporated in the analysis. Clearly two alternative interventions that are similar in every way, except that one requires more time to travel to obtain health care, are not equally desirable.

Once it is recognized that time costs must be included, the question for cost-effectiveness methodology is whether they should be included as monetary costs (i.e., in the numerator of the C/E ratio) or as decrements to utility (i.e., in the denominator). Placing the costs in both locations, of course, would amount to double-counting; if the financial implications of lost time are reflected in the utility weights assigned to health states in the calculation of QALYs, then it would be incorrect to count the lost productivity again as costs in the numerator. In that case, only the costs borne externally to the individual whose health is affected, such as frictional costs to the employer, would be counted additionally in the numerator. If, however, respondents to the utility questions are specifically instructed *not* to consider loss of income when assessing their preferences for health states, then the full time costs must be counted in the numerator. We return to the question of which time costs to place in the numerator or denominator after discussing two pertinent theoretical issues: whether and under what conditions it matters, in principle, if time costs go in the numerator or the denominator, and the conceptual basis for assigning monetary value to time costs.

Does it matter whether time costs are valued in dollars or QALYs?

Garber and Phelps (1995) show that under conditions of perfect markets, the cost-effectiveness method leads to the same decision rules for allocating health resources whether one places time costs in the numerator or the denominator of the C/E ratio. The optimal resource allocation can be achieved by comparing C/E ratios with a threshold value representing the willingness to pay for additional QALYs; interventions with C/E ratios lower than this threshold will be accepted and interventions with C/E ratios higher than this threshold will be rejected. Garber and Phelps show that, under specific conditions, the position of the C/E ratio above or below the threshold is the same whether time costs are valued in the denominator as a decrease in the number of QALYs produced or in the numerator by a dollar value. For an activity whose utility is considered equivalent to death (i.e., whose quality-of-life weight is 0), their result requires that the opportunity cost of time equals the willingness to pay for additional QALYs. For other activities—i.e., whose quality-of-life weight is positive—their result requires that the opportunity cost equal the willingness to pay to improve the quality of life from that experienced in the activity to the level corresponding to a value of unity on the QALY scale. Thus an activity that imposes no disutility (i.e., no decrement in the QALY) has zero opportunity cost.

Are these results heavily dependent on the assumptions underlying the model? As Garber and Phelps (1995) acknowledge, the two methods will not produce equivalent results if the wrong valuation of time is used in either the denominator or the numerator. For example, for reasons discussed below, wages can be used as a proxy for the opportunity cost of time under certain conditions. However, for most people work is not the equivalent of death; on a scale from death to unrestricted leisure in full health, working while otherwise healthy might be assigned a relatively high weight. Therefore, it would be incorrect simply to subtract time spent in a doctor's waiting room from the number of QALYs gained in the denominator of the C/E ratio, unless that time was considered to be equivalent to death. (See Chapter 4 for a discussion of the meaning and sources of health-related quality-of-life weights.) In the numerator, the wage rate would understate the true opportunity cost of time if some of the compensation for the work does not take the form of wages. For example, a manager might accept a lower salary if it meant that she would get a corner office, extensive secretarial support, and flexibility in work hours; a machinist might decline more lucrative job opportunities to take a position that included substantial on-the-job training and offered better opportunities for future advancement. The disparity between wages and opportunity costs poses a challenge that must be surmounted if time costs are to be included in the numerator of the C/E ratio.

Other deviations from the underlying assumptions of perfect markets can mean that health interventions will be ranked differently if time costs are placed in the numerator rather than in the denominator of the C/E ratio. However, under the same circumstances C/E ratios may no longer be valid guides to the alternative ranking of interventions. For example, income taxes cause wages to deviate from opportunity costs. Leisure time is not taxed, and the worker deciding how many hours to work considers *after-tax* wages, but the employer bears the full cost of the pretax wages. Tax rates and subsidies that differ across people and across inputs into health care greatly complicate the determination of the socially optimal types and levels of medical interventions to use.

The Garber-Phelps model refers to an individual allocating his or her own lifetime resources, and not to resource allocation at the population level. If society applies different cost-effectiveness criteria (dollars per QALY) to each individual, based on their own willingness to pay for QALYs, then the conditions leading to the equivalence between including time costs in the numerator and denominator may be satisfied. However, if C/E ratios are applied to populations, the two approaches will yield equivalent rankings only if the monetary value of time (and QALYs) is the same for everyone.

Thus, the theoretical framework suggests that, under certain circumstances, the choice between numerator and denominator for time costs does not matter. However, those ideal circumstances seldom apply, so choices have to be made.

Valuing time costs in monetary terms

Placing the time costs in the numerator presupposes that there is a method for converting time costs into dollar values. The dollar valuation of time is a central theme of labor economics: It is key to understanding such phenomena as unemployment, job turnover, hours of work, and retirement. The central concept, as described above in the context of valuing health resource costs, is that of *opportunity cost*, or the value of time in its best alternative use. The fundamental assumption of this literature is that people will take their opportunity cost into account when allocating their time, choosing to devote it to the activities that produce the greatest utility. They will work an extra hour, for example, if the compensation they receive exceeds the value they place on their time in other activities.

The well-established basic theory, along with variants that take into account forms of ''market imperfection,'' have been subjected to empirical analysis and can shed some insight into the valuation of time costs for cost-effectiveness analysis. The *labor–leisure tradeoff*, which is at the heart of the theory of labor supply, illustrates the method used to value time that is not spent at work: if there is perfect competition; if workers and employers are perfectly well informed; if the worker has declining marginal utility of leisure time (i.e., the more time spent away from work, the lower the value of each incremental increase in leisure time) and diminishing marginal utility of income; and if the quantity of labor supplied in the market is continuously variable, then the worker ''consumes'' leisure time up to the point at which the value of an additional hour of leisure equals the (hourly) wage that he or she can receive by working.

Although only chimerical markets may satisfy all the conditions of perfect competition that underlie the simplest, idealized model of value of time, in mainstream economics all efforts to value time build upon the concept of opportunity cost. Even in settings in which market imperfections are prominent and empirical tests of the theory are infeasible, the concept has direct, concrete implications. For example, it leads to the conclusion that the value of time is not near zero for people who are retired or otherwise out of the labor force. Economists would infer, for example, that people who choose to retire place a higher value on time spent in leisure activities or "household production" (which encompasses diverse activities such as child raising, food preparation, and cleaning) than they place on wages they could receive if they continued in their current job. Although it is not easy to infer the exact value of their time (i.e., the wage rate that would induce them to continue to work), there is no reason to believe that the number is negligible.[9]

If we accept the principle that time costs should be valued by their opportunity costs, then it follows from the theory that the time of people with differing opportunity costs should be valued differently. To the degree that wages reflect opportunity cost, the time of persons in demographic groups that tend to have lower-paying occupations would be valued less. It remains controversial whether it is ethically acceptable, for example, to value the time of women less than that of men in CEAs, although this is the implication of the theory.[10] Like the issue of whether to count the QALYs of disabled persons the same as those of nondisabled persons, ethical concerns may sometimes override the strict interpretation of the theory. We return to this question in Chapters 4 and 6.

Should time costs go in the numerator or denominator?

Despite the practical difficulties, then, there is at least a conceptual basis for valuing time costs in either dollar terms or in utility terms so that it will often be possible to choose either to place such costs in the numerator or the denominator of the C/E ratio. In some circumstances, however, it is clear that the numerator and denominator are not equally appropriate for this purpose. For example, the common practice in dealing with lost earnings due to death is unambiguous. The value of lost life is included in natural units (adjusted or unadjusted) in the denominator of the C/E ratio precisely to distinguish it from CBA, in which the value of life is monetized. Subtracting from the numerator to reflect a monetary valuation of savings due to deaths averted clearly amounts to double-counting.[11]

In contrast to the handling of lost productivity due to death, there is no convention guiding the placement of lost productivity due to morbidity in the numerator or denominator of a CEA. However, the principle of not double-counting is also relevant in considering morbidity costs. In principle, the answer depends, at least in part, on the framing of the question used to elicit utility weights for health states. If we choose the convention of eliciting utility weights for health states in such a way that the opportunity cost of morbidity time is in the denominator, this principle dictates that the monetary value of this time should not also be placed in the numerator. If we choose the opposite convention, and explicitly exclude monetary costs from consideration in the utility assessment procedure by stating that the respondent would be compensated financially for lost earnings, then these costs must be in the numerator. We consider these two situations in turn.

First, consider the situation in which the preference weights for health states are assessed under the assumption that the respondent receives full monetary compensation for the loss of work time directly resulting from impaired health status. In that case, the full societal cost of that time must be included in the numerator. If the disutility of work exactly equals the disutility of the illness, then the lost earnings can serve as a measure of the dollar value of the morbidity. Moreover, from a social perspective, the time costs are real even if the worker who is in a hospital or at home with an illness receives sick pay or disability pay; the payments the worker receives are transfer payments, a concept discussed in Chapter 6. Even though the worker may be compensated fully by these transfer payments, society is not, since the disability pay must come out of somebody's pocket. There may be additional frictional or transactions costs that result from the illness—for example, the worker who replaces another who is unable to work may receive as much compensation but be less productive in the position. The productivity loss imposes genuine social costs which, if they are large enough, should be included in the analysis (Johannesson, 1994; Koopmanschap et al., 1995). A similar approach applies to men and women who are not in the labor force—the opportunity cost must be assessed for them just as it is assessed for a worker. If the individual loses leisure time, the appropriate cost is based on the opportunity cost of their leisure time rather than the wage rate. Furthermore, the same principles apply to time costs that result from using health care services.

Second, alternatively, suppose that preference weights are assessed *without* an explicit proviso that there would be financial compensation. In this case, *part* of the cost of the lost time would already be reflected in the (dis)utility weight assigned to the health states that impair ability to work or perform valued leisure activity. The part that would *not* be reflected in the (dis)utility weights, however, pertains to the loss of time per se, independently of any effect on health status. For example, time spent traveling to health care, spent in a physician's office, or recuperating in a hospital or at home, *while otherwise unimpaired in terms of health status*, would not reduce the number of QALYs but would nonetheless represent a time cost. Such time costs would still have to be captured in the numerator, even though the effect of the impaired health status would have been reflected in the denominator.

The quality of time may vary in different activities. Variation in quality of time does not raise major conceptual difficulties, since one can define an opportunity cost for alternative states of health or activities; thus the time spent in a doctor's office may be considered more pleasant than death but less pleasant than work, in which case the dollar value of time in the doctor's office exceeds the wages lost. Appropriate adjustments can be made to the opportunity cost, if time costs are included in the numerator of the C/E ratio, or in the quality adjustments, if they are mediated by health status changes and included in the denominator.

To return to the question of which time costs should be counted as costs (in the numerator) and which should be counted as losses of health-related quality of life (in the denominator), consider two examples. The first example is a major operation which requires a painful period of convalescence during which work is impossible. Should this period be subtracted from the number of life years or QALYs that the intervention produces? Should one place a dollar value on the time spent in recuperation and add it to the costs in the numerator? Or should some costs appear in the numerator and others in the denominator? If the utility weights are elicited under the assumption of full compensation for lost earnings, then the loss of QALYs will reflect only the pain itself and not the opportunity cost of the time. In that case, to fulfill the requirement that all resource costs be included in the analysis, the full societal cost of that time must be included in the numerator. Hence, the lost productivity (as a proxy for the opportunity cost of the time) would be included in the numerator as a component of the costs. If, alternatively, the utility weights are elicited without any implication of financial compensation for lost time, then it may be inferred that the loss of utility due to the inability to work has been captured as a loss of QALYs; to count the lost earnings in the numerator would be double-counting in this case. In the latter case, only the frictional, or transitional, costs of lost productivity should be included in the numerator (Johannesson, 1994; Koopmanschap et al., 1995).

As a second example, consider the valuation of time spent in an exercise program. If the individual values the time spent exercising as equivalent to time spent in other leisure activities, then the time cost is zero. If the time spent exercising is valued as equivalent to time spent at work, then the time cost is equal to the opportunity cost of leisure, as measured by lost earnings. If exercise is considered so onerous that it impairs health-related quality of life, then its cost would exceed the opportunity cost of leisure. The issue of numerator versus denominator rests on whether the time spent in exercise is incorporated into the calculation of QALYs. If so, and if exercise results in an impairment (or improvement) of health-related quality of life, then the opportunity cost of the time per se must still be counted in the numerator.

Thus, while the handling of time costs associated with mortality is relatively clear in CEA, the costs of other patient time consumed could be incorporated into either the numerator (as a monetary cost) or the denominator (as a decrease in QALYs). Either approach is theoretically justified, and either is feasible. The social welfare approach indicates only that these time costs, like other resource use, should be included. Further guidance is provided by the principle of not double-counting, which requires that if such costs are incorporated in the denominator they should not appear in the numerator (or vice versa) and by the motivation to achieve consistency across C/E ratios, which requires that a decision be made as to which costs are included in the numerator and the denominator of Reference Case C/E ratios.

What about time spent by family members or paid helpers, either as part of treatment or consequential to the illness? The social welfare framework clearly implies that such costs must not be ignored. The above logic implies that when unpaid work is performed by people who are not in the labor force, the value of the time should again be based on opportunity cost. Insofar as QALYs usually refer to health outcomes for the patient receiving treatment, the time costs borne by others do not appear in the QALY weights;

hence, to ensure that it is not overlooked, caregiver time that is not incorporated in the QALY measure should be valued in dollar terms and included in the numerator of the C/E ratio.

It must be noted that when CEAs are conducted from perspectives other than societal, the answer to the question of what belongs in the numerator and what belongs in the denominator could be different. For example, the "costs" from the point of view of a government agency that administers a health program might be limited to the payments it makes; if it pays for a visiting nurse, the cost will be included in the numerator of the C/E ratio, but if services are provided by a family member or the patient, the time costs might be ignored (or treated as a reduction in the number of QALYs produced). But our focus is on the social perspective, in which all costs count. Thus we cannot avoid making a decision about whether to put time costs in the numerator or the denominator of the C/E ratio.

Summary: theoretical considerations in handling time costs

1. *Mortality costs.* By definition in CEA, mortality is incorporated into either life years or QALYs as the effectiveness measure. Therefore, it would be double-counting to include a monetary value for lost life years in the numerator of the C/E ratio. To do so,would be tantamount to performing a complete cost-benefit analysis in the numerator, which would render the C/E ratio meaningless.

2. *Morbidity costs and time spent receiving care.* Under specific circumstances, it can be shown that it does not matter whether time costs are incorporated in the numerator (in dollar terms) or in the denominator (in QALYs) of the C/E ratio, as long as the practice is consistent. A choice about the best practice must be made, however, both for those occasions when these circumstances are not valid and to ensure consistency across cost-effectiveness estimates.

As discussed in Chapter 4, standardization of QALYs can be achieved only if the denominator is used solely to represent health-related quality of life and not the value of time per se. If this argument is accepted, and, therefore, the value of time spent receiving health services is excluded from the denominator, then it must be placed in the numerator. This would imply that the monetary value of time spent receiving health services must be placed in the numerator of the C/E ratio. To the extent that these activities also result in an impairment of health-related quality of life which is reflected in, *and measured as*, a loss of QALYs, these reductions in QALYs can be included (in the denominator); their consequences must not, however, be doubly counted in the numerator as opportunity costs in excess of the cost of time per se. These time costs should appear regardless of whether they arise from the illness, are associated with receiving health care, or are part of recuperation.

If the full consequences of morbidity to patients, including lost productivity and leisure, are included in the QALY measure in the denominator, then they must not be double-counted in the numerator. Under these circumstances, only the costs borne by persons other than the patient, such as frictional costs to employers and co-workers due to disability, should be included in the numerator. If the full consequences of morbidity to patients are not included in the denominator—for example, if preference weights for QALYs are assessed under the explicit assumption that the individual will be financially compensated for lost ability to work—the monetary value of that financial compensation must be included among the time costs in the numerator.

The panel's recommendations on these issues are contained in Chapters 4 and 6.

3. *Placing a dollar value on time.* When it is necessary to value time to include in the numerator, each hour should be valued at its opportunity cost. The wage rate can be used as a proxy for the opportunity cost of time for employed persons, but it does not adequately reflect the value of time for persons engaged primarily in leisure or in activities for which they are not compensated.

Unrelated Future Costs of Health Care

One of the most persistent of the unresolved issues in the application of cost-effectiveness analysis is the handling of so-called "unrelated" future costs of health care. Should health care costs that result solely from the fact that a successfully treated patient lives longer be attributed to the health intervention? Suppose, for example, that we contemplate instituting a suicide prevention program in a high school. It is highly effective and reduces teenage suicides by 50%. Students who would otherwise have died now lead lives of average length and have medical care utilization comparable to those of average persons their age. Should the future costs of health care that they consume be counted as costs of the intervention? The literature contains diametrically opposed opinions on this issue. Weinstein and Stason (1977) and Drummond et al. (1987) have argued that they should be counted while Russell (1986) has argued that they should not. Adherents to the former view argue that insofar as health care expenditures rise when people live longer, the true cost of the intervention exceeds the simple expenditures for the treatment. According to the alternative view, however, health care is but one of many costs of living longer: If we count future health care costs in added years of life, why not also count future expenditures on food, clothing, and shelter as part of the cost of the intervention?

Garber and Phelps (1995) claim that the method of accounting for truly "unrelated" future costs of health care does not matter, under the circumstances described above, in the section on time costs. In defining "unrelated" costs, they consider those future costs of care that are conditionally independent of expenditures on the intervention under consideration, as in the suicide prevention program.[12] They further assume that the future stream of health expenditures meets certain optimality conditions. These assumptions imply that the decision to include or exclude the unrelated costs merely changes every cost-effectiveness ratio, as well as the cutoff cost-effectiveness ratio, by a constant amount. Then it does not matter whether the cost-effectiveness analysis incorporates changes in future unrelated costs of health care, as long as the practice is entirely consistent. The calculated cost-effectiveness ratio for any intervention that prolongs life, of course, will be greater if these costs are included, but the ranking of interventions will not be affected.

An important limitation of this theoretical result is that it applies only when comparing programs targeted at persons with the same remaining survival, that is, persons of the same age who are not known to differ in ways that would cause their age-specific risks of death to diverge. Otherwise, the amount by which the cost per life year will increase when these costs are included will not be constant but will depend on the age-specific pattern of health care costs.

Many interventions can be expected to alter future patterns of health care significantly, so future costs of health care cannot be considered conditionally independent of current expenditures. Failure to measure or anticipate such effects will alter not only the estimates of the effectiveness of the therapy but also the estimates of the long-term costs. It is fair to ask whether the pattern of future expenditures is ever truly unaffected by an intervention that has a large impact on longevity. Often we don't know and can't easily find out; for example, an unanticipated long-term side effect of a drug usually takes years to be discovered, and a cost-effectiveness analysis cannot be expected to reveal such consequences of treatment if clinical studies do not.

Even if there are no long-term side effects of therapy, it is possible that no costs will be truly unrelated because any treatment that has a sizable impact on mortality acts (by reducing ''competing risks'') to change the rates of other diseases. For example, if we were to cut heart disease death rates by a large amount, such as 50%, we would increase the prevalence of cancer solely because people who would have died of heart disease, the most common cause of death among adults, now live to die of other common diseases. If cancers are associated with more expensive treatments, and if we were to treat such costs as unrelated, we would fail to anticipate a potential increase in total health expenditures that reductions in heart disease mortality would provoke. Such arguments are quantitatively important only when an intervention is highly effective and in a population with high mortality rates, because competing risk effects essentially represent the product of two (small) mortality terms, and for most preventive interventions in the general population such effects are negligible.

To illustrate the importance of including costs of ''unrelated'' diseases whose incidence is affected by competing risk, consider the following hypothetical scenario. Suppose, for purposes of illustration, that all causes of death are associated with ''terminal care'' costs of $10,000. This cost is incurred, for example, in attempting to save a patient with a fatal heart attack or metastatic cancer. In performing a cost-effectiveness analysis of an intervention to prevent heart attacks (such as cholesterol lowering), suppose the costs of ''unrelated'' health care in the added years of life were excluded.

Then, the $10,000 saved by preventing a fatal heart attack would be credited to the intervention, but the $10,000 cost of dying from cancer would not be counted. Such an analysis would be predicated on an illusory saving of $10,000—the unavoidable cost of terminal care in this illustration—when in fact this cost is merely shifted by the intervention from one disease to another.

Toward a resolution of the dispute over future costs

To clarify the issues, we define three categories of induced costs that may or may not be germane in a cost-effectiveness analysis. These are: (1) costs related to the intervention, which are incurred during years of life that would have been lived without the intervention; (2) costs unrelated to the intervention, which are incurred during years of life that would have been lived without the intervention; and (3) costs that occur in years of life added (or subtracted) by the intervention. The third category may be subdivided further into three subcategories: (a) health care costs for the disease or diseases affected by the intervention, (b) health care costs for other diseases, and (c) nonhealth costs such as food, shelter, and clothing.

Costs in category (1), related diseases in the original life span, are not controversial; they must be included in the analysis. Analyses of cardiovascular prevention programs must include the costs or savings of treating heart attacks and strokes if these events are affected by the program. Likewise, costs of treating complications of treatment must be included.

Costs in category (2), unrelated health and nonhealth costs occurring during the original life span, are also not controversial. By definition, these costs are the same with and without the intervention. They cancel from the calculation of incremental cost in the numerator of the C/E ratio and, therefore, may be excluded. Furthermore, because their measurement may induce error in the estimation of costs with and without the intervention, it is usually preferable to exclude them.[13]

Category (3) is more complicated. First consider category (3)(a), costs for diseases related to the intervention but occurring in added years of life. These are typically included in cost-effectiveness analyses. For example, if a coronary bypass operation or a cholesterol-lowering intervention delays a fatal heart attack by 5 years, the costs of treating coronary events that occur during those 5 years are included. Likewise, the costs of an ongoing treatment during added years of life, such as lifelong antihypertensive therapy and its side effects, are always included.

Next consider category (3)(b), costs for diseases unrelated to the intervention and occurring in added years of life. This has been the source of much controversy. As a first step, we argue that in practice—that is, under usual circumstances—it matters whether these costs are included or excluded from all analyses if cost-effectiveness ratios are to be comparable. One important reason is that health care costs are not independent of age. Adding an 80th year of life truly costs more to maintain in good health than adding a 20th year of life. Thus, if different interventions add years of life for different age groups, a set of C/E ratios calculated including these costs could be ranked differently from a set calculated for the same interventions if these costs were excluded.

Setting aside the fact that these costs vary with age, the Garber-Phelps model might seem to suggest that these costs could be either consistently excluded or consistently included without changing the ranking of C/E ratios. However, in order to apply this principle correctly, one would have to note that some of the costs in category (3)(a) are actually "unrelated" by the Garber-Phelps definition. For example, persons who are not candidates for a cholesterol-lowering intervention may nonetheless experience cardiovascular costs in future years of life. These age-specific "background" costs of coronary heart disease are no different conceptually from the costs of clearly unrelated diseases such as arthritis and Alzheimer's disease; they may be consistently included or consistently excluded without changing C/E rankings, but the key is consistency.

This means that if we choose to exclude the costs of "unrelated" diseases, we would also have to exclude the "unrelated" component of the costs of "related" diseases. To fail to do so would create an uneven playing field for comparing interventions into different diseases: Life-prolonging heart disease interventions would be burdened with *all* of the future costs of heart disease, while suicide prevention programs would not. There are practical and conceptual problems in disentangling the "related" and "unrelated" components of costs for "related" diseases, both of which are included in category (3)(a). The comprehensive exclusion of future "unrelated" costs would therefore be difficult, if not impossible, in practice.

We turn finally to category (3)(c), nonhealth costs in added years of life. Theoretically, these costs should be included, if health care costs in added years of life are included. However, if these nonhealth costs meet the Garber-Phelps definition of "unrelated," then their consistent inclusion or exclusion would only add or subtract a constant from the C/E ratio. Whether nonhealth costs are truly "unrelated," or at least approximately so, is an unresolved empirical question. If it were true, for example, that non–health care consumption is more closely constant with age than health care, then the constant added for consumption in each year of life at different ages would be, approximately, truly constant across ages. The question then becomes whether the Garber-Phelps result allows us to exclude these nonhealth costs without affecting the ranking of C/E ratios.[14] The Garber-Phelps argument does not, however, apply to health care costs, because they are not nearly constant with age and because a portion of the apparently related costs is, in fact, unrelated in complex and often unknown ways and would have to be excluded along with the costs of unrelated diseases in order to achieve consistency.

Like other costs and consequences, the rule of reason applies to these health care costs in added years of life. If they are small compared to the magnitude of the C/E ratio, they can be omitted without affecting the conclusions of the analysis.

Discounting

The practice of discounting health care expenditures—adjusting the dollar amounts to reflect the time value of money by assigning lower values to dollars paid in the future than to dollars paid in the present—has never been controversial. In modern economies people pay interest when they borrow money and receive interest payments when they lend or save. Thus, a dollar paid in the future is worth less than a dollar today, and for health interventions whose costs are spread over many years or whose savings are spread over many years, the practice of discounting is essential.

Discounting is more controversial, however, when it is applied to health effects. At first glance, it is not obvious why health effects that are obtained in the future should count less than immediate health effects. Is it less valuable to avert a heart attack 10 years from now, for example, than a heart attack next year, if they have the same impact on health-related quality of life and on life expectancy? Economists who work on cost-effectiveness analysis have long accepted that health effects should be discounted in the same way that the dollar expenditures are and that the same discount or interest rate should be used. Others have argued that a year of life is a year of life, whether it occurs today or in the future, and therefore health effects should not be discounted.

The social welfare foundation of CEA depends heavily on the fidelity with which an outcome measure, such as QALYs, approximates utility. QALYs are construed to have a particular functional form, usually with constant-rate discounting; a zero rate of time discount is a special case. Whether QALYs serve to approximate utilities when the personal rate of time preference is set to zero is an empirical question. If individuals place the same weight on future events as on those that will occur soon, or if they are as happy to receive a reward in the future as now, then a zero rate of time discount may be consistent with utility maximization. If they apply positive rates of time preference, the social welfare foundation only applies if the QALYs include nonzero time discounting.

An empirical question—What are appropriate rates of time preference?—thus drives the theory regarding discounting. The empirical literature on rates of time preference involves determining the rate at which individuals trade off future gains (or losses) against current gains (losses) from either their response to surveys (which ask them to consider a set of hypothetical alternatives) or from observations of their actual behavior (particularly with regard to life-saving investments or financial behavior). This issue is explored more fully in Chapter 7. In brief, estimates of personal rates of time preference vary widely, but it appears that few people have a rate of time preference near zero. In fact, much of the literature implies that the rates of time preference are implausibly large, suggesting that individuals place far greater weight on costs and benefits that occur soon as compared to delayed costs and benefits, regardless of the domain of the question (i.e., financial tradeoffs or health tradeoffs).

Even if one accepts the need for discounting, there is substantial disagreement about whether the same rate of discount should be applied to nonmarket outcomes as to market outcomes. For example, if a person is willing to save money at a 5% annual interest rate, does it imply that the same individual will trade off the benefits of preventive therapy for current risks at the same 5% annual rate of discounting? Much of the conventional wisdom suggests that the same discount rate should be applied to all outcomes, but cogent arguments have been made that when a market good that can serve as a close substitute for a nonmarket good (such as health) is not readily available, rates of time preference need not be uniform across goods and services. Thus the welfare-economic foundations suggest that discounting is ordinarily appropriate, but it does not always provide unambiguous guidance to the particular discount rate to use.

When viewed in terms of welfare-economic foundations, the argument for discounting health effects rests on the implicit assumption that a rich and virtually continuous set of opportunities exists for exchanging money for current and future health effects. This assumption is needed so that individual marginal rates of substitution between current and future health equal societal rates of time preference. Because such opportunities to buy and sell health are not infinitely rich in an individual's lifetime, we observe wide variations between individual discount rates for health (Redelmeier and Heller, 1993), some of which are different from societal discount rates. The implications of interindividual variation in rates of time preference, and the interpretation of empirical time preferences estimates, are discussed in detail in Chapter 7.

We defer our recommendations regarding the practice of discounting in CEA until Chapter 7, where we elaborate further on the theoretical and empirical basis for discounting future costs and health consequences and for choosing a discount rate.

Conclusion

Cost-effectiveness analysis is, in the end, a pragmatic approach to measuring relative value for money in health care. It evolved as a practical response to the need to allocate limited resources for health care, not as a practical implementation of social welfare theory. Nevertheless, decision-making rules based on cost-effectiveness criteria can, under some circumstances, be directly justified on the basis of social welfare theory. Exploration of these foundations offers more than an intellectual justification for the techniques of C/E analysis because, insofar as the technique is viewed in isolation from any theoretical foundation, the answers to thorny questions in its application—such as whether to discount future health outcomes and how to account for time costs—are often arbitrary. The theoretical foundations can expose the implications of alternative responses to these questions and reveal that some practices are more useful and readily justified than others. In the subsequent chapters of this document, we describe issues that arise in different aspects of cost-effectiveness analysis. Some of the areas of uncertainty that we describe can be resolved by exploring the theoretical foundations. In other cases, the theoretical foundations help us understand what the results of cost-effectiveness analysis mean, what uses they have, and what their limitations are.

Notes

1. The "human capital" method, which values health according to the economic productivity of individuals, is still used, but it has been shown not to be consistent with welfare-economic theory (Mishan, 1988). In any case, the human capital method raises at least as many objections as the more theoretically sound willingness-to-pay method.

2. The modification by Johannesson et al. (1994) is that the constant proportional tradeoff assumption and risk neutrality should apply to discounted life years rather than to undiscounted life years.

3. It is possible to modify the analysis so that risk neutrality is not required. However, much of the power and simplicity of CEA are lost when risk neutrality is violated.

4. This standard result of public finance has been explained in a number of articles and textbooks; see, for example, Harberger (1971) or Mishan (1988).

5. In this sense, health would satisfy Rawls's (1971) definition of a "primary good."

6. Note that each individual's utility may depend on the well-being of others; thus, individual utilities could, for example, reflect altruistic values. Thus, individuals maximizing utility from behind the veil of ignorance might choose a more egalitarian distribution of well-being than if their concept of well-being were purely individualistic.

7. No individual economic agent, either seller or buyer, has sufficient market presence to affect the market price. This rules out monopoly (single seller) and oligopoly (small number of sellers), and also monopsony (single purchaser).

8. For a discussion of what to do when the price varies with the amount consumed, and of the role of taxes and other distortions, see Thompson (1980) and Gramlich (1990). Although most of their discussions are in the context of cost-benefit analysis, many of the solutions also apply to cost-effectiveness analysis.

9. The literature that addresses these issues includes work by Becker (1964), Ghez and Becker (1975), Mincer (1974), Heckman (1974), and MaCurdy (1981). Research on labor supply and the value of time are reviewed in the book by Killingsworth (1983).

10. It is possible that women receive greater nonpecuniary compensation for their time than men, for example, in the form of flexible hours, or less stressful jobs which facilitate child care responsibilities. If those factors fully explained the wage differential between men and women, then after adjusting for these factors the valuation of the opportunity cost of time might be the same for both. This remains an unresolved empirical question.

11. Although most analyses do not include lost earnings due to earlier death as part of the numerator of the cost-effectiveness analysis, some studies and government agencies list these figures as either the indirect costs of treatment or (reduced) indirect costs of disease. This practice, however, often amounts to conducting a cost-benefit analysis, since the dollar valuation of early death averted is a measure of the dollar benefit of treatment. If the analyst has such data, and if the dollar losses averted are valid measures of the benefits of prolonging life, it would seem that there is little reason to perform a cost-effectiveness analysis instead of a cost-benefit analysis.

12. Formally, costs in period 2 (C_2) are defined as "unrelated" to costs in period 1 (C_1) if $dC_2/dC_1 = 0$ (Garber and Phelps, 1995, p. 6). "Related" costs are not explicitly included in the Garber-Phelps model.

13. This issue of measurement error is particularly germane in the context of clinical trials. To include clearly unrelated diseases or unrelated costs that may be larger in magnitude than the related costs would greatly reduce the precision of estimation of the incremental cost between interventions. However, if there is uncertainty as to what costs are "related," it may be prudent to measure them nonetheless.

14. The same rationale permits the exclusion of external benefits from continued productivity during added years of life. Specifically, individuals who live longer would transfer a portion of their productivity to the rest of society, through taxes and other mechanisms, in part to finance health care. However, these benefits, like the nonhealth costs of added life expectancy, are "unrelated" in the sense of Garber and Phelps, and may therefore be excluded as long as this practice is consistently followed.

References

Arrow, K.J. 1963. Uncertainty and the welfare economics of medical care. *American Economic Review* 53:941–73.

Becker, G.S. 1964. *Human capital*. New York: National Bureau of Economic Research.

Culyer, A.J. 1991. The normative economics of health care finance and provision. In *Providing health care*, ed. A. McGuire, P. Fenn, and K. Mayhew. Oxford: Oxford University Press.

Drummond, M.F., G.L. Stoddart, and G.W. Torrance. 1987. *Methods for the economic evaluation of health care programmes*. Oxford: Oxford University Press.

Drummond, M., G. Torrance, and J. Mason. 1993. Cost-effectiveness league tables: More harm than good? *Soc Sci Med* 37:33–40.

Garber, A.M., and C.E. Phelps. 1995. Economic foundations of cost-effectiveness analysis. National Bureau of Economic Research.

Ghez, G.R., and G.S. Becker. 1975. *The allocation of time and goods over the life cycle*. New York: National Bureau of Economic Research.

Gramlich, E.M. 1990. *A guide to benefit-cost analysis*. Englewood Cliffs, NJ: Prentice-Hall.

Harberger, A.C. 1971. Three basic postulates for applied welfare economics:An interpretive essay. *J Economic Literature* 9:785–97.

Harsanyi, J.C. 1955. Cardinal welfare, individualistic ethics, and interpersonal comparisons of utility. *J Political Economy* 63:309–21.

Harsanyi, J.C. 1953. Cardinal utility in welfare economics and in the theory of risk taking. *J Political Economy* 61:434–35.

Heckman, J.J. 1974. Shadow prices, market wages, and labor supply. *Econometrica* 42:679–94.

Hirshleifer, J., and J.G. Riley. 1992. *The analytics of uncertainty and information*. Cambridge, England: Cambridge University Press.

Holloway, C.A. 1979. *Decision making under uncertainty: Models and choices*. Englewood Cliffs, NJ: Prentice-Hall.

Johannesson, M. 1994. The concept of cost in the economic evaluation of health care: A theoretical inquiry. *Int J Technol Assess Health Care* 10:675–82.

Johannesson, M., J.S. Pliskin, and M.C. Weinstein. 1994. A note on QALYs, time tradeoff, and discounting. *Med Decis Making* 14:188–93.

Kamlet, M.S. 1992. *The comparative benefits modeling project: A framework for cost-utility analysis of government health care programs*. Washington, DC: U.S. Department of Health and Human Services, Public Health Service.

Killingsworth, M. 1983. *Labor supply*. Cambridge: Cambridge University Press.

Koopmanschap, M.A., F.F.H. Rutten, B.M. van Ineveld, and L. van Roijen. 1995. The friction cost method for measuring indirect costs of disease. *J Health Econ* 14:171–89.

MaCurdy, T.E. 1981. An empirical model of labor supply in a life-cycle setting. *J Political Economy* 89:1059–85.

Mincer, J. 1974. *Schooling, experience, and earnings*. New York: National Bureau of Economic Research.

Mishan, E.J. 1988. *Cost-benefit analysis* 4th ed. London: Unwin Hyman.

Nord, E. 1992. An alternative to QALYs: The saved young life equivalent. *BMJ* 305:875–77.

Phelps, C.E., and A.I. Mushlin. 1991. On the (near) equivalence of cost-effectiveness and cost-benefit analyses. *Int J Technol Assess Health Care* 7:12–21.

Pliskin, J.S., D.S. Shepard, and M.C. Weinstein. 1980. Utility functions for life years and health status. *Management Science* 28:206–24.

Raiffa, H. 1968. *Decision analysis*. Reading, MA: Addison-Wesley.

Rawls, J. 1971. *A theory of justice*. Boston: Harvard University Press.

Redelmeier, D.A., and D.N. Heller. 1993. Time preferences in medical decisionmaking and cost-effectiveness analysis. *Med Decis Making* 13:212–17.

Russell, L.B. 1986. *Is prevention better than cure?* Washington, DC: Brookings Institution.

Scanlon, T.M. 1982. Contractualism and utilitarianism. In *Utilitarianism and beyond*, ed. A. Sen and B. Williams. Cambridge: Cambridge University Press.

Sen, A. 1995. Rationality and social choice. *American Economic Review* 85:1–24.

Sox, H.C., Jr., M.A. Blatt, M.C. Higgins, and K.I. Marton. 1988. *Medical decision making*. Boston: Butterworths.

Thompson, M.S. 1980. *Benefit-cost analysis for program evaluation*. Beverly Hills, CA: Sage Publications.

Weinstein, M.C., and W.B. Stason. 1977. Foundations of cost-effectiveness analysis for health and medical practices. *N Engl J Med* 296:716–21.

Weinstein, M.C., H.V. Fineberg, A.S. Elstein, H.S. Frazier, D. Neuhauser, R.R. Neutra, and B.J. McNeil. 1980. *Clinical decision analysis*. Philadelphia: W. B. Saunders Company.

Williams, A. 1993. Cost-benefit analysis: Applied welfare economics or general decision aid. In *Efficiency in the public sector*, ed. A. Williams and E. Giardina. London: Edward Elgar.

3

Framing and Designing the Cost-Effectiveness Analysis

G.W. TORRANCE, J.E. SIEGEL, and B.R. LUCE

Before undertaking a cost-effectiveness analysis (CEA), the analyst must decide on an overall approach to the study and on specific aspects of the study design. The early conceptualization and planning steps are essential for focusing the study on relevant research questions, maintaining the focus of the study as it progresses, and avoiding analytical pitfalls midway through an analysis.

In this chapter, we discuss framing and designing the cost-effectiveness analysis. Framing a study involves making a series of decisions that collectively define and describe the study to be undertaken. Designing the study involves planning the approach to the analysis, including determining the types of data to be used and the means for incorporating these data into the CEA.

Framing the Study

To assess the impact of an intervention, cost-effectiveness analysis describes and contrasts the costs and outcomes of a "treatment" course of events that would be expected to occur with the intervention and the costs and outcomes of a "comparator" course of events without the intervention. This general approach has many variations: More-intensive forms of an intervention can be compared with less-intensive forms (with the less-intensive form serving as the comparator); different types of prevention or of treatment can be compared for the same health problem; prevention of a problem can be compared to treating it.

Analysts approach a cost-effectiveness study with a general conception or question about the cost of an intervention and its impact on health outcomes. To move from this

54

general idea to the concrete details necessary to calculate a cost-effectiveness ratio, the analyst addresses a series of decisions that constitute the study frame.

Objectives of the CEA

Broadly speaking, the goal of cost-effectiveness analysis is, as discussed in Chapter 1, to inform a policy maker or others involved in health care decisions about the value of a particular health care program. For a specific study to be relevant, it must take into account the policy context and the controversies that relate to decisions about the use of the program. It must address an appropriate audience, and it must be conducted from a viewpoint relevant to that audience. Before beginning a study, it is thus essential to assess the decision-making process related to the intervention and to have an idea about how the study will contribute to this process. Examination of the decision context allows the analyst to clarify the objectives of a particular study.

A number of questions should be considered. Is there a specific decision motivating the analysis, or is the analysis intended to contribute to a general policy discussion? Who are the decision makers who will make or participate in decisions regarding the program? What groups will influence the decision by providing information directly to decision makers or by developing their own recommendations? What issues are of concern to these parties?

For example, an analyst considering a study about breast cancer screening might predict that, at some future time, decisions about screening for breast cancer will be constrained by the benefit packages offered by insurance organizations. Her purpose might be to assess the cost-effectiveness of screening strategies based on the latest evidence of screening and treatment effectiveness to inform benefits policy. The analyst would note that decisions about screening have traditionally been made by individual physicians and patients based on the recommendations of groups such as the American Cancer Society, the National Cancer Institute, and the U.S. Preventive Services Task Force. New policies may draw on these existing recommendations, and it is likely that these groups as well as physician organizations will have input in future developments regarding screening benefits.

Understanding the decision context will guide the choice of audience and the perspective of the study. These choices will, in turn, affect many of the other decisions made in designing the study. As noted in Chapter 1, we recommend that studies intended to inform resource allocation decisions (or to be comparable with those that do) take a societal perspective; a specific decision context should not induce the analyst to undertake an inappropriately narrow analysis. However, the objectives of an analysis may prompt the inclusion of other viewpoints as well. In addition, the decision context may affect the alternatives assessed or the comparisons made within an analysis.

As the above example demonstrates, cost-effectiveness analyses often address emerging issues and often are intended to supply information for future debates. In these cases, just as when an analysis pertains to a current and identifiable policy debate, envisioning how the study will be used and establishing its objectives in advance of undertaking the analysis serve to define and focus the study.

For the analysis of both emerging issues and existing programs or practices, cost-effectiveness analyses can be either "what is" studies or "what if" studies, depending on the data available for the analysis and its quality. Much of this chapter is directed at the "what is" type of study, where reasonably good data can be obtained or estimated on costs and outcomes. However, some studies must be undertaken well before good data are available if they are to address relevant policy questions in a timely manner. "What if" studies can investigate the magnitude of costs that an intervention can generate and/or the level of effects that are necessary in order for the intervention to meet acceptable standards of cost-effectiveness. This type of study is also called a *threshold analysis*, because it determines the thresholds with regard to costs and effects that the intervention must achieve to be acceptable. It should be noted that while "what if" studies can be done according to most Reference Case recommendations, inadequate evidence of effectiveness generally precludes comparison of the results of these studies with those of Reference Case analyses.

Cross-study comparisons for resource allocation

One of the ways that a cost-effectiveness study can be used is as an input into resource allocation decisions concerning a wide spectrum of alternative programs. The cost-effectiveness information bearing on these decisions will include the evidence regarding cost-effectiveness of each program and comparisons across studies. Tables summarizing the results of relevant cost-effectiveness studies can facilitate such comparisons. A common table format lists the results of multiple studies in descending order of cost-effectiveness. These tables are sometimes called cost-effectiveness "league tables"— after the tables used to rank teams in British soccer leagues (Mason et al., 1993; Drummond et al., 1993).

In the past, when comparisons across programs have been attempted (Torrance and Zipursky, 1984; Williams, 1985; Russell, 1989; Schulman et al., 1991), one of the major problems has been the noncomparability of methods across studies (Drummond et al., 1993)—an obstacle that provided the impetus for our Reference Case recommendations, as noted in the Introduction to this volume. Although tables comparing cost-effectiveness ratios across studies have been imperfectly realized, the basic idea is sound. Tables properly constructed from studies using standardized, comparable methodology can provide valid information to inform resource allocation decisions.

The large number of possible incremental comparisons within a cost-effectiveness table must be interpreted carefully. In particular, cost-effectiveness ratios for the interventions listed should reflect differences in cost and effectiveness as measured against an appropriate comparator, using established methods for calculating incremental cost-effectiveness ratios. These methods are described in more detail in Chapter 9.[1] It is also important that table entries carefully identify the important features of each intervention being considered and its comparator. For example, the entry "annual mammography screening for breast cancer for women 40–49 as compared with biannual screening" provides information needed in the interpretation of a cost-effectiveness ratio, in contrast to "annual breast cancer screening," an entry which would allow considerable opportunity for misinterpretation.

The ideal table of cost-effectiveness ratios would list all existing and potential programs, at all feasible levels of program scale and intensity, for all population and patient groups, compared to all feasible alternatives. This table would provide complete cost-effectiveness information for decision making from which a technically optimal allocation of resources could be identified, given a budget constraint.[2] Of course, the creation of an such an ideal, truly comprehensive cost-effectiveness table covering all health-improving interventions would be an enormous undertaking, well beyond what is currently realistic.

In practice, the usefulness of a cost-effectiveness table depends on the richness of detail provided and its relevance to the decision under consideration. The inclusion of a full range of program options enables a decision maker to identify the most appropriate alternatives rather than generalizing from the cost-effectiveness ratios for a generic program. However, a table alone cannot convey many of the caveats and explanations contained in a journal article. For example, the sources of cost or effectiveness data, the results of sensitivity analyses, and the source of preference weights are not accessible in a table format. For this reason, cost-effectiveness tables must be interpreted with caution.

The creation of tables that contain adequate information to inform resource allocation decisions remains an important challenge for the future. Some past projects that have assembled CEA results have retrospectively standardized the analyses included in a table to the extent possible by redoing them using a common discount rate, calculating incremental C/E ratios, and even by reprogramming models to standardize a range of assumptions (Brown and Fintor 1993; Tengs et al., 1995). With consistent use of a standard Reference Case analysis, much of this work could be avoided in the future. However, when nonstandard analyses are used—as will be the case if existing analyses are included—this extra attention to standardization will greatly improve the resulting table.

Audience for the Study

Who is the target audience for the study? When specific decision makers are responsible for a decision, these individuals will normally be the primary audience to whom the study is addressed. Some decision makers will have specific requirements or formats for studies to be submitted to them. For example, several countries are developing guidelines for the listing of new pharmaceuticals on government formularies. These guidelines specify such features of the study as the comparison program and the viewpoint the study should adopt (Henry, 1992; Canadian Coordinating Office for Health Technology Assessment, 1994).

Often, there is no single identifiable decision maker. A CEA may be intended to influence opinion on a subject or simply to add to the weight of information on an intervention. For example, the National Cholesterol Education Program (NCEP) publishes widely used guidelines for the management of elevated cholesterol, but it is individual physicians and patients—or sometimes formulary committees—who make the treatment decisions. As another example, medical specialty societies such as the American College of Physicians frequently issue practice guidelines that may be influenced by information in a CEA. A CEA may be intended to inform the recommending groups and/or the relevant medical practitioners directly.

Primary audiences for a CEA may include managed-care organizations, government entities such as Congress, the Public Health Service, or state health departments, as well as individual health care providers. Often there are additional decision makers who can use the same or similar information. Such secondary audiences may be groups who are not decision makers but have an interest in the study results, such as patient advocacy groups, the press, the research community in the public and private sector, or the general public.

In framing a cost-effectiveness analysis, it is important to determine the audience for the study before the analysis is begun. A CEA on fortifying cereal grains with folic acid to prevent neural tube defects in newborns might consider its primary audience to be a federal government task force charged with formulating regulations concerning food supply fortification. A potential side effect of a fortification policy is the masking of vitamin B_{12} deficiency, a disorder most common among the elderly. As a result, one secondary audience might be geriatricians. Since there are limited data on the prevalence of vitamin B_{12} deficiency, the analyst might identify epidemiologists or research funding agencies as other secondary audiences potentially interested in conducting additional surveys in this area.

The identification of these audiences will affect the analyst's strategy and methodological choices. In this example, the analyst would consider the debates occurring in each of these groups and the data cited in these debates. Consideration of the audience will also affect the issues highlighted in the report of the CEA.

Types of Analysis

Before undertaking an analysis, the analyst should determine the type of analysis or analyses that will best illuminate the subject of the study. Many different forms of information can contribute to a decision. These may include a set of cost-effectiveness and related studies.

Cost-effectiveness analysis should be distinguished from other closely related types of analysis. Not all of these approaches are widely used, but we outline them here because they are conceptually separate and complementary forms of analysis. They are cost-minimization analysis, cost-consequence analysis, and cost-benefit analysis. (See earlier discussion of cost-benefit analysis in Chapter 2.)

Cost-minimization analysis (CMA)

Cost-minimization analysis is a form of cost-effectiveness analysis in which the effectiveness of the program and the comparator are presumed to be equal. In this case, the decision simply revolves around the costs. Although the effectiveness of alternative programs is rarely exactly equal, this assumption may be a reasonable approximation in some cases.

Cost-consequence analysis (CCA)

Cost-consequence analysis is a disaggregated type of study that makes few assumptions and puts a relatively greater burden on the consumer of the analysis. The costs and consequences of the program compared to one or more relevant alternatives are computed separately and listed. The analysis itself does not combine these components, for example, by totalling across different types of costs and savings (such as medical costs, patient out-of-pocket costs, and costs of patient time), nor does it indicate the relative importance of the various outcomes. This option is left to the user of the study.

CCA is based on the premise that users of the study can and should make the value judgment tradeoffs necessary to integrate a disparate list of pros and cons (costs and consequences) of the various alternatives and reach a final decision. One concern is whether these individuals—whether they be clinicians, elected officials, health services managers, or others—are the right source of values across outcomes. An additional practical issue is whether decision makers can cope with the cognitive burden of making all the necessary value judgments and tradeoffs (Miller, 1956).

Cost-effectiveness analysis (CEA)

In cost-effectiveness analysis, the added costs and health outcomes associated with a program are used to calculate the incremental cost-effectiveness ratio relative to some comparator. Health outcomes can range from intermediate outcomes, such as millimeters-of-mercury blood-pressure reduction or disability days averted, to more distal outcomes such as lives saved, life years gained or quality-adjusted life years (QALYs) gained. The QALY (or analogous measure) is the most comprehensive measure of outcome used in CEA, incorporating both quality and survival information.

The particular type of cost-effectiveness analysis that uses QALYs is sometimes referred to as cost-utility analysis (Drummond, et al., 1987; Freund and Dittus, 1992; Torrance, 1986; Torrance 1995) and sometimes included under the rubric of cost-effectiveness analysis (Weinstein and Stason, 1977; Eisenberg, 1989). We will use the latter convention, describing these analyses as cost-effectiveness analysis with QALYs as the measure of effectiveness.

Cost-benefit analysis (CBA)

In cost-benefit analysis the incremental consequences are expressed in dollar terms, so the overall analysis of a program's costs and effects can be conducted entirely in dollars. The most common methods of assigning dollar value to health consequences are willingness to pay and human capital. Willingness to pay can be assessed directly by survey, using an approach known as *contingent valuation*, or it can be inferred from decisions actually made that involve tradeoffs between health and money. Human capital essentially values health in terms of the productive value of people in the economy. A CBA determines the net social benefit of the program: the incremental benefit of the program less the incremental costs, all measured in dollars. A positive net social benefit indicates that from the CBA perspective, the program is worthwhile.

CBA results are sometimes expressed as a benefit/cost ratio (incremental benefits divided by incremental costs). This approach is not recommended, because the inconsistent placement of costs in the numerator versus the denominator results in different ratios (Stokey and Zeckhauser, 1978). For example, the costs of averted illness could be viewed as a benefit (in the numerator) or as a negative cost (in the denominator), and the choice would affect the result of the analysis. Calculating net benefit circumvents this pitfall.

Because CBA entails valuing all outcomes in monetary terms, in principle it allows for comparisons across health and other sectors such as the environment, education, and defense spending. For example, a local government could use CBA to inform a decision about whether to use tax dollars for a road improvement program that saved commuting time, reduced pollution, and improved access to recreational facilities versus a health initiative offering free vaccinations and other programs to promote child health and welfare. But the advantages of CBA come at the expense of difficult measurement issues, such as the assignment of dollar values to lost life, illness, clean air, and leisure activities.

Cost-consequence analysis, cost-effectiveness analysis, and cost-benefit analysis are not mutually exclusive. Cost-consequence analysis is a natural part of both cost-effectiveness analysis and cost-benefit analysis, and much of the information obtained for a cost-effectiveness analysis can be used in a cost-benefit analysis. In many cases the effort required at the margin to add an additional analytic technique is small. Analysts are encouraged to present the data using a variety of analytic techniques. It is particularly useful to present a cost-consequence analysis as part of the descriptive material supporting a cost-effectiveness analysis.

Perspective of the Analysis

Cost-effectiveness analyses can be undertaken from a number of different perspectives. The broadest is the comprehensive societal perspective, which incorporates all costs and all health effects regardless of who incurs the costs and who obtains the effects.

The "societal" perspective is defined by the jurisdiction of the decision maker and the applicability of the decision. Often, it is delimited by national borders; however, it should not be confused with the "governmental" perspective, which may include only a subset of costs. Other perspectives that can be used in CEA include those of the health care institution (hospital or clinic), the third-party payer, and the patient and family.

The choice of the study perspective is an important methodological decision because it determines what costs and effects to count and how to value them. The appropriate perspective depends upon the objective of the study. For studies addressing the broad allocation of resources, we recommend that the societal perspective be used, as discussed in Chapter 1. The societal perspective includes all health care costs, social services costs, spillover costs on other social sectors such as education, and costs that fall on the patient and family. This perspective assures that all resource costs are included in the analysis, even when shifted among hospitals, insurers, patients, and other parties—as is often the case in health care.

Decision makers dealing with choices affecting organizations or specific interest groups may often wish to conduct CEA from the narrower viewpoint of the entity of interest. Fortunately, doing a CEA from one perspective does not preclude using other perspectives as well. The preferred approach when a specific viewpoint is needed (such as that of a health care organization or the patient and family) is to conduct the CEA and present results both from the broad societal perspective and from the narrower perspective relating to the particular interests of that actor. We recommend this approach in general for cost-effectiveness studies, and in particular for studies dealing with publicly funded programs.

It should be noted that the decision to use the comprehensive societal viewpoint has important methodological ramifications. It means that all costs and all effects should be incorporated no matter who pays the costs or who receives the effects. For example, if the program has an effect on the number of children with learning disabilities, costs or benefits to the educational system are counted. It means that all types of resources of value to society should be included; thus, patient's time costs (lost work time, lost leisure time) are counted, as discussed earlier and in Chapter 6. It means that opportunity costs are the appropriate method of valuation (see Chapter 2), and it means that the general public is the appropriate source of preferences for health outcomes (see Chapter 4).

Defining the Program or Intervention

The program to be analyzed in the CEA must be clearly specified. The program may include a large number of variations; for example, variations in the frequency of an intervention, in the ages and types of patients involved, or in the presence of comorbidities or risk factors. Screening for breast cancer can consist of self-examination, clinical examination, and mammography, in various combinations. Clinical screening can be conducted at different frequencies—every year, every 2 years, or less often. Screening strategies can vary for women in different age groups (40–49 versus 50–65) and even for different risk groups within ages. Thus, there may be many "programs" that are being evaluated. This is entirely appropriate, as one of the strengths of cost-effectiveness analysis is its ability to demonstrate the relative cost-effectiveness of programs given a wide range and variety of options. However, it is clearly essential in framing the study to define precisely what programs and program variations are to be included.

In general, the definition of the program should make clear to consumers of the analysis whether or not the cost-effectiveness results will apply to specific real-world programs. That is, the components of the program should be well-enough specified so that the audience of the study can compare the subject of the CEA to other programs and know whether their cost-effectiveness is likely to be similar or very different. For example, a smoking cessation intervention could be based in a community center or in a hospital outpatient clinic; it could utilize counselors or physicians; it could consist of a single counseling session or weeks of group meetings. Only if the analyst specifies these components can the consumer of the CEA know the extent to which the results apply to, for example, the smoking cessation program run within his own local hospital clinic.

The types of program characteristics that will be important depend on the analysis. Some aspects of the program that the analyst should consider are: the specific technologies used, the type of personnel delivering the service or treatment, the site of delivery, whether the service is "bundled" with other services, and the timing of the intervention. The target population, discussed separately below, is also a critical aspect of the program definition.

Target Population for the Intervention

The target population is the population for whom the program is intended.[3] Depending on the program, this may be individuals of a given age and sex, individuals living in a particular region, those with a specific disease, those with a certain risk profile, or groups defined by combinations of these characteristics. The target population can have a dramatic effect on the cost-effectiveness of an intervention.

The choice of target population will generally depend on the context of the analysis. For example, an analysis of public health programs designed to screen and treat medically underserved populations for high cholesterol in a defined geographic location would have a much different target population than an analysis focusing on alternative treatments for persons already identified with high cholesterol.

A target population can be divided into effectiveness subgroups, identifiable groups that would be expected to experience a different level of effectiveness from the program, on the basis of previous research. For example, the sensitivity of mammography screening is greater for elderly women than for younger women as a consequence of age-related changes in breast tissue. As a result of this improved test performance and the increasing incidence of breast cancer with advancing age, screening the elderly will yield a greater number of cases detected compared to screening nonelderly women. Although the elderly have a lower life expectancy, the cost per quality-adjusted year of life gained could be lower for this subpopulation than for other groups—a counter-intuitive possibility that the analyst would likely wish to explore by dividing a broad target population into the relevent age subgroups for analysis (Brown, 1992a,b).

There may also be ''cost subgroups'' within a target population. A cost subgroup is a particular subgroup that would be expected to have different resource consumption or savings as a result of the program. Due to economies of scale, a smoking cessation program for pregnant women conducted in an urban setting might be less costly per person than the same program in a rural area where there were fewer pregnant women, and, as a result, fewer participants attending the program.

Subgroups with differential effectiveness and/or with differential costs will, in general, have differential cost-effectiveness. It is important in framing the study to identify such subgroups and to determine the extent to which subgroup analyses will be undertaken. Subgroup analyses may be more relevant to the decision maker, but this advantage must be balanced against the decreased precision of available data. For example, many clinical trials do not have sufficient power to provide strong evidence on the differential effectiveness of an intervention in various subgroups. Often, statistical and/or simulation modeling is needed to infer the value of interventions in subgroups. (See Chapter 5.)

In addition to effectiveness and cost subgroups, the target population may contain preference subgroups—groups that have significantly different preferences for the relevant outcomes. For example, hormone replacement therapy lowers the risks of heart disease and osteoporosis in postmenopausal women, but evidence suggests that it increases the risk of uterine and, possibly, breast cancer. Some individuals may be particularly averse to the quality of life associated with the manifestations of osteoporosis or heart disease, while others might particularly fear the symptoms and circumstances accompanying cancer. When these preferences are reflected in the quality-of-life measure in a CEA, they will lead to differences in the cost per QALY result for the subgroups. The analysis might demonstrate that a particular program is much more cost-effective for individuals with a certain preference structure than for those with a different preference structure. Thus, it may be important to include preference subgroups within the target population in the analysis.

Comparison Program

Selection of the appropriate comparator is crucial in a cost-effectiveness study. In theory, if study resources were unlimited, the ideal approach would be to identify all

possible program variations applicable to the particular problem and all possible comparator programs and their variations, including a "do-nothing" option. Costs and
effects would be gathered on all of these programs. The incremental cost-effectiveness
algorithm (Torrance, et al., 1972; Weinstein, 1990) would be used to analyze the results
and to present the findings to the decision makers. (See Chapter 9.)

In reality, resources for undertaking cost-effectiveness analyses are limited, and normally studies must be much less ambitious. As a rule and as a minimum, studies from
the societal perspective should compare the intervention to existing practice for addressing the health problem (the status quo). The question being addressed is, What is
the cost effectiveness of replacing existing practice with the new program? If an intervention is *not* compared with the existing practice, the results can be deceptive. For
example, if a new drug treatment for hypertension is compared to "no treatment," it
will appear more cost-effective than it should. This comparison does not reflect the
value of an incremental change in practice.

Using the status quo as a primary comparator raises the problem of defining it. The
status quo is often not a single approach but a mixture of different approaches. The
alternative to bone marrow transplant for advanced breast cancer may be a variety of
different treatment regimens, depending upon the treatment center involved. Similarly,
the alternatives to folic acid supplementation of the food supply would include counseling to improve women's intake of dietary folate and physician advice to use vitamin
supplements.

When the status quo is a mixture of different interventions, there are two possible
approaches in selecting the comparator for the analysis. One approach is to select each
intervention, or at least the main ones, as comparators and use multiple comparators in
the analysis. This has the advantage of identifying the cost-effectiveness of all the
interventions, but it has the disadvantage of requiring extensive data on each intervention, which may not be readily available. It also presupposes that the interventions are
truly alternatives, in the sense that any of the them can be given to any of the patients.

The alternative approach is to use the status quo mixture of interventions as a single
comparator. This approach may better match the data, particularly if the costs and
outcomes for the comparator have come from actual community practice. It may also
correspond better to the reality of the decision situation, especially if the patients who
would receive the program under study would come randomly from the various treatments of the status quo. The two approaches address different questions. The first
approach addresses the question, Assuming that patients could receive any of the current
interventions of the status quo, or the new intervention under study, which would be
recommended using cost-effectiveness analysis? The second approach addresses the
question, What is the incremental cost-effectiveness ratio of a shift in practice from the
current mixed status quo approach to the new intervention under study? The analyst
may select either approach, or even both approaches, as appropriate to match the needs
of the decision maker and the availability of data and analytical time.

Comparing a new intervention with current practice is useful for evaluating the impact of replacing an existing program with an alternative, which is often the goal of a CEA. However, if exisiting practice is relatively cost-ineffective, the new program can look better than it would if compared to other real options. In essense, the program is being compared to a "straw man" rather than to truly desirable choices. Unfortunately, we may not know whether or not the status quo is cost-effective in its own right, since, more often than not, existing practice has not been subjected to careful evaluation.

To circumvent the problem that existing practice may not be the most suitable comparator, an analysis should investigate a range of other alternatives. These may include the best available alternative (as defined by clinical guidelines or some appropriate authority), and particularly any viable low-cost alternatives. A "do-nothing" option (an option defined in a relative sense as not doing the type of intervention in question, as opposed to the absolute absense of care) is usually important to consider. In some cases, the "do-nothing" approach will be existing practice, but in others it will be a distinct option—one which provides a comparator for the status quo option as well as the new intervention. Thus, if the investigator wishes to undertake a broader analysis, assessing the status quo in addition to the new intervention, a "do-nothing" option is needed.

Adding comparator programs to the analysis is equivalent to considering these programs as new alternatives. For example, technically the problem is the same whether one thinks of the "do-nothing" alternative as an additional comparator program or as an additional candidate program to replace existing practice. The inclusion of a range of other alternatives, as discussed here, may be particularly appropriate when a broad set of interventions is considered in a policy context. It falls to both analysts and policy makers to recognize incentives and traditions contributing to the status quo and to ensure that the benefits of alternative approaches are not lost from view.

The Comparator in Programs of Varying Intensity or Duration

Programs often vary in intensity, defined by frequency of screening, dosage of treatment, or positivity criteria applied to a screening test. When there are variations on the intensity of a program, each variation on the program that is more intense is compared to the next-less-intense option being considered. That is, it is important to use the next-less-intense option as the comparator in order to calculate the incremental cost-effectiveness of the options, as discussed earlier. For example, annual screening with mammography for breast cancer should be compared to biannual screening, which in turn should be compared to screening every 3 years. If a biannual option is available, it is the cost-effectiveness of one additional screening in a 2-year period that is at issue in comparisons between the biannual and annual options. If annual screening were instead compared to no screening, this average cost-effectiveness ratio would credit the annual program for benefits that could have been obtained by the less-intensive screening plans.

In programs of varying intensity, the analyst is also faced with specifying the program options—which, in reality, are part of a continuum of options—that will be compared. In the mammography example above, a CEA could compare mammography every 1, 2, or 3 years, or it could compare mammography every 1, 3, or 5 years. The options selected (or developed) for inclusion may have a significant affect on the results. Annual screening will appear more cost-effective when it is compared to screening every 3 years than when it is compared to screening every 2 years. Moreover, if screening every 2 years is a feasible option, the comparison against every 3 years is incorrect and misleading.

We recommend that the analyst use the principle of including in the analysis all the frequencies (or levels of intensity in other dimensions) that are really feasible. This determination will be a matter of judgment. For example, if an annual screening program is an option, should screening every 6 months also be included? What is the least intensive version of the program to be considered in the analysis—that is, the one to be compared to "no program"? Should it be screening every 5 years, every 7, or once in a lifetime? The analyst will have to decide at what point comparisons are no longer realistic and when programs differ little enough in their effect that finer distinctions will not offer much additional insight. In addition, the analyst will want to be alert to the possibility of using the study to *design* protocols that will be good policy choices. An analysis that assesses an option of screening at an odd interval or of screening only once every 3 years once a series of negative annual tests is obtained may place new and better options into policy consideration.

Boundaries of the Study

In framing a cost-effectiveness analysis, the analyst must consider the boundaries, or scope, of the study. Spillover effects ripple out from every program. The question is how far to follow such ripples. The primary goal of a smoking cessation program for pregnant women is good health for the unborn child. Smoking during pregnancy can cause low birthweight, respiratory distress syndrome, and other problems for the infant. In addition, a smoking cessation program would clearly affect the health of the mother, and a CEA presumably would include effects on the mother's probability of developing lung cancer, heart disease, and other smoking-related illness. However, the scope of the study could be broader still. For other children in the family, the risks associated with the mother's second-hand smoke will be eliminated if she quits smoking. A spouse's health may also be protected, or he may himself be influenced to quit smoking. Should the analyst track down these impacts or not? In theory, they are all relevant, but part of framing the study is to draw practical limits around the analysis.

Two aspects of scope can be differentiated. The first concerns the groups of people to be considered in the analysis. A childhood illness or disability will likely require parents to spend time away from work. Infectious diseases, such as human immunodeficiency virus (HIV), tuberculosis, and measles, are transmitted across populations and, over time, a single case can ultimately affect very large numbers of individuals. Many interventions—bone marrow transplant for breast cancer patients, removal of lead paint—will have their greatest effect on the health of the index patient but will also affect the well-being of the family, other relatives, friends and neighbors. In the extreme, through altruism, entire communities can be affected.

The analysis should generally encompass all populations where effects are notable. However, if the effects on a particular group are small relative to the major costs and health outcomes considered in the analysis—that is, if they would have a negligible impact on the study results—they can reasonably be excluded. As part of the definition of the boundaries of the study, the analyst should clearly delineate the groups of people included in the analysis and explain the exclusion of other affected groups.

Although the societal perspective prescribes that consequences for all affected persons be included in the analysis, it has not in fact been standard practice to include health-related quality-of-life effects on persons other than the individuals directly affected by the intervention. Thus, in an analysis of Alzheimer's disease, the analyst might well include the costs of caretaking provided by a spouse or children and the health-related quality-of-life impact on the individual suffering from the disease, but would not include the effects of the illness on the health-related quality of life of family members.

To date, little research has been conducted on health-related quality-of-life effects for family members, and little precedent exists for including these effects in CEA. However, as the research base develops, we encourage analysts to think broadly about the people affected by the intervention and to begin to include health-related quality-of-life effects of significant others in sensitivity analyses when they are important.

A second aspect of scope involves the types of health outcomes to be counted. A study may focus primarily on life years gained, or it may also incorporate health-related quality of life. Health-related quality of life itself can incorporate many domains of health, including physical, mental, and emotional health. (See Chapter 4.) In framing the analysis, the analyst should decide which of these types of health outcomes are most appropriate for inclusion in the study.

Nonhealth effects can also be important. For example, a program that prevented neural tube defects would reduce costs for the special education and other services needed by those with spina bifida. An environmental cleanup might have effects on property values as well as health effects, and a drug abuse prevention program might have effects on the criminal justice system. Depending on the extent of nonhealth effects, the analyst may wish to consider cost-benefit analysis as an alternative or a supplement to CEA.

Defining the boundaries of a study can be thought of as drawing a circle around the study to contain it. Any study can become a career in itself if the investigator chases down every ripple and linkage. In circumscribing the study, the analyst must attempt to balance the need to capture all significant effects of the intervention that will be relevant to the decision maker with the need to contain the study to the form of a manageable and feasible project.

Time Horizon

The time horizon of the analysis for a cost-effectiveness study should extend far enough into the future to capture the major health and economic outcomes—both intended effects and unintended side effects. As a result, some analyses follow patients for the duration of their lives. For certain interventions, such as the removal of environmental toxins, the effects of a program may run even longer, requiring a time horizon that extends for generations.

Frequently, the appropriate time horizon extends beyond the availability of primary data, and modeled data must be used in the analysis. It is often useful to analyze the data using several time horizons: a short-term horizon that includes only primary data and a long-term horizon that also incorporates modeled data. An analysis of smoking cessation programs for pregnant women that used a short time horizon, for example, could focus on the success of these programs in helping mothers quit smoking for the duration of their pregnancy. The study would focus on the health outcomes for the infant. A longer time horizon would be able to incorporate the health benefits for the mother as well. However, this analysis would need to model the long-term success of these programs and the effects on the health of the mother of having stopped smoking for short and long periods of time.

It is particularly important to extend the analysis far enough in the future to capture important lifesaving effects. For example, consider an analysis of a cholesterol-lowering program based on a clinical trial with a 5-year follow-up period. If only years of life within the 5 years were included, then any differential between programs in survival beyond the 5-year period would be lost. The gain in life years for the group with the higher 5-year survival would be grossly underestimated. Hence, at a minimum, modeling should be used to estimate gains in life expectancy due to differential survival.

When a positive discount rate is used, as is recommended for the Reference Case Analysis (see Chapter 7), the time horizon of the study will in many cases be effectively limited by the discount rate. That is, costs and effects occurring far in the future will change the cost-effectiveness ratio very little.

Designing the Study

The Analysis Plan

Designing the data collection and analytic plan for the CEA involves three basic steps. First, the analyst must develop a conceptual model describing the intervention and its effects on health outcomes. Essentially the model describes the course of events with the intervention compared to that without the intervention. Second, the analyst must determine how to collect the data on costs, health effects, and preferences for health effects for the intervention and the relevant comparators from the perspectives selected for the study. The tasks required for this step vary greatly depending upon whether, and to what extent, the analysis will collect primary data, use existing data (e.g., performing secondary analyses on data from administrative data bases or published reports), or estimate parameters using mathematical models. Finally, the analyst must develop the analytic methods to combine the information appropriately into a cost-effectiveness analysis.

The Conceptual Model

The conceptual or schematic model serves as a guide to the conduct of a cost-effectiveness analysis. In concrete and well-defined steps, the conceptual model outlines an "event pathway" stemming from the use of the intervention (or affected by the intervention) and linking the intervention to health outcomes. It reflects the analyst's conception of how the intervention is used and the manner in which it affects the course of the disease of interest, its treatment, and the health status of the target population and other affected individuals.

The conceptual model includes all relevant effects of the intervention being considered and the alternatives to it—side effects and other events induced by the interventions, as well as intended effects. For example, a conceptual model of a breast cancer screening intervention would allow for falsely positive and falsely negative as well as correct results of screening and would identify the possible events following each of these results. The model would outline disease-related and clinical events in the screened population (stages of cancer, surgery, medical treatments) within the bounds of the scope, time horizon, and other aspects of the study frame. A conceptual model of a bicycle helmet program would trace the possible types of bicycle accidents, the potential range of injuries with and without the protection of a helmet, and the lifetime sequelae of these injuries.

While the event pathway is generally constructed to represent health effects, depicting health states and events that have an impact on health, it also reflects the cascade of cost implications resulting from an intervention. The same events that cause changes in the health state of an individual generally trigger costs. The screening intervention that uncovers disease, for example, requires a visit to a clinician or other screening site, expends the patient's time, and uses health care resources including a clinician's time and laboratory tests. When costs arise from an event that is not explicit in a "clinical" event pathway—such as when a person moves from an acute care facility to a rehabilitation hospital without a change in health status—it is often useful to represent the change as a separate step or "state" in the pathway.

Decision trees or probability trees are widely used to diagram the conceptual model. The intervention and each comparator can be represented by main branches in the tree, and subsequent events, including probabilistic events, can be depicted by the further branches and twigs of the tree. Decision trees are a convenient graphic for displaying the probability of various outcomes, the costs associated with various clinical events, and preferences for the different outcomes.

Implications for the analysis

Aspects of the conceptual model will affect the analyst's range of choice regarding the inputs to the cost-effectiveness analysis and, to some extent, the methods for conducting the analysis. It is useful to consider these aspects of the conceptual model as it is being designed—and to structure the conceptual model to undergird a workable study.

The manner in which events and health states are defined in an event pathway has far-reaching implications for the conduct of the analysis, because the event pathway specifies the types of data to be used. For example, if a model of a smoking cessation program links "smoking history" states to ultimate survival, the data requirements will be different from a model linking smoking history to cardiac events and cancer and then linking these events to survival.

The time periods during which movement along the event pathway occurs are also part of the conceptualization of the analysis. The appropriate time period—that is, the size of a unit of time in the model, as distinct from the time horizon of the analysis—depends on the intervention under study and the conditions it affects. For many conditions, the basic unit of 1 year provides sufficient detail. For some conditions, however, important changes in a patient's condition, including his or her chances of survival, may occur in just a few days or weeks. In these cases, the time period used will generally be shorter, as in analyses relating to treatments of conditions such as AIDS. For still other conditions, a mixture may be necessary: Events in the immediate aftermath of the condition and its treatment may require short periods of time to define health states and their probabilities, while later events may be adequately represented by probabilities that change from one year to the next.

The definition of health outcomes in the conceptual model has an important effect on the types of preference weights that can be used to assign quality-of-life values in the study. If the analyst intends to use an existing system of preference weights to calculate QALYs—as will often be the case—the model must use health states that can be "mapped" to that system. For example, if the system has an average weight for "kidney failure," it would only be necessary to know the impact of an intervention on that state. But, if the system had weights for different health states associated with kidney failure, it would be necessary to know the distribution of those health states for a population with kidney failure. (See Chapter 4.)

The conceptual model, as noted above, outlines the full range of events stemming from the intervention. Because it will guide the analysis, it should be considered in great detail, including costs and effects at all levels of importance. However, in most cost-effectiveness analyses it is not efficient, nor would it be financially feasible, to measure and include every relevant effect and cost in the analysis itself. Any cost or outcome that is not appreciable in the context of the analysis need not be included in the analysis. After constructing the conceptual model, therefore, the analyst should consider the importance of components of the analysis, using a "rule of reason" to determine whether an element should be included, excluded, or further investigated to determine its importance.

As the analyst learns more about the details of the analysis, including the data available and the software to be used, the conceptual model can be reevaluated and refined; the process of designing a study is generally an iterative one. The feasibility of gathering primary data and the availability of secondary data on event probabilities, health outcomes, and resource use all affect the ultimate form of the analysis. For example, the types of data on survival, health care utilization, and cost available for smokers might determine the choice of models in the smoking cessation example discussed earlier.

In most analyses, the conceptual model will be incorporated into a mathematical or simulation model for use in actually calculating net cost and net effectiveness for the population, subgroup, or individual undergoing the intervention. (See Chapter 5.) In developing the conceptual model, it is useful to consider the technical form of the analysis so that the steps can be readily translated into this operational form.

Collecting the Data

As part of the design of the CEA, the analyst must decide what types of data to include in the analysis. The analyst can collect primary data on costs, effects, and health states. Secondary data, obtained from studies in the literature, from databases, or from other sources of existing data can be used instead of, or in addition to, primary data.

The estimates of resource consumption and health effects of relevance for the analysis are those for the population or group that is actually affected by the health intervention.[4] For example, a program requiring extra prenatal visits would consume the time of women of childbearing age, and the analyst's task is to estimate the value of this time as accurately as possible. Similarly, a study of a screening program in California would incorporate cost estimates (e.g., for clinician visits) reflective of opportunity costs (wages) in California as well as effects expected in California.

As discussed in Chapters 4–6, when population-specific estimates are used in an analysis, the results of the study may diverge from what they would have been for a broader population in ways that the researcher believes to be ethically controversial. So, for example, while most analysts would not consider the difference in life expectancy between adults and children a source of discrimination against adults, assigning different time costs to employed and unemployed individuals is much more controversial. In these cases, the analyst may want to conduct sensitivity analyses to demonstrate the effect of group-specific estimates. In planning data collection, the analyst will want to consider whether ethically sensitive issues will arise and be prepared to collect both group-specific data and data for a broader population.

Cost and effectiveness data

Ideally, data on the costs and effects of an intervention should both be collected from the same properly designed primary study. However, for a variety of reasons discussed in this section (and in Chapter 5), this ideal is frequently not a feasible design for a cost-effectiveness analysis given the goals of the analysis and the financial constraints for most studies. In general, primary designs are most feasible for interventions with short-term effects—for example, a new therapy to treat migraine headaches.

When a primary cost-effectiveness study is not feasible, effectiveness and cost data can be gathered from separate sources. These sources may be primary or secondary, and they may employ a variety of study designs. For effectiveness data, prospective sources are often, although not always, preferred. Data on resource use are infrequently gathered in formal trials, so other secondary sources such as adminstrative or claims databases are far more commonly used.

When data are gathered from separate sources, the analyst will generally rely on mathematical or simulation models to combine the information into a structure based on the conceptual model. As a rule, interventions with long-term consequences (including most prevention programs) require synthesis of data from diverse studies and a modeled projection of outcomes into the future. For example, a CEA on breast cancer screening might draw evidence from primary studies to estimate the probability of detecting cases of breast cancer and link this information to evidence from other studies to model the natural history of disease and treatment following detection.

Primary research designs: *piggyback studies.* The most common primary study design used in CEA is one in which economic and additional health outcomes are ''piggybacked''—added onto—a randomized controlled clinical trial (RCT). For example, drug companies have broadened phase III pivotal drug trials designed to obtain efficacy and safety data for submission to the FDA to obtain these types of data. Less commonly, economic and health outcomes have been included in early stage or post marketing studies of drugs. In addition, interest in incorporating economic evaluation into National Institutes of Health (NIH)-sponsored trials of health care interventions is growing rapidly (McCabe and Friedman, 1995).

Typically, data on health care utilization are collected during the RCT, and sometimes after the trial. Utilization information includes, for example, the number of hospital admissions and lengths of stay, tests and procedures, physician visits, and drugs prescribed. Patients are often surveyed to measure changes in quality of life and time costs for cost-effectiveness analysis. Health-related quality of life information is sometimes assessed directly via questionnaire.

Piggyback studies of pharmaceuticals are now common in clinical trial programs throughout the world. The advantages are several. First, since many of these studies build on an existing RCT, the piggyback design can itself be relatively efficient. Second, it obtains timely cost-effectiveness data. Since cost-effectiveness information is generated concurrently with the clinical information, it is available at the time of regulatory, coverage, and pricing decisions. A third advantage of the piggyback design is its credibility in the biomedical community. This design is usually randomized, double-blinded, and controlled. The design has high internal validity, minimizes bias, and has tight protocol control. Finally, relevant information on health-related quality of life, preferences for health states, and time loss can be collected along with data on costs and effectiveness.

However, piggyback designs are not without problems, primarily because the studies are usually designed to study safety and efficacy, not cost-effectiveness. Like other RCTs, they tend to have low external validity due to restrictive inclusion and exclusion criteria and the specialized clinical settings where the studies are often conducted. (See Chapter 5.) They are likely to include protocol-induced costs for required hospitalization, extra physician visits, or special tests, all of which distort estimates of the health and economic effects under real-world conditions.

Statistical significance for economic results is generally difficult to achieve in a piggyback trial. This is the case even when the mean difference in the cost of interventions is large, because study power, and thus sample size, is typically calculated using clinical endpoints that tend to have a much lower variance than economic endpoints. Ultimately, in cost-effectiveness studies, statistical significance is not critical; rather, the most important factor is whether the precision around the estimates of costs, effects, and cost-effectiveness ratios is sufficient for the decision at hand. (See Chapter 8.) However, while the economic data in piggyback trials provide useful information on cost, this information may not be as convincing to consumers of the study as the traditional measures of statistical significance obtained in the trial for intervention effectiveness. It would be possible to conduct a piggyback trial large enough to establish statistically significant differences in the costs of alternatives, but the cost of expanding the trial could be substantial and would need to be weighed against the benefit of this additional information as well as against the ethics of prolonging a trial beyond the point where effectiveness has been established in order to collect more precise estimates of costs.

Primary research designs: cost-effectiveness trials. An alternative to the piggyback option is to design an RCT expressly for cost-effectiveness purposes: the cost-effectiveness trial (Revicki and Luce, 1995). This option is one in which the trial itself is specifically designed to study cost-effectiveness, as opposed to efficacy. Typically, patients are randomly assigned to a study group, often comparing one course of therapy to usual care or another active control. Few additional constraints are imposed.

It is important to note that because the cost-effectiveness trial examines an intervention in a real-world health care context, the question addressed is whether the decision to use the technology is a cost-effective one—taking into account current medical practice, health care policies, patient compliance, and other factors—rather than whether the technology of interest is potentially cost-effective under some ideal set of circumstances. In this sense, cost-effectiveness trials differ from most clinical trials, which generally obtain efficacy rather than effectiveness data.

The cost-effectiveness trial has a number of advantages. Although external validity may be limited by specific features of the study, such as the practice setting or the geographic location in which the trial is conducted, the validity will generally be higher than in piggyback trials, because the trial is designed to reflect more closely average patients being treated under average clinical conditions. As with the piggyback trial, data on health-related quality of life, preferences for health states, and time costs can also be included.

An important disadvantage of this option is its cost. These studies tend to be larger than traditional clinical trials, although less expensive per patient due to the lower intensity of the protocol. The cost-effectiveness trial is more expensive than the piggyback design because an entire clinical trial must be funded. There are also concerns of timing and timeliness. These trials are lengthy, and, because of their protocols, they usually cannot begin until a commercially marketed technology is near approval or after it has been launched. However, if the technology has already been proven efficacious, it may be impractical or unethical to assign individuals to a control group receiving an alternative intervention.

Cost-effectiveness trials have lower internal validity than the piggyback design because the relaxed protocol constraints permit the introduction of potential confounding variables such as patient cross-over, bias due to lack of blinding, and variations in practice patterns.

Secondary research designs. Although primary cost-effectiveness studies are today increasingly being used for the evaluation of new and important drugs, funding is often not available for the primary study of other new interventions, and it is seldom available for existing ones. For technologies already in the inventory of health care, cost-effectiveness analysis is most frequently conducted using existing data.

Existing data for use in a CEA can be derived from a variety of research designs, including RCTs, observational (epidemiologic) studies, databases, and synthesis methods. Often, cost and effect data or event probability data have to be obtained from more than one source. The advantages and disadvantages of each type of study design from the perspective of cost-effectiveness analysis are discussed in Chapter 5 (for effectiveness data) and in Chapter 6 (for designs commonly used to assess resource utilization).

One example of a cost-effectiveness analysis drawing on secondary data uses a retrospective cohort design to analyze existing resource use data, obtaining corresponding data on effectiveness from other secondary sources, such as RCTs reported in the literature. The retrospective cohort analysis examines health care utilization or costs for a patient cohort that has experienced a given intervention and a cohort that has not, comparing the two. The retrospective cohort design requires large and comprehensive data sets to allow statistical control for any possible confounding variables such as age, sex, severity of disease, comorbid conditions, and competing risk factors. The data may be derived from medical chart review or from existing computerized administrative records such as an insurance claims file. For example, Geweke and Weisbrod (1982) used Medicaid data to compare insurance expenditures for peptic ulcer disease before and after the introduction of cimetidine, a drug used to treat the disease. The insurance data reflected the substitution of drug treatment for ulcer operations and hospitalization.

The retrospective cohort design has several advantages. It is relatively inexpensive, and it can be done fairly quickly because the data are already available. It also maximizes external validity, since one is analyzing what actually transpired in the community setting. The retrospective cohort design's main problem, and it can be a serious one, is selection bias: Those who received the intervention likely differ from those who did not, and this difference may not be completely correctable by statistical control. Also, the data may not be well suited for the cost-effectiveness analysis, because they were initially gathered for other purposes. There may be particular problems in obtaining appropriate outcome data. For example, a claims history may capture utilization of hospital services but give no indication of patient outcome—not even survival, let alone quality of life. Also, some types of costs may not be included in the data set; for example, payer-based data sets frequently do not include out-of-plan or noncovered services. Finally, retrospective data will sometimes include only billing data rather than indicating the quantity of specific services consumed.

Modeling designs. Cost-effectiveness analyses almost always employ mathematical or simulation modeling to some extent. We distinguish ''modeling designs,'' where the model, as opposed to a specific study, is the primary feature of the analysis.

There are two main groups of models, clinical decision-analytic models and epidemiologically based models. Clinical decision-analytic models portray medical practice and the clinical decisions pertaining to an intervention. They are frequently used to evaluate these decisions, tracing the implications of the choices within the model. Decision-analytic models are usually appropriate for studies addressing the cost-effectiveness of clinical interventions for treating present disease.

Epidemiologically based models track risk factors and the course of disease. Clinical decisions are not explicitly modeled, although they are often embedded in the assumptions regarding, for example, life expectancy and costs associated with a health state. Instead, the intervention is represented as a change in probabilities of movement through the event pathway. Epidemiologically based models are suited for evaluating interventions affecting future disease, including primary prevention efforts, such as smoking cessation, or secondary prevention, such as treatment of elevated cholesterol.

Modeling designs draw heavily on existing literature as a source of secondary data on costs and intervention effects relevant to the subject of study. They may also incorporate available primary data. When few studies have been done, estimates and projections based on expert opinion or the mathematical modeling of specific components of the analysis are used as inputs to the model.

Modeling is useful when primary data (such as RCT data) are scant, and these designs are virtually required when extremely long periods must be studied, such as for interventions to prevent heart disease or cancer. They offer a means to combine data from disparate sources to depict the cascade of events resulting from an intervention. Models are useful for scenario building and for exploring the future implications of alternative policies. For example, drug manufacturers have begun to use models to predict cost-effectiveness early in the drug development cycle as a guide to the potential value of their investments. In addition, models are often employed when the analyst wishes to extrapolate results from one setting to another.

Modeling designs are important for assessing unique composite programs, such as school health or lead abatement programs, that may combine elements of many interventions. For example, estimating the cost-effectiveness of new school health programs might require the analyst to combine information on dietary counseling, smoking cessation programs, and family planning services. If the program has already commenced, the analyst may be able to obtain some information, such as the program structure, startup costs, or space requirements, directly from the program. If the analysis is entirely prospective, the CEA will generally project the cost-effectiveness of a prototype program.

Model-based CEAs can be an inexpensive and quick way of estimating cost-effectiveness when compared to alternatives requiring primary data collection. However, elaborate models are generally required to simulate an intervention's effects in a thorough and credible fashion, as required for publication. Models have clear limitations. Estimates incorporated into the analysis may be inaccurate, whether derived from data or based on expert opinion. Because of the complexity of many models, biases may not be readily apparent to readers of the study. For this reason, decision makers responsible for pricing and reimbursement decisions, promotional claims, or other decisions requiring conservative judgments have been critical of cost-effectiveness analyses relying on models.

Combination designs. The last CEA design option—and probably the most common—combines the various methods discussed above. Often, these designs begin with primary data—for example, from a clinical trial. These data may be sufficient to make circumscribed inferences regarding health and economic consequences, but a model is required to extend the analysis beyond the original setting and time frame to estimate ultimate patient outcomes and cost-effectiveness. Combination designs may look similar to modeling designs, which also combine models with data. For conceptual purposes, however, we define pure modeling designs as either those containing only secondary data—or, if primary data are used, as designs in which they are not the major empirical basis for the analysis.

A combination design would be used, for example, to examine the long-term effects of an intervention to maintain stable blood sugar levels in people with diabetes. The original study might have been designed to show statistically significant differences in diabetic events or changes in the vasculature of diabetics, as compared to a standard treatment regimen. The cost-effectiveness analysis would use a model to extrapolate from the changes in these intermediate outcomes to predicted changes in the incidence of heart disease, high blood pressure, and renal failure in diabetic patients. These health effects would be associated with changes in health-related quality of life and life expectancy. Research documenting these final outcomes in patients undergoing the intervention would be decades away. The model would account for such variables as predicted changes in patient compliance with the treatment regimen over time and compliance levels in different patient subgroups. Therefore, a cost-effectiveness study might include the clinical (and possibly economic) results from the primary study at hand, results from other clinical research previously reported, and modeling for future health events and their costs.

Data on preferences

Like data on costs and health effects, the preference weights used to quality adjust life years in the denominator of the C/E ratio can be obtained from primary or secondary sources. Preference weights can be obtained along with cost and effectiveness data from subjects in a clinical trial. In this case, patients can give preference weights for their own health states and for other states relevant to the study but hypothetical to the patient at the time of the interview.

Analysts can also obtain preference weights for a cost-effectiveness study from existing studies that have collected data on preferences for health states. There may be other studies of the same disease that have already established preference weights for the relevant health states. Alternatively, condition-specific weights may be judged suitable for the study (Gold et al., personal communication).

Another option that is being widely used in clinical trials consists of gathering primary prospective data on the health status of patients in the trial using a generic health state system (e.g., the Quality of Well-Being Index [Kaplan and Anderson, 1988] or the Health Utilities Index [Feeny et al., 1995; Torrance et al., 1995]) that already has preference weights available. The actual health status of the patients can then be scored with the preestablished preference weights, eliminating the need to undertake primary measurement of preferences.

Computing Cost and Effectiveness

The final aspect of study design to be considered concerns the means for calculating cost and effectiveness. Because of the number of calculations required, especially when multiple event pathways are involved, CEAs frequently employ computer spreadsheets, decision-analytic software, or simulation software. Analysts can write their own computer programs or make use of existing software that incorporates Monte Carlo simulation, state-transition models, or decision tree models (including influence diagrams), eliminating the need for extensive original programming. The characteristics and requirements of mathematical models used can influence the types and form of data that will be needed and are therefore usefully considered along with other aspects of study design early in the development of a CEA.

The basic core of any cost-effectiveness analysis is an incremental comparison of an intervention with a comparison program. Here the term *incremental* is used, rather than *marginal*, to denote two aspects of appropriate comparisons in cost-effectiveness analyses. First, the comparison is always between two discrete alternatives. That is, two programs or two interventions are compared; there is no attempt to develop smooth continuous functions with continuously changing marginal cost-effectiveness at every point on a hypothetical continuum. Second, the appropriate incremental comparisons for cost-effectiveness are sometimes comparisons between entirely different programs and sometimes comparisons between different levels of intensity within the same program. Only the latter fits the usual definition of marginal. In this way, incremental is a

Table 3.1 Incremental Comparison

Let
IC = Incremental Cost
IE = Incremental Health Outcome (e.g., QALYs)
C/E = Cost-effectiveness ratio

TC_1 = Total cost, in present value terms, for treatment program
TC_2 = Total cost, in present value terms, for comparison program

E_1 = Total health outcome, in present value terms, for treatment program
E_2 = Total health outcome, in present value terms, for comparison program

$C1_1$ = total medical costs, in present value terms, for treatment program
$C1_2$ = total medical costs, in present value terms, for comparison program

$C2_1$ = total nonmedical costs, in present value terms, treatment program
$C2_2$ = total nonmedical costs, in present value terms, comparison program

$C3_1$ = cost of total working time lost in treatment, in present value terms, treatment program
$C3_2$ = cost of total working time lost in treatment, in present value terms, comparison program

$C4_1$ = cost of total leisure time lost in treatment, in present value terms, treatment program
$C4_2$ = cost of total leisure time lost in treatment, in present value terms, comparison program

$C5_1$ = future medical costs, other conditions, present value, for treatment program
$C5_2$ = future medical costs, other conditions, present value, for comparison program
Then
$TC_1 = C1_1 + C2_1 + C3_1 + C4_1 + C5_1$
$TC_2 = C1_2 + C2_2 + C3_2 + C4_2 + C5_2$

$IC = TC_1 - TC_2$
$IE = E_1 - E_2$
$C/E = IC/IE$

broader term, which includes marginal, but is restricted in the usage here to the discrete case. The formulation for this basic case is given in Table 3.1.

Conclusion

Framing and designing the study are the crucial first steps in undertaking a cost-effectiveness analysis. Framing involves making a series of decisions which lay out in broad outline the methodology of the study. This is a critical step that is often given inadequate attention; time spent here will be more than saved later in avoiding methodological quandaries, quagmires, and ad hoc methodological decisions. Designing the study requires the analyst to "fill in" the study frame, making the practical decisions that will determine the structure of the analysis and the data to be used.

The major elements to be considered in framing and designing the study have been presented in this chapter. Analysts are encouraged to address all of these issues before beginning a cost-effectiveness analysis.

Recommendations

1. Cost-effectiveness analysis, cost-consequence analysis, and cost-benefit analysis are complementary, rather than mutually exclusive, forms of analysis. The use of one does not preclude the use of any of the others.

2. CEA is most widely useful for resource allocation when conducted from the societal perspective. When the primary purpose of a CEA requires a perspective other than societal, analysts are urged to present a Reference Case analysis (societal perspective) in addition for comparabiity with other studies.

3. All aspects of the interventions that may affect their cost or effectiveness should be defined for the analysis. These will include the target population and such features of interventions as the specific technologies used, the type of personnel delivering the service or treatment, the site of delivery, whether the service is "bundled" with other services, the frequency of the intervention, and its timing.

4. The Reference Case analysis should compare the health intervention of interest to existing practice (the "status quo"). If existing practice appears not to be a cost-effective option itself, relative to other available options, the analyst should incorporate other relevant alternatives into the analysis, such as a best-available alternative, a viable low-cost alternative, or a "do-nothing" alternative.

5. When varying levels of program intensity are relevant, alternative program options (for example, as defined by variation in duration or frequency of the intervention) should be included in the analysis and compared using the incremental cost-effectiveness algorithm.

6. Boundaries of a study should be defined broadly enough to encompass the range of groups of people affected by the intervention and all types of cost and health consequences.

7. The time horizon adopted in a CEA should be long enough to capture all relevant future effects of a health care intervention.

8. Decisions about costs and health effects to include in a CEA, such as the precision with which costs and effects are measured, the time horizon of the study, and the definition of the study boundaries, should strike a reasonable balance between expense and difficulty on one hand, and potential importance in the analysis on the other.

9. Costs and outcomes that are insignificant in the context of the analysis can reasonably be excluded.

10. The estimates of resource consumption, effects, and preferences of relevance for a CEA are those for the population or group that is actually affected by the health intervention.

11. In some instances, when population-specific estimates are used in an analysis, the results of the study may diverge from what they would have been for a broader population in ways that are ethically controversial. In these cases, sensitivity analysis should be used to demonstrate the effect of group-specific estimates.

Notes

1. Additional references are Torrance et al. (1972) and Weinstein (1990).

2. Even without a budget constraint, the information in the table could enable all programs and program increments to be ranked in order of incremental cost-effectiveness for use as an input into the resource allocation decision making process.

3. It should be noted that the target population is not necessarily the only group experiencing the effects of the intervention. See later discussion of the boundaries of the analysis.

4. Estimates of preferences for health states, for reasons discussed in Chapter 4, are those of the broader community in Reference Case analyses.

References

Brown, M.L. 1992a. Sensitivity analysis in the cost-effectiveness of breast cancer screening. *Cancer* 69(suppl):1963–67.

Brown, M.L. 1992b. Economic considerations in breast cancer screening of older women. *J Gerontol* 47(suppl):51–58.

Brown, M.L., and L. Fintor. 1993. Cost-effectiveness of breast cancer screening: Preliminary results of a systematic review of the literature. *Breast Cancer Res Treat* 25:113–18.

Canadian Coordinating Office for Health Technology Assessment (CCOHTA). 1994. *Guidelines for economic evaluation of pharmaceuticals: Canada*. Ottawa: CCOHTA.

Drummond, M.F., G.L. Stoddart, and G.W. Torrance. 1987. *Methods for the economic evaluation of health care programmes*. Oxford: Oxford University Press.

Drummond, M., G. Torrance, and J. Mason. 1993. Cost-effectiveness league tables: More harm than good? *Soc Sci Med* 37:33–40.

Eisenberg, J.M. 1989. Clinical economics: A guide to economic analysis of clinical practice. *JAMA* 262(20):2879–86.

Feeny D., W. Furlong, M. Boyle, and G.W. Torrance. 1995. Multi-attribute health status class-sification systems: Health utilities index. *PharmacoEconomics* 7:490–502.

Freund, D.A., and R.S. Dittus. 1992. Principles of pharmacoeconomic analysis of drug therapy. *PharmacoEconomics* 1:20–29.

Geweke, J., and B.A. Weisbrod. 1982. Clinical evaluation vs. economic evaluation: The case of a new drug. *Med Care* 20:821–30.

Gold M.R., P. Franks, and K. McCoy. 1994. Condition weights for chronic diseases from a nationally representative sample. *Med Decis Making* 14:431 (abstract).

Henry, D. 1992. Economic analysis as an aid to subsidisation decisions: The development of Australian guidelines for pharmaceuticals. *PharmacoEconomics* 1:54–67.

Kaplan, R.M. and J.P. Anderson. 1988. A general health policy model: Update and applications. *Health Serv Res* 23:203–35.

Mason, J., M. Drummond, and G. Torrance. 1993. Some guidelines on the use of cost effective-ness league tables. *BMJ* 306:570–72.

McCabe, M.S., and M.A. Friedman. 1995. Introduction to the National Cancer Institute economic conference: The integration of economic outcome measures into NCI-sponsored thera-peutic trials. *Monographs. J Natl Cancer Inst* 19:vii.

Miller, G.A. 1956. The magical number seven, plus or minus two: Some limits on our capacity for processing information. *Psychol Rev* 63:81–97.

Revicki, D.A., and B.R. Luce. 1995. Methods of pharmacoeconomic evaluation of new medical treatments in psychiatry. *Psychopharmacol Bull* 31:57–65.

Russell, L.R. 1989. Some of the tough decisions required by a national health plan. *Science* 246:892–96.

Schulman, K.A., L.A. Lynn, H.A. Glick, and J.M. Eisenberg. 1991. Cost-effectiveness of low-dose zidovudine therapy for asymptomatic patients with human immunodeficiency virus (HIV) infection. *Ann Intern Med* 114:798–802.

Stokey, E., and R. Zeckhauser. 1978. *A primer for policy analysis.* New York: W. W. Norton.

Tengs, T.O., M.E. Adams, J.S. Pliskin, D.G. Safran, J.E. Siegel, M.C. Weinstein, and J.D. Gra-ham. 1995. Five-hundred life-saving interventions and their cost-effectiveness. *Risk Anal* 15(3):369–390.

Torrance, G.W. 1995. Designing and conducting cost-utility analyses. In *Quality of life and pharmacoeconomics in clinical trials*, ed. B. Spilker, 1105–11, Philadelphia: Lippincott-Raven.

Torrance, G.W. 1986. Measurement of health state utilities for economic appraisal: A review. *J Health Economics* 5:1–30.

Torrance, G.W., W. Furlong, D. Feeny, and M. Boyle. 1995. Multi-attribute preference functions: Health utilities index. *PharmacoEconomics* 7:503–20.

Torrance, G.W., W.H. Thomas, and D.L. Sackett. 1972. A utility maximization model for eval-uation of health care programmes. *Health Serv Res* 7:118–33.

Torrance, G.W., and A. Zipursky. 1984. Cost-effectiveness of antepartum prevention of Rh im-munization. *Clin Perinatol* 11:267–81.

Weinstein, M.C. 1990. Principles of cost-effective resource allocation in health care organiza-tions. *Int J Technol Assess Health Care* 6:93–103.

Weinstein, M.C., and W.B. Stason. 1977. Foundations of cost-effectiveness analysis for health and medical practices. *N Engl J Med* 296:716–21.

Williams, A.H. 1985. Economics of coronary artery bypass grafting. *BMJ* 291:326–29.

4

Identifying and Valuing Outcomes

M.R. GOLD, D.L. PATRICK, G.W. TORRANCE,
D.G. FRYBACK, D.C. HADORN, M.S. KAMLET,
N. DANIELS, and M.C. WEINSTEIN

Once the framework and design of a cost-effectiveness analysis have been conceptualized, the next step is to develop estimates of the numerator and denominator of the cost-effectiveness ratio. Estimation of the numerator is discussed in Chapter 6. In this chapter and in Chapter 5 we discuss issues pertaining to the denominator term, which is the difference in effectiveness between an intervention and the alternatives to which it is compared. The panel's recommended approach to estimating the denominator is to use a system of generic health states and values to describe and measure the outcomes. Using this approach involves the following steps: (1) identifying the relevant outcomes in terms of generic health states (including death); (2) describing the elements of health states and their possible course over time for individuals who receive the intervention and for those who receive each alternative; (3) combining the elements of each health state into a single number reflecting the value assigned to that health state; (4) integrating the values assigned to the health states with the quantity of life (expressed as life expectancy, duration of survival, or interval of observation) associated with each state; (5) estimating the probabilities of each outcome; and, finally, (6) using the outputs of step (4) and step (5) to compute a numerical average outcome for each of the alternatives being compared.

This chapter addresses the first four steps described above, detailing how health outcomes are conceptualized for purposes of CEA. Chapter 5 completes the process of estimating the denominator by describing how probabilities of outcomes are determined and used to complete the effectiveness estimate in the cost-effectiveness ratio.

In order to make our discussion accessible to readers from different disciplinary backgrounds, we define terms in specific ways throughout this book. This is of particular importance in this chapter, where the language has been derived from many different intellectual traditions, and there is extraordinary variation in the literature in the manner in which a number of important terms are used. While we have not sought to redefine terms— indeed, many of the authors describe similar concepts differently—we hope that the language used here will help clarify some of the important issues in this aspect of CEA methodology.

Within the context of CEA, health outcomes are the end result of the evaluated intervention and its alternatives with regard to the health status of a population from the time of the intervention until death (or the end of the observation period). Numerical judgments of the desirability of a set of outcomes are called "preferences," "values," or, within neoclassical economic theory and decision science, "utilities." The most commonly understood use of the term "utility" is preference, and unless characterized differently, the terms "preference," "value," and "utility" are used interchangeably throughout the remainder of this chapter. For differentiation, when we wish to refer specifically to utilities measured under uncertainty according to the axioms of expected utility theory (von Neumann and Morgenstern, 1947) we use the term "von Neumann-Morgenstern (vNM) utilities." "Health status," "functional status," and "health-related quality of life" are often used interchangeably in the literature. Here we will use "health state" or "health status" to describe the health of an individual at a particular point in time. These health states may be modified by the impairments, functional states, perceptions, and social opportunities that are influenced by disease, injury, treatment, or health policy (Patrick and Erickson, 1993). We will use "health-related quality of life" (HRQL) to connote the values assigned to different health states. Thus HRQL will indicate the relative desirability of measured or estimated health states.

This chapter reviews outcomes that are relevant for use in CEA. It discusses how health-related quality of life can be combined with survival or life-expectancy data in order to merge morbidity and mortality impacts into a single measure. It reviews different approaches for describing health states and discusses the rationale for assigning values to health states. The chapter considers whose preference judgments for outcomes are germane, and in what setting; it examines different methods used to elicit preferences; and it concludes by suggesting that a standardized catalogue of preference-weighted health states could advance the field through improving the comparability of cost-effectiveness analyses.

The Outcomes of Interest in Cost-Effectiveness Analysis

All CEAs involve the selection of relevant health outcomes for the health interventions being compared. For example, a CEA of cholesterol screening, comparing a particular screening protocol with a well-defined "usual care" alternative, might select the health outcome to be studied as any of the following: the number of cardiac events averted per patient per year, the expected years of life gained per patient, or the number of quality-adjusted life years gained per patient.

Table 4.1 illustrates the wide variation of outcomes used as the measure of effect in selected cost-effectiveness studies. Many studies have used increased life expectancy or expected life years saved as the sole, or primary, outcome for the analysis. For example, Goldman et al. (1991) found that using cholesterol-lowering agents in 55–64-year-old men, with an initial cholesterol level of >300, had a C/E ratio of $49,000/year of life saved. Years of life gained provides a convenient metric for many cost-effectiveness analyses and therefore remains the most widely used type of outcome measure.

In many cases, however, years of life gained is an insufficient outcome measure in CEA. Richer descriptions than years of life are frequently relevant in considering the effects of a health intervention. In industrialized nations, where length of life has shown steady increases over the past century, it is the improvement in quality of life produced by health care inputs that is often the truer gauge of how well the health care system is performing. For example, in evaluating the effectiveness of cholesterol screening, mortality from heart disease is certainly an important outcome. But simply counting deaths, or even life years gained, may leave out other important health outcomes, such as the morbidity repercussions of angina and heart attacks, as well as the psychological concerns that may accompany a diagnosis of hypercholesterolemia. All of these outcomes may be highly relevant in assessing the value of an intervention.

Moreover, it is necessary to consider not only the health outcomes directly related to the condition under study but also the side effects from the intervention. For example, people being treated for elevated cholesterol levels may also experience premature onset of cataracts, with loss of visual acuity. These would be missed if only morbid events of the cardiovascular system were measured. Finally, event counts severely limit the degree to which CEAs of dissimilar conditions can be compared. As Moriyama (1968) pointed out many years ago in discussions of health status measurement, total "case counts" lead one to question how "one equates a case of congenital anomaly with a case of senile psychosis."

In deciding which outcomes are appropriate for a particular CEA, investigators should ask the following questions: (1) What are the potential differences between groups with respect to the main effects of the intervention? (2) What are the potential side effects or unintended consequences of the intervention? and (3) What are the outcomes of interest to consumers, patients, families, clinicians, decision makers, and society at large? Measures that capture both quantity (duration) of life and quality of life, as described below, are best suited for use in a Reference Case analysis.

The Health-Related Quality-of-Life Continuum

In order to capture health outcomes beyond simple survival it is necessary to obtain information on the health-related quality of life associated with different interventions.

Table 4.1 Outcomes and Methods of Valuation Used in Example Cost-Effectiveness Studies[a]

Authors Subject	Method of Valuation	Concepts and Domains	Outcomes
Boyle et al., 1983 Neonatal intensive care of very-low-birthweight infants	Health Utility Index, Primary data collection	Physical function, psychological function, social function, impairment, death & duration of life	Quality-adjusted life years, life years
Dasbach et al., 1991 Diabetic retinopathy	0/1[b]	Good sight, bad sight	Sight years
Eddy, 1989 Screening for breast cancer	0/1	Mortality/survival	Life years
Eddy, 1991 Screening for cervical cancer Common screening tests	0/1	Mortality/survival	Life years
Edelson et al., 1990 Monotherapies for hypertension	Investigator assigned[c]	Mortality/survival	Quality-adjusted life years, life years
Fahs et al., 1992 Cervical cancer screening for the elderly	0/1	Mortality/survival	Life years
Goldman et al., 1991 HMG-CoA reductase inhibition	0/1	Mortality/survival	Life years
Gottlieb et al., 1983 Glaucoma screening	Investigator assigned	Impairment	Quality-adjusted years of vision
Hatziandreu et al., 1988 Exercise as health promotion	Investigator assigned[c]	Holistic, physical-symptom-defined or disease-defined states; mortality/survival	Quality-adjusted life years, life years, cases, deaths
Hinman and Koplan, 1984 Pertussis vaccine	No quality adjustment, cost-benefit analysis considering only direct medical costs	—	Cases

85

Table 4.1 Outcomes and Methods of Valuation Used in Example Cost-Effectiveness Studies[a] (*Continued*)

Authors Subject	Method of Valuation	Concepts and Domains	Outcomes
Hutchinson and Stoddard, 1988 *Primary tetanus vaccination in the elderly*	0/1	Mortality/survival	Life years, lives, cases
Koplan et al., 1979 *Pertussis vaccine*	No quality adjustment, cost-benefit analysis considering only direct medical costs	—	Cases
Littrup et al., 1993 *Prostate cancer*	No quality adjustment, cost-benefit analysis considering only direct medical costs	—	Cost/cancer compared to cost of screen techniques
Mandelblatt and Fahs, 1988 *Cervical cancer screening in low-income elderly women*	Investigator assigned[c,d], 0/1	Holistic, physical-symptom-defined or disease-defined states; mortality/survival	Quality-adjusted life years, life years
Oster et al., 1986 *Nicotine gum*	0/1	Mortality/survival	Life years
Sisk-Willems et al., 1980 *Pneumococcal pneumonia*	Other literature—QWB	Physical function, social function, impairment, death & duration of life	Quality-adjusted life years
Stason and Weinstein, 1977 *Hypertension*	Investigator assigned	Holistic, physical symptom-defined or disease-defined states	Quality-adjusted life years

Source		Mortality/survival	Life years
Taylor et al., 1990 *Cholesterol reduction*	0/1		Life years
Thompson et al., 1988 *Auronofin*	Other literature—QWB validated by primary data collection on other health states	Physical function, social function, impairment, death & duration of life states	Change in quality of life
Torrance and Zipursky, 1984 *Antepartum prevention of Rh*	Investigator assigned	Holistic, physical symptom-defined or disease-defined states	Quality-adjusted life years, life years, cases, lives
Tosteson et al., 1990 *Screening perimenopausal white women for osteoporosis*	Investigator assigned[c,d]	Holistic, physical symptom-defined or disease-defined states	Quality-adjusted life years, life years
Weinstein and Tosteson, 1990 *Hormone replacement*	Investigator assigned[c,d]	Holistic, physical symptom-defined or disease-defined states	Quality-adjusted life years, life years
White et al., 1985 *MMR immunization*	No quality adjustment. Benefit to cost (B/C) ratio where B/C = (disease costs without immunization program – disease costs with an immunization program)/costs of the immunization program	—	Cases

a. The sources in this table represent examples from the peer-reviewed literature of cost-effectiveness and related analyses of preventive services.

b. 1 = full presence of attribute, 0 = absence of attribute (when applied to mortality 1 = alive, 0 = dead).

c. Some or all of the investigator-assigned weights were borrowed from other literature.

d. Some or all of the investigator-assigned weights were evaluated by experts.

Cost-effectiveness analysis requires that HRQL be placed onto a continuum and that changes on this continuum be followed for the duration of survival. This continuum, shown in Figure 4.1, is anchored at the top by an optimal level of HRQL assigned the value of 1.0 and at the bottom by a level of HRQL judged equivalent to death, assigned the value of 0.0.

"Optimal health" is an abstract notion. It has been interpreted to mean "normal good health," "free of all disease, symptoms, or dysfunction," and "health as good as you can imagine it." This notion of optimal health is neither the absolute upper limit, nor the average. No matter how optimal health is defined, there will always be those exceptional individuals who exceed the definition. However, the population average falls short of optimal health. Thus, in practice, few health interventions will have the capacity to restore people to a HRQL value of 1.0. At the other end of the scale, although death may be considered the minimal level of health for many people, states of health such as coma, constant pain, or severe cognitive dysfunction may be considered by some to be worse than death. In this case the minimal level is designated at a negative value such as −0.50. Empirical work supports the notion of states that are seen as worse than death (Patrick et al., 1994).

The area under the curve in Figure 4.1 represents the duration of an individual's life, as modified by the changes in health and well-being experienced over a lifetime. Figure 4.1 is a display for a single individual; however, the same graph can be used to measure and report the health of a population. A number of terms have been coined to describe the area under the curve, including *quality-adjusted life years* (QALYs), *well years,*

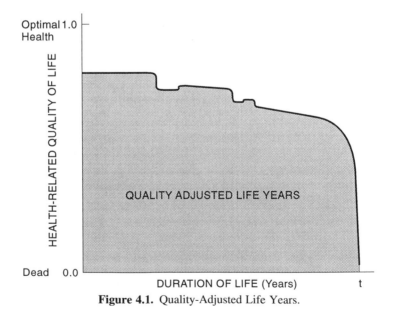

Figure 4.1. Quality-Adjusted Life Years.

years of healthy life, quality-adjusted life expectancy, health-adjusted person years, and *health-adjusted life expectancy.*

Combining Duration of Life with Health-Related Quality of Life

Comparing programs across populations, illnesses, and interventions requires that duration of life and HRQL be combined into a single summary measure. In practice, this is handled by combining quality and quantity into a one-dimensional measure of overall effectiveness such that more is better. It is important to understand, however, that even with a single measure of effectiveness, the tradeoffs between quality and quantity still exist; they are simply hidden from view. They are buried within the method for combining quality and quantity, and different methods imply different approaches to the tradeoff question.

The conventional QALY measure—in which each health state is assigned a numerical weight, regardless of the length of time spent in the state or the sequence of health states experienced—is only one of several possible methods of assigning values to lifetimes of varying HRQL. It is currently the method of choice because of its relative simplicity and ease of implementation. The ethical and behavioral assumptions underlying QALYs have been described in Chapter 2. Here we begin with the most general approach to assigning numerical values to lifetimes of varying HRQL and then turn to conventional QALYs and a few alternatives.

Lifetime Health Paths

In the most general case, each individual is born and lives out a lifetime that consists of moving through different health states over time until death. Each individual has a different path through these health states that terminates at a different time of death. For example, consider a perinatal intervention designed to improve the health of a newborn. Without the intervention the average newborn faces a probability distribution of possible paths through life. With the intervention, the person faces a different, hopefully improved, probability distribution of paths. How should we assess the different paths, and the different probability distributions over paths, remembering that each path consists of both quality and quantity of life?

In the ensuing discussion, we consider the task of evaluating preferences for the paths themselves, rather than individual health states along the paths. This task in its most general form is extremely taxing, because each sequence of health states over a lifetime must be evaluated holistically. This is the reason that the QALY approach—which reduces the task to assigning values to individual health states—is so appealing.

Two special paths represent the extremes of possible health outcomes and they bound the range of effectiveness scores for possible health paths. One is the path that consists of immediate death at birth. The other is the path that consists of "optimal" health for a "full" lifetime. (The problem with the latter is how to define a full lifetime. This might be done by assigning an arbitrary maximum lifetime, for example, 100 years. It might be done empirically by asking the general public to rank healthy lifetimes of different lengths, and selecting the most preferred length [Sutherland et al., 1982]).

The valuation task is to assign numbers to the various paths, and to probability distributions over the paths (1) such that better paths and better probability distributions have higher numbers—that is, more is better—and (2) such that the numbers have interval scale properties—that is, equal intervals on the scale (e.g., 0.1–0.2, 0.8–0.9) have an equivalent interpretation. These two requirements stem from the fact that the numbers will be used in cost-effectiveness analyses to compare the aggregate consequences of alternative health programs.

The first requirement, *more is better*, is self-evident, because the numbers are used to define the effectiveness of programs. The second requirement, *the interval scale property*, is necessary because the CEA approach cannot discriminate, for example, between a gain from 0.1–0.2 and a gain from 0.8–0.9 and treats all numerically identical gains as equal. Thus, it is important to ensure that when the numbers are first derived, equal numerical differences represent equal preference differences.

One of the properties of an interval scale is that it can have numbers arbitrarily assigned to any two defined points on the scale and the rest of the scale follows. For example, temperature is measured on an interval scale, with freezing point and boiling point of water arbitrarily assigned numbers 0 and 100 on the Celsius scale and 32 and 212 on the Fahrenheit scale. One can convert between these two interval scales quite simply using what is called a positive linear transformation.

Putting this all together suggests the following. Using the two extremes of outcome paths as the reference points for the interval scale of preferences over lifetime health paths, the number 0.0 is assigned to the path "immediate death" and the number 1.0 is assigned to the path "optimal health for a full lifetime." An instrument with interval-level scaling properties measures preferences for the other paths relative to these two reference points. In addition, if the analyses will require preferences for probability distributions over paths as well as for paths themselves (which, in general, they do), one would have to either measure preferences for all required probability distributions over paths (a nearly impossible cognitive task) or measure preferences for paths only, but using an approach that supports the probabilistic combination of results (for example, the "standard gamble" approach, discussed later in this chapter).

Note that the system described above can accommodate "paths worse than death." Just as setting the freezing point of water at 0.0 does not preclude negative temperatures—similarly, setting the preference for "immediate death at birth" at 0.0 does not preclude negative preferences for paths worse than death.

At this point in the discussion we have interval-scaled numbers for paths of different duration and quality on a scale with reference points at 0.0 and 1.0 as described above.

Because the numbers have been measured such that they have interval scale properties, they can be multiplied by any positive constant without changing the basic nature of the scale. If these numbers are multiplied by the years established as a full life (e.g., 100 years), or by its present-value equivalent (31.6 years, using a 3% annual discount rate), the result now has the dimension of years. Specifically, the result can be interpreted as a quality-adjusted life year (QALY) figure for each path which is an interval scale. This approach, which is empirically daunting, may be as close to a "gold standard" as one will get for the measurement of preferences and the calculation of QALYs. One aspect of this general approach, focusing on the valuation of health paths rather than health states, is a key feature of the healthy-years equivalents (HYEs) method (Mehrez and Gafni, 1989).

The technique may not be very practical, however, for two reasons. First, in most studies there will be a large number of lifetime paths that would require preference measurements. Second, the measurement of preference for each path would be cognitively very demanding because it would require the respondent to assess an entire complex path in one summary judgment. The task can be simplified by directly measuring preferences, and thus QALYs, for single health states assuming that they lasted a lifetime, and computing QALYs for paths of changing states based on the preference scores for the component states. (See, for example, Boyle et al., 1983.) The computation uses the conventional QALY calculation (described below), which can be equivalently seen as a weighted average of the lifetime QALYs for each state, with the weights based on the time spent in each state.

Conventional QALYs

In the conventional approach to QALYs the quality-adjustment weight for each health state is multiplied by the time in the state (which may be discounted, as discussed in Chapter 7) and then summed to calculate the number of quality-adjusted life years. The advantage of the QALY as a measure of health output is that it can simultaneously capture gains from reduced morbidity (quality gains) and reduced mortality (quantity gains), and integrate these into a single measure. A simple example is displayed in Figure 4.2, in which outcomes are assumed to occur with certainty. Without the health intervention an individual's health-related quality of life would deteriorate according to the lower curve and the individual would die at time Death 1. With the health intervention the individual would deteriorate more slowly, live longer, and die at time Death 2. The area between the two curves is the number of QALYs gained by the intervention. For instruction purposes the area can be divided into two parts, A and B, as shown. Then part A is the amount of QALY gained due to quality improvements (i.e., the quality gain during time that the person would have otherwise been alive anyhow), and part B is the amount of QALY gained due to quantity improvements (i.e., the amount of life extension, but factored by the quality of that life extension).

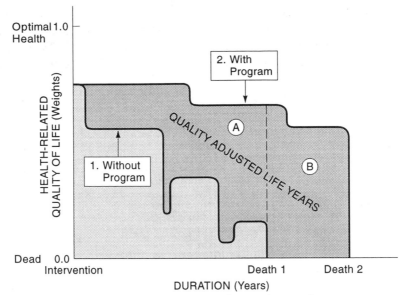

Figure 4.2. QALYs gained from an intervention.

Of course, much more complicated cases can be handled. The curves may cross each other. For example, many cancer treatments cause a QALY loss in the short term in order to achieve a QALY gain in the longer term. The curves may also be identical for a long time after an intervention and only diverge in the distant future. An example of this pattern could be a hypertension drug that is well tolerated and has no side effects but eventually averts serious cardiovascular events.

More important, uncertainty with regard to both survival and HRQL can be handled by calculating the expected, or average, number of QALYs under each intervention. Under uncertainty, the curves in Figure 4.2 can be interpreted as the expected, or average, HRQL at each point in time. The area under the curve represents, therefore, the average number of QALYs, or quality-adjusted life expectancy (QALE).

Calculation of QALYs

Conceptually, the QALY calculation is straightforward. Referring to, Figure 4.2, the QALYs gained are the area under curve 2 less the area under curve 1. The area under each curve is simply the sum of the quality weights for the various health states on the curve (the path) multiplied by the duration (in years or fractions of years) of each health state. This is the number of QALYs gained without discounting.

Because individuals and society prefer gains of all types, including health gains, to occur earlier rather than later, future amounts are multiplied by a discount factor to adjust for this time preference. The technique of discounting, which is described in detail in Chapter 7, essentially consists of taking amounts that will occur in the future and converting them to equivalently valued amounts at the present time. This is done by multiplying the number of QALYs in each future year by the factor $1/1+r^t$ where r is the chosen annual discount rate (e.g., 0.03) and t is the number of years between the present and the given future year.

Alternatives to QALYs

The QALY concept is not without controversy. For a sample of the debate see Donaldson et al. (1988), Weinstein (1988), Loomes and McKenzie (1989), Mehrez and Gafni (1989), Carr-Hill (1989), Cox et al. (1992), Gafni and Birch (1993), Mehrez and Gafni (1993), Culyer and Wagstaff (1993), Fryback (1993), Johannesson et al. (1993), Broome (1993), and associated comments and rebuttals. The critics range from those who argue that the QALY approach is needlessly complex and should be replaced by simpler disaggregated measures (Cox et al., 1992) to those who claim that the QALY approach is overly simplistic and should be replaced by more complex methods which are descriptively superior (Mehrez and Gafni, 1989, 1993; Gafni and Birch, 1995). Several alternatives to QALYs have been suggested, and two are described briefly below.

Healthy-Years Equivalents (HYE), the more general approach to assigning preferences to lifetime health paths, have been suggested as an alternative to QALYs (Mehrez and Gafni, 1989, 1993; Gafni and Birch, 1995). HYEs are calculated by measuring the utility for each possible health path of changing health states and converting this utility through a second measurement into its HYE. There are two essential components to the HYE approach. One is the measurement of preferences over complete life paths, rather than over discrete health states. The second is the use of a two-stage standard gamble assessment procedure in the measurement process.

There is little dispute over the desirability of the first component of the HYE approach. Measuring preferences over lifetime paths of outcomes is conceptually highly attractive. It is, however, empirically daunting. The issue is, to what extent are the simpler methods of conventional QALYs an acceptable approximation for the more complex methods of path-based lifetime QALYs? Although there are some studies in the field that address this issue, there is scant evidence to date.

There is considerable dispute over the second component of the HYE approach. Critics have argued that the use of the two-stage standard gamble is unnecessarily complicated and is equivalent to a much simpler one-stage time-tradeoff question (Buckingham, 1993; Johannesson et al., 1993). The developers of the HYE approach dispute this (Mehrez and Gafni, 1993; Gafni and Birch, 1995). Empirical evidence is currently unavailable.

Responding to concerns of some authors (Harris, 1987) that it is unethical to consider the value of a life to be less because a person is disabled, *saved young life equivalents* (SAVEs) have been proposed for use in lieu of QALYs (Nord, 1992a). The unit of value is measured by determining the equivalence between the health *gains* afforded by the program (rather than the health state) under study, and a standard measure is defined as the saving and restoring to full health of one young life. That is, the effects of the program under study would be judged to be equivalent to a certain number of SAVEs. The distinguishing feature of the SAVE approach is that it is changes in health status that are valued; both the baseline health state (e.g., the prospect of imminent death) and the improved health state (e.g., survival with or without permanent disability) enter into the valuation, rather than assigning value to health states themselves. The measurement strategy in SAVEs is constructed to yield social values for health gains for individuals. All programs would be measured in terms of their equivalent SAVEs, and this would be the common metric of program output, replacing the QALY.

Both of these potential alternatives to the QALY are still at the early stages of investigation and debate. In the meantime the conventional QALY remains the dominant approach, and we therefore recommend that in a Reference Case analysis morbidity and mortality consequences of an intervention be incorporated into a single measure by the use of QALYs.

Before leaving this overview of QALYs, it should be noted that if the overall QALY measure is to be an interval scale, for reasons discussed earlier, the quality weights must also be interval scaled. Furthermore, if death is to have a score of 0, the weight assigned to the state of death must be 0. These observations lead to the recommendations that to satisfy the QALY concept the quality weights must be (1) interval scaled and (2) measured or transformed onto the interval scale where the reference point "death" has a score of 0.0 and the reference point "optimal health" has a score of 1.0.

Health Status Measures

Capturing health status is a first step in creating a QALY. To illustrate the different ways that health states may be recorded, take as an example a woman with breast cancer, and consider how her experience might be presented:

> Three years after radical mastectomy for breast cancer, a 55-year-old former professional tennis player is without pain related to her surgery, but has developed moderate arthritic pain in her shoulders. In addition, as a consequence of her breast cancer surgery, she has muscle weakness that affects her right arm. Because of the combination of the arthritis and the muscle weakness, she can no longer play tennis, an activity that gives her a good deal of satisfaction. She dislikes the tamoxifen she is on as "it reminds me every day I have cancer," and this is somewhat distressing to her. She was divorced 18 months ago, and cannot retire early, as she had planned before the divorce.

This written description, termed a ''scenario,'' is an abstraction of the reality of the patient, and reading the scenario is not equivalent to seeing and interviewing the patient herself. The scenario emphasizes certain things that its author feels are important to understanding the health state. Not all health-state describers would present it in the same way, nor would they necessarily choose to describe the same elements of health. Similarly, researchers studying outcomes associated with treatment of breast cancer would not all decide to measure the same aspects of health status (e.g., some would not use measures that would capture the effects of comorbidities such as this patient's arthritis).

Deciding what aspects of the health state should be included in such a scenario, or which aspects should be observed and measured in patients being observed, is an area of controversy. Table 4.2 lists the various health concepts and domains that many researchers agree should be included in a comprehensive general description of health status. ''Indicators'' and ''measures'' provide operational definitions of concepts and domains. (We use the terms ''concepts'' and ''domains'' in this chapter to describe generic elements of health status. They have also been called ''attributes'' or ''dimensions'' because of their roles in constructing multiattribute utility measures.)

Note that domains are not always independent and may interact with one another; for example, minor physical symptoms may produce little psychological or social deficit, while major chronic physical impairments can (but don't always) produce profound

Table 4.2 Core Concepts and Domains of Health-Related Quality of Life

Concepts and Domains	Indicators
Health perceptions	Self-rating of health; health concern, health worry
Social function	
Social relations	Interaction with others; participation in the community
Usual social role	Acute or chronic limitations in usual social role (major activities) of child, student, worker
Intimacy/sexual function	Perceived feelings of closeness; sexual activity and/or problems
Communication/speech	Acute or chronic limitations in communication/speech
Psychological function	
Cognitive function	Alertness; disorientation; problems in reasoning
Emotional function	Psychological attitudes and behaviors
Mood/feelings	Anxiety; depression; happiness; worries
Physical function	
Mobility	Acute or chronic reduction in mobility
Physical activity	Acute or chronic reduction in physical activity
Self-care	Acute or chronic reduction in self-care
Impairment	
Sensory function/loss	Vision; hearing
Symptoms/impairments	Reports of physical and psychological symptoms, sensations, pain, health problems or feelings not directly observable; or observable evidence of defect or abnormality

Adapted from Patrick and Erickson (1993).

psychological and/or social dysfunction. Researchers interested in specific effects of the disease process under study may augment this list with additional measures thought to be sensitive to changes in particular diseases.

Health status measures are systems that are used to define and describe health status. A *health status profile* is an instrument that describes the health status of a person on each of a comprehensive set of domains. For example, the Medical Outcomes Study SF-36, a commonly used health status profile, addresses eight domains (Ware and Sherbourne, 1992). The Sickness Impact Profile (SIP) covers four broad concepts incorporating 12 domains (Bergner et al., 1981).

A comprehensive set of concepts and domains covering the major aspects of health status, each operationalized by a measurement method, collectively forms a classification scheme for describing and cataloguing health states. The potential number of health states catalogued by a highly detailed classification scheme with many domains, each divided into many levels, is vast, because each individual can be described by a distinct combination of levels on the different domains. In practice, measures of health status and health-related quality of life frequently draw on a common set of domains for which there is broad consensus regarding their importance to health.

Which health status measures to adopt and which domains to include in a particular inquiry depend on the objectives of measurement and the particular concerns of the users, including patients, clinicians, researchers, policy analysts, and funding sponsors. In addition, not all measures of health states are appropriate for CEAs, as we discuss next.

Why Value Health Outcomes?

A health outcome is a path of health states evolving over time, often over the lifetime of the individual. Developing a single numeric score for the health outcome involves developing a score for each health state and combining that score with duration in order to determine the number of QALYs created. Because each health state is comprised of different health domains, developing a score for the state requires a process that combines the effect of each domain into a single metric.

For example, let us return to the tennis-playing patient who, desiring a return to her game, seeks treatment for arthritic pain. A clinical investigator might choose to measure outcomes that assess components of two domains: pain (impairment) and physical function. A brief description of the individual's health state at baseline, known as a *taxonomic health-state description*, is as follows:

> **Health State A**
> pain: moderate pain in shoulders
> physical function: able to conduct normal work and self-care activities but
>   cannot play tennis

Now assume that this woman participates in a treatment regimen with a nonsteroidal antiinflammatory medication that is useful in controlling her arthritis but which, as a side effect, gives her gastritis with accompanying stomach pain. At the 3-month follow-up, her health state, described in the same terms and taxonomic form, is reported as follows:

Health State B

pain:	mild pain in shoulders
	moderate abdominal pain
physical function:	able to play tennis

Is this woman "better off" at the 3-month follow-up than she was at baseline? If so, how much better off? There are two distinctly different and alternative approaches for addressing this question. *Preference*-based methods ask subjects to make judgments regarding the value of particular health states and use these judgments to produce a score. *Nonpreference* approaches use methods that assign scores to individual components of the health state and then sum the component scores to a total score.

The method of summated ratings of health status, from the psychometric tradition in psychology, provides the basis for the most commonly used nonpreference-based methods of weighting. Nonpreference models assume that individual components of health status may be measured by asking a series of questions ("items"), each pertaining to an aspect of the health domain, and then further assume that a sum of answers across the items is approximately linearly related to the attribute. Generally, each item is given equal weight. In effect, this approach assumes that the number of items on each dimension provides an adequate reflection of the importance of the various domains contained in the questionnaire.

Often, summated rating scales are comprised of items using a Likert response scale, such as: 1 = All of the time, 2 = Most of the time, 3 = A good bit of the time, 4 = Some of the time, 5 = A little of the time, and 6 = None of the time. But other responses to items may be obtained, such as strength of agreement, extent to which the state describes an individual, and binary responses of agree/disagree or yes/no and so on. An aggregate score is obtained across items by summing the numerical ratings for the items and converting them to a 0–100 scale. Scores between these values represent the proportion of the total possible score achieved.

Let us return to the question of whether the previously described woman is actually better off. In our example, a nonpreference-based scale would provide a numeric measure for each of the two domains (pain and physical function) and sum them to get an overall score for this individual. In this case, the pain score would combine a decreased score for joint pain with an increased score for abdominal pain. This new pain score would be added, with equal weight, to the new, improved score for physical impairment. But without knowing how important each type of pain and each component of her health state (physical function and pain) is to her overall experience of health, it is difficult to make a judgment as to whether she is in fact better off. A more meaningful answer would seem to depend upon the importance the individual places on having less joint pain and being able again to play tennis, as compared to having moderate abdominal pain. The definition of ''better off'' would depend on her views on the relative importance of these two domains, as well as the different components of the domains.

In short, simply summing up numerical weightings across questions on a health assessment scale does not guarantee that changes in scores will coincide with changes in health status that are seen as better off or worse off by patients or by the general public. This is a major problem for use of summated rating instruments in creating QALYs. First, it is unlikely that individuals give equal weights to all components of a health state. Second, when one is considering resource allocation, it is important to know what values people attach to different health outcomes in order to provide, as efficiently as possible, more of the outcomes that are desired and fewer of those that are not. For these reasons, nonpreference-weighted measures are viewed as inappropriate for use in cost-effectiveness analysis. For example, the MOS SF-36 (Ware and Sherbourne, 1992), a nonpreference-weighted measure that is widely used in measuring changes in health status in clinical settings, is not currently suitable for CEA.

Preference-weighted HRQL methods assign scores or ''weights'' to health states by collecting information regarding individual and population preferences for particular health states. In all of these methods, the domains of which HRQL is comprised are valued with respect to one another by collecting information about a set of health states that contain different levels of experience within the domains. For example, in the woman with breast cancer and arthritis, her preferences for different kinds of pain, and for pain versus physical function, underlie her expressed preferences for health states which consist of different combinations of pain and physical function. By collecting information about her preferences for these health states, we can infer her underlying weights and tradeoffs for the health-state domains.

Methods used for gathering preferences derive principally from utility theory, as discussed in Chapter 2. Psychological scaling methods developed from psychophysics (judgments of sensation) are also used to assign preferences to health states. Decision-analytic methods that incorporate aspects of both economic and psychological methods are also being used for preference assignment. We return to discussions of these methods later in the chapter.

Whose Preferences Should Be Used in CEA?

Once health states have been defined for a cost-effectiveness analysis, numerical preference judgments about the relative desirability of these states are required. The goal in collecting preferences should be that an assessment accurately reflect the desirability of the baseline health state as well as the desirability of those that are likely to occur with and without the evaluated intervention(s). However, because preferences for health states represent values rather than objective measures of functional capacity and there is no such thing as a "correct" value, the question of whose preference scores are suitable for use in CEAs becomes an important one.

In practice, preference scores are obtained in different ways depending on the design of a study (e.g., primary data collection in a clinical trial versus secondary analyses conducted from existing databases), and its purpose and perspective (e.g., is the study comparing different methods of treating the same condition or is it designed to consider an intervention in the context of overall resource allocation?). Current practice as to whose preferences are used in valuing outcomes ranges from patients experiencing the health states (and their surrogates), to health professionals, to community samples of the general public. In this section we discuss theory-based, ethical, and pragmatic concerns that direct the choice of whose preferences are best suited for use in CEAs that are designed to inform different types of decision making.

Preferences for Use in the Reference Case

We begin with a look at whose preferences are most suitable for a Reference Case analysis which is designed to make comparisons across types of interventions and across populations. A variety of considerations push in different directions with respect to the use of community-based versus patient preferences.

In Chapter 1 we concluded that the societal perspective is the appropriate one for decision making concerning health care resources in the public interest. A logical extension of that reasoning would suggest that the best articulation of society's preferences for particular health states would be gathered from a representative sample of fully informed members of the community. Only with preferences so gathered could we begin to scale the differences between "optimal health" and a large array of conditions (with their accompanying health states) on an interval scale.

It can be argued, however, that persons experiencing a particular health state are better suited to provide an assessment of the value of that health state. Judgments about the relative value of a health state may depend on the goals and expectations people have for themselves. When the ill or the elderly alter their expectations and goals and accommodate to the limitations imposed by a functional disability or a set of symptoms, their overall utility for that condition is likely to be higher than a nondisabled sample of the community who lack understanding of the adjustments that are possible in what appears, from the outside, to be a diminished health state. The public may well harbor stereotypes and biases that are incorporated into their preferences for health states, based on the assumption that their overall utility would be less than it would be were they to make some reasonable accommodation.

However, the public may well be reflecting the objective fact that the range of capabilities for people having certain conditions and disabilities is lessened compared to the normal range. It would be inappropriate to lose sight of the fact that although high utility is achievable for someone who is objectively disabled, a more plausible goal, from the societal perspective, should be to minimize disability and maximize full function in all health domains.

Given arguments on both sides, what help does theory give us in deciding whose judgments should be considered most "valid" for use in CEAs? If we return to our previous discussions of the "veil of ignorance" (Chapters 1 and 2), where a rational public decides what is the best course of action when blind to its own self-interest, aggregating the utilities of persons who have no vested interest in particular health states seems most appropriate.

Practical concerns must, however, be considered in seeking rational judgments about preferences for health states. To inform public policy decisions, one would wish to have judgments that are informed, unbiased, and competent. Problems emerge in meeting these measurement criteria simultaneously both for persons who are experiencing the health state and for those who are not.

In assessing health states, a community sample may be asked to consider a not-heretofore-experienced health state as well as to perform the unfamiliar task of comparing and rating health states against one another. The level of understanding of the nature of particular health states by members of the general public or by others who are not experiencing the health state is not always accurate and can be heavily influenced by "cues" in how the assessment procedure is done (McNeil et al., 1982). Although efforts can be made to provide in-depth descriptions of the health state, lengthy descriptions can result in cognitive overload, and the health states, even if described in detail, remain hypothetical.

The judgments of persons experiencing the health states might also be viewed as unreliable in some instances. For persons experiencing cognitive or emotional impairment, or in children, the task of making an assessment and using probabilities and numerical judgments may make those who are experiencing the health state poor subjects. Moreover, those experiencing an acute condition may not be best able to make well-considered judgments of how severe the state actually would be in the long run. They may not be "neutral" judges.

If we knew that there were no differences in the preference structure of people with and without a defined constellation of limitations, then whose preferences to measure would not be an issue. Some evidence suggests that people's values for generic health states are remarkably consistent (EuroQol Group, 1990; Froberg and Kane, 1989b,c; Balaban et al., 1986; Llewellyn-Thomas et al., 1984; Boyle and Torrance, 1984; Patrick et al., 1985; Hadorn and Uebersax, 1995). Llewellyn-Thomas, et al. (1993) determined that subjects' pretreatment ratings for the states produced by radiation for cancer did not change after they actually entered those states. This provides support of the view that people can visualize at least some specific health states relatively well. Other literature, however, tends to support the finding that people who have a disease or condition will value that associated health state higher than those who have not experienced it (Sackett and Torrance, 1978; Najman and Levine, 1981; Epstein et al., 1989; Slevin et al., 1990). We assume that the preferences of affected and unaffected individuals for a particular health state will, in general, differ somewhat and base our reasoning and recommendations on this assumption.

Do Community Preferences Discriminate Against Persons Who Are Ill or Have Disabilities?

Positing differences between patient and community preferences requires us to examine the critical issue of whether using community rather than patient preferences discriminates against the aged, the ill, or persons with disability in CEAs designed to inform resource allocation. Note that the discussion here does not address the larger issue of whether or not QALYs per se discriminate against these vulnerable groups. As we have noted in Chapters 1 and 2, lifesaving interventions in populations having reduced HRQL and life expectancy because of illness, disability, and age yield fewer QALYs than they would in a young or "well" population. In this section we look specifically at the issue of whether the use of community preferences for health states (rather than the preferences of people actually experiencing the health states) is discriminatory. As described below, we believe that the use of community preferences is less likely to discriminate against persons with illness or disability than the use of their own preferences. We use specific examples of disability and illness here, but the points are generalizable.

Consider an example in which persons who are paraplegic assign a more favorable value to a health state that includes wheelchair dependency than does a community sample while assigning values that are equivalent to the overall community's to all other health states. The community sample would be a representative one and as such would actually contain some paraplegic persons, but only in proportion to the prevalence of that disability in the general population. Consider then an intervention (e.g., coronary artery bypass graft surgery [CABG]) that is targeted at all persons who experience ischemic chest pain. In calculating the cost-effectiveness of the intervention using community judges the analyst would use the average gain in HRQL experienced by all members of the community who improve from a health state that reflects the decrements associated with angina to a health state that is unencumbered by the functional limitations and symptoms of angina. Hence all persons who undergo successful CABG, including those who are paraplegic, will be credited with the average gain as valued by the full community. From a resource allocation perspective, the cost-effectiveness ratio for interventions directed at conditions unrelated to those experienced by a disabled or ill group of individuals would be exactly the same for the chronically ill or disabled as for the general population.

Where the cost-effectiveness of a therapy to cure paraplegia is itself being evaluated, using population-based preferences in the Reference Case is likely to result in *greater* estimated effectiveness for paraplegic persons than would be the case if their own preference scores were used. If wheel-chair dependent mobility is systematically rated lower by a community sample (whose average self-rated HRQL is 0.9) than by those who require wheelchairs, the gains possible from the intervention become larger when the perspective is that of the general population, and the cost per QALY gained decreases. For example, suppose that community judges would rate a health state that includes the functional limitations associated with paraplegia as 0.4, while paraplegic persons rate the same state as a 0.6. A cure for paraplegia would produce a gain of 0.5 (the difference between 0.9 and 0.4) using the values of community judges and only 0.3 (0.9 versus 0.6) using those of judges who are paraplegic. The increased QALYs produced using the assessments of the general population will produce more QALYs (at the same cost) and hence will make cure of paraplegia more "cost-effective" than if the preferences were elicited by paraplegic persons. The same conclusion is reached when the cost- effectiveness of a therapy to *prevent* paraplegia is being evaluated: The gain will be greater using the preferences of the general community rather than the preferences of paraplegic persons. This example, like the previous ones, provides no evidence that using community versus patient preferences discriminates against the ill or disabled. An interesting illustration of this principle is discussed in the evaluation of the Oregon Medicaid proposal by the Office of Technology Assessment (OTA). The OTA report notes 12 conditions among 28 where those "experienced" with the condition rate it as significantly more desirable than those who are not experienced. The results of using the "experienced" weights would have to give less priority to amelioration of those conditions (OTA, 1992).

Populations With Different Preferences

We suggest that preferences from the general population rather than preferences of particular subgroups should be used in a Reference Case CEA. This holds when the condition/health state under consideration is related or unrelated to the intervention being evaluated. It holds whether the intervention is health-improving or lifesaving. It is important, however, to make a distinction between preferences that are used in CEA and those that are used in bedside decision making. Simply because a CEA provided evidence that treatment of angina with CABG is a relatively "good" investment does not imply that all patients with angina, irrespective of clinical condition, should receive surgery. An individual's capacity to benefit from treatment is always influenced by age or underlying condition, and in a clinical setting, the preferences and health status of individual patients may well argue for approaches that differ from those suggested by a CEA that has been crafted to inform resource allocation decisions.

Many researchers take exception to the idea of an "average" preference, even in the case of resource allocation decisions. What should be done in the situation where the existence of preference subgroups within a community sample could substantially change the favorability of a cost-effectiveness ratio? For example, investigators have shown that the benefits of transurethral surgery for benign prostatic hypertrophy (BPH) depend heavily on the preferences men have for the symptoms of the disease—nocturia, urinary frequency—as compared to the possible side effects of the intervention—incontinence and impotence (Barry et al., 1988). Assuming for the moment that there were no significant risk of death from surgery, the relative preferences men have for urinary frequency and nocturia, versus those for a small risk of postintervention incontinence and impotence in the face of symptom resolution, would determine the magnitude of change in the denominator of a cost-effectiveness ratio. If some men will always assign a higher utility to a health state involving urinary frequency than to one with incontinence, the net cost per QALY gained for transurethral surgery will always be very high. However, if the preferences of another group of men suggested that the gain in utility for a health state free of nocturia and urinary frequency (permitting them, for example, to continue work or leisure activities that do not readily allow for voiding) is great enough, transurethral surgery could be quite "cost-effective." Taking the "average" preferences of the population into account might miss the reality for two distinct preference subgroups.

The magnitude of that difference in preference when calculated separately (not averaged with the overall population) might well result in a cost per QALY that would be much lower than one that was based on averages. For example, if the cost of transurethral surgery is $20,000 and the average QALY increment gained by the procedure for the population overall is 0.1, the C/E ratio for the intervention would be $200,000/QALY. However, the preference subgroup described above might report a utility gain of 0.5, decreasing the C/E ratio to $40,000/QALY, a far better value.

Suppose that a cost-effectiveness table was then created that compared the treatment of all conditions and the decision made that if a cost-effectiveness ratio was higher than x dollars per QALY the treatment would no longer be available. Which C/E ratio should appear in the table? The concerns raised by the existence of population subgroup preference structures would be difficult to surmount if in fact a treatment that was cost-effective in a population subgroup was denied to it.

We therefore view subgroup preference structures as important complements to informing decision making for resource allocation purposes. While we do not view subgroup preferences as feasible for the purpose of the Reference Case, we suggest that when investigators are aware of systematic differences in preference scores for particular populations that might bear significantly on the final C/E ratios, these considerations should be highlighted in sensitivity analyses and discussions of results.

Use of Patient Preferences

Many analysts will have legitimate reasons for using patient preferences in certain types of CEAs. For example, when an analysis is designed to evaluate alternative interventions for the same condition, use of patient preferences is not only legitimate; it may be preferred. This type of analysis is not primarily intended for resource allocation decisions over a wide universe of illnesses or conditions but rather as a way to assess the most efficient way to create health given a circumscribed condition and a selection of treatment choices. In general, however, because of its reliance on patient preferences, it will not be a Reference Case analysis.

For example, developers of a formulary for a managed care organization might wish to assess which drugs would be most cost-effective in the treatment of high blood pressure. Here, the question is not whether to treat high blood pressure, but rather how to treat it least expensively while achieving a beneficial effect. Effect here would include not only control of blood pressure (and hence the decrease in premature cardiovascular deaths) but also how the medication influences health-related quality of life.

Two considerations support the use of patient preferences in this setting. First, no other conditions are under consideration in this evaluation, and comparisons of the medication- or hypertension-related health states with respect to other health states becomes irrelevant. Second, finely tuned assessment techniques and measurement instruments that are designed to capture the nuances of particular drug- or hypertension-associated states are likely to better capture pre- and posttherapy effects.

While patients can provide helpful information when used in this manner, we emphasize that patient preferences should *not* be seen as equivalent to community preferences, and they are therefore not the optimal ones for use in the Reference Case.

Practical Considerations

Reality dictates that we address the issue of availability of information on preferences. Often investigators will not be doing primary data collection; their analyses will be built from models that use extant sources. These analyses require either the use of previously collected preference weights or a mechanism to efficiently estimate preferences. Health professionals, knowledgeable about the nature of the health state, can provide considered judgments about the likely gains from an intervention.

Two methods that rely on expert opinion are available. The direct scoring of the utility of the underlying condition and that of the expected outcome of the treatment have been done by health professionals. Health professionals have been seen as credible sources of preference scores because they have witnessed a particular condition or health state in scores or hundreds of patients and are able to provide a considered judgment about the true long-run effect of the health state on a patient. Health professionals may, however, give too much weight to functional status and inadequately take into account more subtle and subjective influences of an illness (e.g., emotional problems, pain and discomfort) when attaching a value to a condition-related health state. In addition, health professionals do not constitute a representative cross section of the general public with regard to age, income, and socioeconomic class, and therefore systematic biases may be built into these surrogate preferences. Using health professionals, then, to directly *value* health states is regarded as an unsatisfactory method of obtaining preferences.

Alternatively, health professionals can describe the baseline and intervention-attributed health states of the CEA in terms that allow mapping to a set of community-based preference scores (e.g., as gathered for the EurQol, Health Utilities Index, or Quality of Well-Being instruments). Here they function in the preferred role of ''describer'' rather than as a ''judge'' of health states. An example of how experts may be used to describe outcome health states for particular conditions which can then be mapped to community preferences is illustrated in the neural tube defects example found in Appendix B.

Another consideration pertains when preferences have been gathered in a patient group because of convenience and are then used as approximations for the preferences of the community. For example, in prospective clinical studies two methods are commonly used for obtaining health-state preferences. The first approach directly measures patient preferences for baseline and outcome states. While these preferences would be useful in CEAs that compare interventions for the same condition, they are not ideally suited to a Reference Case analysis, where community preferences for health states are the relevant ones. The second, and preferred approach is to have patients describe their health states in terms of a health-state classification system that has already been weighted by a representative community sample. These two approaches are described in more detail in the next section.

In clinical trials, when possible, the direct assessment of patient preferences, in addition to collecting information on health states in a form that allows for community weighting, will expand the data available for use in Reference Case analyses. In addition, information that deepens an understanding of the relationship between community and patient preferences will be developed.

Concerns have been raised about the representativeness of existing community-based preferences. Two widely used classification schemes, the Quality of Well-Being Scale, and the Health Utilities Index, provide scores based on samples of residents of San Diego, California, and Hamilton, Ontario, respectively. Neither of these may be entirely relevant for the general U.S. population. While concerns with respect to representativeness may be exaggerated given the stability of preferences for generic health states across different groups of people when measured with the same instrument (Balaban et al., 1986; EuroQol Group, 1990; Froberg and Kane, 1989c), some discrepancies have been noted between scores for QWB health states when gathered from community samples in San Diego when compared to scores of Oregonians (OTA, 1992). However, one set of interviews was conducted face to face, while the other was telephone-administered. Unresolved questions with respect to the comparability of one community's weights with those of another suggests that collecting preferences from a representative sample of the U.S. population for health state classification instruments suitable for Reference Case analyses should be a priority for the field.

Conclusion

This section has reviewed theoretical and practical concerns regarding whose preferences to use in different types of CEAs. The goal in collecting preferences should be
an assessment that accurately reflects, in a manner consistent with required measurement
properties, and from the appropriate viewpoint, the relative desirability of health states
that arise from an intervention.

For studies designed to compare alternative therapies for a patient group in a setting
where resources have already been allocated to the treatment of their condition, patient
preferences should be used. Reference Case analyses done from the societal perspective
for purposes of resource allocation should use the health-state preferences of a well-
informed, cognitively robust, unbiased community sample. Although pristine weights
are currently unavailable, primarily because of the difficulty of ensuring that the subjects
are indeed perfectly informed, preferences from a community sample are, on balance,
the most appropriate source. Techniques that create a better understanding in the general
public of the experience of differing health states will be highly useful in strengthening
this field.

There will be times when a satisfactory source for community preferences is unavailable for use in a Reference Case analysis. In these cases, patient preferences may
be used as an approximation. The manner in which they might differ from community
preferences should be discussed and, where relevant, sensitivity analyses that reflect
likely differences should be included.

Finally, the health-related quality of life of those whose lives have been saved or
extended by a health intervention may be influenced by characteristics such as the age,
gender, race, or socioeconomic status of the population involved. This may affect a
Reference Case analysis in ways that are ethically problematic. In these instances, we
recommend that sensitivity analysis be conducted to indicate explicitly how the analysis
is affected by these characteristics.

Preference Classification Systems

In practice, preferences may be located on the HRQL continuum using one of two
methods. If the researcher is collecting primary data, individuals experiencing a condition, or ones to whom a condition is described through a scenario, can be asked to
rate health states directly onto the continuum through one of several self-weighting
methods. These methods, which include rating scales, paired comparisons, time tradeoff, and standard gamble methods, are described in more detail in the next section.
Alternatively, individuals experiencing a health state can be asked questions that locate
their health state on each attribute in a comprehensive classification scheme. Preference
scores for the classification scheme gathered previously from other populations may
then be used to assign values to the health states.

Assigning Preference Weights to Health States

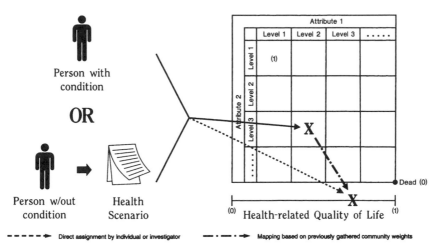

Figure 4.3. Assigning preference weights to health states.

Figure 4.3 represents two methods for placing a health state onto a 0–1 scale of HRQL. In one instance, individuals directly assign values to a described or experienced health state. In the second instance individuals are placed in a "cell" within a health-state classification system for which preference scores have been previously determined, based on information gathered from another population.

Many CEAs are secondary analyses—that is, they rely on previously published data (e.g., on effectiveness, or costs) and modeling assumptions made by the analyst, rather than on primary data. In secondary analyses the investigator must first describe the health states of interest (often this involves a small number of archetypal states associated with the condition) and then impute preferences or utilities for these by extrapolating or interpolating previously published data. In the depiction of Figure 4.3, the analyst must describe the likely health states of patients in the language of the classification scheme (e.g., "at 1 year post breast cancer surgery, 40% of patients will be in cell 1,1; 40% will be in cell 3,1; 19.5% will be in 3,3; and 0.5% will be "dead") and then apply previously published preferences scores corresponding to these states.

Table 4.3 summarizes the domains included in a number of generic instruments that can provide preference weights for use in secondary analyses. Appendix 4.1 includes additional information about these instruments. All of these measures include some combination of health perceptions—of physical, social, and psychological function and of impairment—but no two measures share identical domains. Absent in many of these measures is the ability to collect information on the dimension of mood or emotional function. In the scenario presented in the section on health status measures, restoring the ability of the breast cancer survivor to play tennis might well result in substantial

Table 4.3 Principal Concepts and Domains of Health-Related Quality of Life Contained in General Preference-Weighted Instruments for Assessing Quality-Adjusted Life Years

					Instrument				
	Disability Distress Index	EuroQol	15D	Health Utility Index			Years of Healthy Life HP2K	Quality of Well-being Scale	Quality of Life and Health
Concept				Mark I	Mark II	Mark III			
Health perceptions			**				**		**
Social function									
Social relations		**		**				**	
Usual social role		**		**					**
Intimacy/sexual function									
Communication/speech			**		**	**			
Psychological function									
Cognitive function			**		**	**			
Emotional function		**		**	**	**			**
Mood/feelings									**
Physical function									
Mobility	**	**	**	**	**	**		**	
Physical activity	**	**	**	**		**	**	**	**
Self-care		**	**	**	**	**			**
Impairment									
Sensory function/loss			**		**	**			**
Symptoms/impairments	**	**	**		**	**		**	**

Adapted from Patrick and Erickson (1996)

improvement in her mood. Failure to use a measurement system that recognizes that dimension could markedly distort the interpretation of the effects of her therapy. The paucity of instruments that capture mood and psychological dysfunction has been an impediment to conducting CEAs that use QALYs as an outcome measure for mental health disorders such as depression and anxiety.

Disagreement remains in the field of CEA as to the scope of the domains to include for description and valuation in preference-based measures. Some instruments are limited to concepts "beneath the skin"—that is, not including any social dimension or description of health that includes social interaction or role definition (Feeny et al., 1995; Torrance et al., 1995b). Many are more expansive and include social role function, i.e., ability to perform major activities such as going to school or working (Drummond et al., 1987; Kaplan and Anderson, 1988). Aspects of the individual's social role may enter the evaluation implicitly, manifesting as an effect on component health domains. In our example of the woman with a mastectomy, the consequences of the health problems may be captured by a health-state classification system that records decrements in aspects of psychological function. If she has emotional or mental health consequences stemming from her divorce, delayed retirement, and inability to play tennis, these effects, rather than the divorce or the requirement to continue work, would be captured in the definition of the health state.

Limiting descriptions to "beneath the skin," or confining them to the individual, has the advantage of eliminating the problem of the environment beyond the individual being considered. However, role function has commonly been included in health state classification systems because it is at the *social* level that illness and disease are recognized within a culture or social system. The Reference Case analysis is built on the assumption that the financial and the health status impact of morbidity are captured in the QALY. (See Chapters 2 and 6 for fuller discussions.) For this reason, role function, that is, assumptions people make with respect to the impact of a health state on work and leisure time, should, at minimum, be implicitly captured by the health-related quality-of-life measurement system used in a Reference Case analysis.

Disease-Specific Measures

Any generic health-state classification system that is general and simple enough to be applied across all diseases and interventions may lack sensitivity to important differences in health status that are salient for particular diseases or interventions. Such differences, while ostensibly small, may be highly relevant for prevention programs that expose large numbers of people to minor side effects (e.g., antihypertensive drugs) or for treatment programs that offer benefits within a domain such as mobility (for arthritis) or pain (for heart disease). Such changes in health may literally "fall between the cracks" in measures as coarse as the Healthy People 2000 Years of Healthy Life (30 states) and EuroQol (243 states) one. Therefore, disease-specific and condition-specific classification systems have an important role to play in CEA, particularly when used in settings where patient preferences are germane. One example of such a disease-specific system is the Q-tility index (Weeks et al., 1994), which is based on a five-item questionnaire used commonly in cancer clinical trials.

Disease-specific classification systems must still satisfy the criteria applied to generic systems to ensure that they are appropriately preference-weighted. In particular, the health states should be framed in the context of overall health, including specification of health status within other domains not addressed in the disease-specific system. For example, the states in an arthritis-specific system should be defined with ''default'' levels of domains such as social and role function even though variations in those domains may not explicitly be captured by the health-state classification scheme used in the disease-specific measure. These disease-specific measures, anchored on a 0–1 scale, could then be mapped to a generic measure that is suitable for use in a Reference Case analysis.

Conclusion

A CEA should be based on a health-state classification scheme which reflects domains (attributes) that are important for the particular problem under consideration. If the CEA is intended for use in a Reference Case, the preference measure used should be a generic one or be capable of being compared to a generic system. Regardless of the instrument chosen for a CEA, health outcomes should be ''health-related'' and not include all the possible effects of an intervention. Nonhealth effects, such as financial consequences that do not flow directly from changes in health status, should be captured in the numerator of the CEA. For example, the cost of time spent traveling to or waiting in the doctor's office should be measured as a cost. However, financial consequences that are directly caused by changes in health status are best reflected in the weights assigned to the health states. For example, patients with arthritis who are unable to work with their hands would reflect their loss of productivity—and, hence, income— in the weights they assign to the pain and loss of dexterity caused by their condition. To the extent that these financial losses are borne by persons other than the patient, they would have to be counted separately among the costs. For further discussion of this issue, see the the discussion of time costs in Chapter 2.

Techniques for Valuing Health States

Many authors have described methodologic issues associated with assigning preference weights to health states or health outcomes (Froberg and Kane, 1989a–c; Torrance, 1986; Patrick and Bergner, 1990; Patrick and Deyo, 1989; Hadorn, 1991), and we do not attempt to reproduce the depth and breadth of the literature and discussion they cover. We focus instead on key issues related to the strengths and weaknesses of methods used for assigning preferences to health states. Our focus is primarily on the measurement of community preferences, since for purposes of resource allocation, the relevant preferences are those of the general public.

When community preferences are required and the outcome health states are gathered prospectively in a clinical trial, the health states must be described and then rated by a representative community sample. When the health states are described in language that is specific to the study, community rating based on the health-state descriptions must follow the clinical trial; this is a cumbersome task and therefore not terribly practical. For this reason, health states are often described using the domains represented in the questions from an established measurement system where community-based preference scores are available as part of the system. For analyses where the investigator does not have access to primary data and health-state outcomes are being modeled, premeasured preferences from one of the generic systems can be used. This section provides information on the characteristics of the methods used to obtain preferences for measures such as those briefly described in Appendix 4.1.

Requirements for Measurement Techniques

In measuring preferences, investigators need to be concerned with a number of issues, including the validity, the reliability, and the feasibility of the task required of the researcher and the respondents. Lastly, the mathematical scaling characteristics of the measurement technique and its suitability for CEA need consideration.

The *validity* of the measurement is the extent to which a technique measures what it is intended to measure. Because there is no set of preferences that can be considered ''true'' or ''right'' for all people, ''criterion validity,'' where one measure is considered the gold standard against which all others are judged, is lacking (Patrick, 1976). Nord (1992b) has suggested that ''reflective equilibrium,'' where people are asked to examine the extent to which the implications of their preferences are in accord with their directly elicited preferences, constitutes a type of criterion validity. Little empirical work has been done in this area, however. Comparisons of results achieved from different methods may be helpful in approaching an understanding of validity; here findings of convergence in preference scores when different methods of measurement have been used may provide reassurance that the underlying construct of preference is being captured. Another measure of validity, ''predictive validity,'' involves testing hypotheses that preferences will predict future health care decisions based on the preferences previously assigned to health states with differing characteristics. For example, people who assign relatively low ratings to health states characterized by significant pain, but not to health states characterized by functional limitation, might be predicted to choose treatments with less-painful side effects, even at the price of incomplete improvement of function, compared to those who place higher value on functional status.

The *reliability* of the measure, its consistency in reproducing repeated measures of a phenomenon by the same individual or across different groups of observers, provides evidence that a concept is understood readily enough by a wide enough range of people to provide stable information. As such, it is necessary, but insufficient, for assessing validity. The reliability of a measurement strategy is evaluated in different ways. "Intrarater reliability" is a measure of the stability of the rating an individual judge gives to the same question that is presented more than once during the same or subsequent administrations. "Test–retest reliability" is a test of reliability that looks at the stability of ratings over a short period of time. Test–retest reliability may be a useful indicator of task comprehension in providing preference weights; concordance of two ratings at separate times can provide evidence that people have constancy in their understanding of the measurement technique as well as of the health state. However, test–retest reliability may be confounded by real changes in preferences for health states that are occasioned by the experience of them. For example, women's preferences for anesthesia during childbirth varied considerably depending on whether the measures were taken during labor or 1 month pre- or postpartum: Test–retest reliability was high for the measures unassociated with labor (Christensen-Szalanski, 1984). Finally, "interrater reliability," a measure of consistency among multiple judges, is generally felt to be less germane as a test of preference reliability, given that preferences, by definition, vary across people.

In settings where judges are providing preferences for hypothetical health scenarios (rather than providing a rating of their own health state), the reliability of ratings is likely to be higher when fewer attributes are included in the health state. Earlier work in the psychometric literature suggests that raters are only able to consider a range of five to nine attributes at one time (Miller, 1956). More recently, Hadorn and Hays (1991) have reported poor test–retest reliability of health-state ratings when more than two or three dimensions were used to define the states.

The *feasibility* of implementing the measurement strategy in primary data collection efforts is also of concern. Considerations included here are the time burden for the respondent and the investigator, and the respondent's cognitive ease in performing the valuation task. Investigators will be concerned with the respondent and interviewer burden in administering particular systems directly, or in mapping primary data into them. The generic preference-weighted systems differ in their data collection demands. The original interviewer-administered version of the Quality of Well-Being Scale (QWB) required up to 15 minutes of questioning to classify the patient into the system. A new self-administered version currently under evaluation takes considerably less time. The Health Utilities Index (HUI) requires 2–3 minutes if interviewer administered or 5–10 minutes if self-administered by the patient. The Quality of Life and Health Questionnaire (QLHQ) and the Years of Healthy Life measure (YHL), consisting respectively of four and eight questions, are quicker still. Investigator experiences with methods designed to directly assess preferences (including standard gamble, time tradeoff, category rating, magnitude estimation, and paired comparisons) have been varied and are discussed later in this section.

Other issues that bear on the feasibility of the measurement task also need to be considered. How well do respondents understand the valuation task? Do attitudes toward risk-taking or choice of comparators influence how a health state is rated? The respondent's cognitive burden, in addition to being a concern for reliability, is also a feasibility issue that has implications for the validity of a measure.

Finally, earlier in this chapter we discussed the requirement for interval-level properties in measures used for cost effectiveness analysis. The *mathematical properties* of the different preference elicitation methods and the implications for their suitability for CEA are of concern to many analysts.

Methods for Assigning Preferences to Health States

Methods of preference weighting have been developed primarily from two theoretical traditions: expected utility theory and psychophysical or psychological scaling methods. The generic systems in Appendix 4.1 weight their component health states using the methods described below.

Utility approaches

The methods derived from expected-utility theory include the *standard gamble* and *time-tradeoff* techniques. The *standard gamble* approach, which is based on the axioms of expected utility theory, has been widely used to measure health state preferences (Torrance, 1986). The technique begins with asking the respondent to consider a hypothetical choice between the certainty of continued life in the health state of interest (one of less than optimal health) and a gamble. The gamble has two possible outcomes. The positive outcome is usually a state of full health (assigned a utility of 1). The negative outcome is usually death (assigned a utility of 0). The probabilities in the gamble are systematically altered (visual aids such as a probability wheel or a chance board are used to illustrate the probabilities) until the respondent is indifferent between the choice of the certainty of continued life in the health state of interest and the gamble. The expected value of the gamble at this point is, by substitution, the utility for the health state of interest relative to full health and death. The standard gamble will accommodate states worse than death. Here the certain state is death, and the choices for which the probability is varied are between cure and a chronic state worse than death.

The *time-tradeoff* method presents the respondent with the task of determining what amount of time they would be willing to give up to be in a better versus a poorer health state (Torrance et al., 1972). Here the choice is between two certain outcomes rather than the certain outcome of the described health state and a gamble between life and death. The time-tradeoff method, also performed with visual aids, asks judges to value the alternatives of being in a less desirable health state (A) for a longer period of time followed by death, versus being in a more desirable state (B) for a shorter period of time followed by death. The time in state B is decreased to a point where the judge becomes indifferent between the alternatives. The preference for state A is calculated as life expectancy at the point of indifference in state B divided by the life expectancy in state A. Time tradeoff can also provide weights for health states worse than death.

Decision theorists and economists have favored either the standard gamble method, because it follows directly from the axioms of expected utility theory, or the time-tradeoff method, which also has theoretical roots in decision theory. They hold that the standard gamble is valid by implication if the basic assumptions of expected utility theory are accepted (Torrance, 1987). In addition, it is argued that preferences are gathered in a setting that mirrors many clinical decisions where judges must make choices under conditions of uncertainty (Ben Zion and Gafni, 1983; Gafni and Birch, 1995; Torrance et al., 1995b). Others have argued that the standard gamble does not correspond to the typical decision-making task in health, where multiple potential outcomes are possible and the choice of two options as certain as death or perfect health are not scenarios that typically confront people (Richardson, 1994). Critics of the technique also argue that the predictions of expected utility theory have not been borne out in empirical trials (Llewellyn-Thomas et al., 1982; Kahneman and Tversky, 1983; Anderson, 1979; Shoemaker, 1982). There is debate also as to whether, when performing CEAs for purposes of informing resource allocation (where preferences for health states are collected from representative populations rather than from patients), considerations of risk are, in fact, germane.

Coefficients of intrarater reliability (0.77) and test–retest reliability (0.80) have been reported for the standard gamble (Froberg and Kane, 1989b). For time tradeoff, intrarater reliability has been reported to range from 0.77 to 0.88 and test–retest reliability in the short term has shown coefficients ranging from 0.63 (at 6 weeks) to 0.87 at 1 week or less (Froberg and Kane, 1989b; Nease et al., 1995). Correlations between standard gamble and time tradeoff have been reported to range from 0.31 (Hornberger et al., 1992) to 0.65 (Read et al., 1984).

There is significant contention with respect to the feasibility of collecting preference weights using the standard gamble. Investigators favoring the approach have argued that when the standard gamble is collected properly, with appropriately designed visual aids and measurement props, it is feasible in general and patient populations (Torrance, 1986). Others have found the approach cognitively demanding for patients and argue that the method is unnatural for many people who are unused to formulating their preferences in terms of gambles. The difficulty with the task is held by some to reduce the validity of the approach.

Both the standard gamble and time-tradeoff methods are structured so that respondents make their choices involving the three health states on an interval-level scale, thereby directly producing preference weights with interval-level scaling properties. Weights derived from both techniques tend to be higher than those generated with many of the other preference-weighting techniques. Empirical work has shown that when individuals are asked to choose between a gain and a loss of similar magnitude, the preference for the gain is much less that the desire to avoid the loss (Kahneman and Tversky, 1983). In the case of the standard gamble, people will almost always choose to remain in a lower state of health—no matter how undesirable it is—rather than accept any substantial risk of death. This conservatism in gambling with respect to death usually results in numerically higher utilities being derived with the standard gamble relative to other techniques.

The time-tradeoff method collapses considerations of quantity of life directly into the measure of health-related quality of life. It thereby directly measures the number of healthy years that are equivalent to a given time in a particular health state. Because this means that the two measurements from which a QALY is formed (effectiveness, and value for a particular health state) are done in the same metric, some authors believe that time tradeoff has a theoretical advantage when compared with other methods of preference elicitation (Nord, 1992b; Richardson, 1994). It has recently been noted that the time-tradeoff question confounds preferences for the health states themselves with time preference; this is because the years of life that are "sacrificed" in the time tradeoff come at the end of the life span and, therefore, may be valued less because they are farther in the future. As a result, time tradeoff values that fail to adjust for time preferences may be biased upward. A method of correcting for time preference in the analysis of time-tradeoff data has recently been suggested (Johannesson et al., 1994).

Time tradeoff and standard gamble have been used in collecting weights for a number of component health states in versions of the HUI. Time tradeoff is currently being used in collecting weights for the EuroQol (Williams, 1995a,b).

Psychophysical approaches

Methods derived from the psychophysical tradition include the *paired-comparison* approach, *rating scale* methods (including *category scaling* and *visual analogue scales*), and *magnitude estimation*. They are discussed below with reference to issues of validity, reliability, feasibility, and scaling properties.

In the *paired-comparison* approach, respondents' preferences for pairs of health states are elicited. Neither health state is rated separately; rather, an ordinal judgment of the comparative desirability of the two states is made. Originally developed as a measurement method by Thurstone (1927), paired comparisons have been utilized in several different versions to assess values for health states. Fanshel and Bush (1970) used paired-comparison techniques to calculate weights for 11 health states. Paired comparisons are held by some to possess properties of face validity, in that people are accustomed to making choices between one of two options. Hadorn and coauthors (1995) report good discriminant and convergent validity in the Quality of Life and Health Questionnaire (QLHQ), a paired-comparison technique. No across-method difference in the 1-week test–retest reliability coefficients was observed for a direct rating technique and a paired comparison approach (Hadorn et al., 1992).

People's comprehension of the task involved in paired comparisons is likely to be good given the familiarity of the method for assessing preferences. When asked how one feels about something, it is natural to ask, Compared to what? The feasibility of the method is constrained, however, by the relatively small number of health states that can be rated using paired comparisons due to the factorial nature of the approach. For example, a set of 10 health states would require a total of 45 paired comparisons in order to cover each possible pair; 100 health states would require 4,950 comparisons. Health-state measures containing several hundred health states, such as the HUI, could not use this method for purposes of preference determination; it is necessarily limited to relatively sparse health-state taxonomies.

In performing a paired comparison task, respondents indicate which of two states is more desirable. These ordinal-level judgments, where health states are rank-ordered but where there is no information provided about how far apart the states are on a continuum, are converted to estimates of interval-level scores through Thurstone's Law of Comparative Judgment, which holds that stimulus differences which are detected equally often are subjectively equal. The QLHQ was developed using a modification of the paired-comparisons procedure that required subjects to indicate the strength of preference of one health state over another using a rating scale presumed to have interval-level properties. A scaling constraint of the original ordinal paired-comparisons procedure is that if there are two adjacent states, A and B, in the preference order such that all subjects always prefer state B to state A, then the scale value for one of these must be assigned arbitrarily since the gap between them is theoretically "infinite." This problem may be particularly encountered with the health states that anchor the health continuum (death and perfect health). The modification of the method for the QLHQ circumvents this scaling problem by assuming that the direct rating of strength of preference has interval-scale properties.

Direct rating methods, including *category rating* and *visual analogue scales*, require judges to assign each health state to one number, usually on a scale from 0 (least desirable or death) to 100 (most desirable or perfect health). Visual aids such as a "feeling thermometer" are used to support this task. Judges are instructed to place health states along the scale according to their relative desirability, typically with the additional instruction that the spacing between each point in the scale should be regarded as equivalent. The preference value for each of the states is simply the value associated with its placement on the scale. States worse than death can be accommodated.

Direct rating methods are referred to as *category rating* when the scale is divided into discrete points, one of which must be chosen (e.g., 0.1, 0.2, 0.3, etc.); they are known as *visual analogue scales* when the scale contains no internal markings and raters are required to place a mark at some point between the two anchor states. Category scaling is considered to be limited by its use of a fixed number of categories in the scaling task; people are held to be capable of making much more accurate judgments of the relative magnitude of stimuli than category scales permit (McDowell and Newell,

1987). *Magnitude estimation*, a related technique, allows judges to compare each state to a selected standard and to report how much "better" or "worse" each state is using unbounded numbers or ratio values. Magnitude estimation assumes that respondents can assess their experience and assign numerical values with interval or ratio meaning. Differences among judges are assumed to be due to random error, and individual estimates are averaged to obtain preference weights (Patrick and Erickson, 1993).

Intrarater reliability of rating scale techniques has ranged from 0.70 to 0.94 with comparable ranges for magnitude estimation (Froberg and Kane, 1989b). Correlation of test–retest reliability at 1 week using a rating scale approach has been reported as 0.77 (O'Connor et al., 1987); at 1 year, another study reported a correlation of 0.49, comparing unfavorably with test–retest reliability of the time-tradeoff technique (Torrance, 1976).

Rating scale methods are highly familiar to most people from a variety of everyday experiences in which they are asked to provide information on an array of experiences (e.g., sporting events, movies, levels of pain) using this technique. It is widely agreed that the cognitive burden of respondents is less than with other techniques. However, empirical work has shown that people have difficulty directly assigning a number to feelings about health states (Patrick et al., 1994). In addition, some investigators have found that individuals are unable to provide an explanation of the relationship of their responses on a rating scale to the concepts of welfare or utility that would be the foundation of decisions about resource allocation (Richardson, 1994).

Rating scales are held to produce interval-level values when respondents are instructed to place the health states on the line such that the intervals between their placement reflect the differences they perceive between the health states. Concerns regarding scaling characteristics of the visual analogue and category rating scales have been raised by the observation that difficulty in making absolute judgments results in the avoidance of the extreme categories of a scale, resulting in a clustering of values that acts to reduce the range of possible responses (Streiner and Norman, 1989). Other empirical work suggests that rating scales provide valid and reliable results when the response continuum is made explicit to subjects (Kaplan and Ernst, 1983).

The QWB uses a rating scale measurement system in estimating preferences.

Choice of Methods

Although methods for assigning weights to health outcomes may meet criteria appropriate to the particular measurement paradigm being used, they often do not yield comparable scores when applied to specific health states or illnesses. A number of investigators have reported discrepant weights for like conditions when different measurement techniques are used (Read et al., 1984; Nord, 1992b; Fryback et al., 1993; Hornberger et al., 1992; Nease et al., 1995). Variations in measured scores across instruments can occur for reasons which include: the sensitivity (or lack thereof) of a measurement strategy to specific domains of health that are affected by an illness; cognitive difficulties the measure presents to the population that is being assessed; the degree to which preferences for health states are affected by risk-taking implicit in the measurement strategy; and the scaling properties particular to the technique used.

Whether there is a "correct" method for assigning numerical scores to health states depends in the first instance on whether there are theoretical reasons for adopting a particular approach. The measurement of health-state preferences for CEA is best accomplished using theory-driven methods that conform to well-articulated methodological standards. The approaches of utility measurement from expected utility theory and the measurement of values arising from psychometrics each represent rigorous systems for assigning weights to health states. All of the techniques described above have been deemed feasible by some investigators for both general and patient populations. However, the methods of category scaling, including rating and visual analogue scales, appear simpler to administer than the tasks of standard gamble, time-tradeoff, and paired comparisons. On the other hand, utilities derived using the standard gamble and time-tradeoff methods are more closely tied by the elicitation technique to the theoretical foundation on which CEA is based. (See Chapter 2.)

In principle, all the described methods have the ability to furnish interval-level data. Direct scaling models such as the standard gamble and the time-tradeoff method assume that judges directly generate an interval or ratio scale. Indirect models require judges to provide information that is ordinal level; the investigator must than apply a set of assumptions that allow the preference scores to be converted to interval level. The methodologic question of which methods produce true interval-level data is an important one from the perspective of the mathematical operationalization of CEA, and further empirical inquiry regarding which methods come closest to embodying this feature will be useful. It bears noting, however, that rating scales, time tradeoff, and standard gamble have not produced scores that are linearly related, (Torrance, 1976; Torrance et al., 1982, 1992). This suggests that each cannot be an alternative transformation of the same underlying interval scale. This conclusion again begs the question, Which is the "correct" scale? Unfortunately, the empirical observations do not settle this issue, either.

The choice of preference measurement method should be based on the decision or problem to be solved, the practical considerations involved in the study, and the use to which data will be put. Methods that involve uncertainty and risk may be suited to clinical applications, where patients are providing information regarding their preferences for health states that they are experiencing, or may be at risk for, due to their condition or therapy. However, it is not clearly the case that incorporation of risk attitudes into the utilities that represent the "quality" dimension of QALYs (where, as noted in Chapter 2, risk neutrality is required in the life years dimension) is necessary for CEA studies designed to inform resource allocation decisions.

Regardless of the valuation method selected, there is wide disagreement about how richly specified generic health states should be. Again, the setting in which it will be used is highly relevant. Rich or complex descriptions, such as those used in the HUI or QWB, are better able to capture the texture of health outcomes and may provide more specific information from which to assign patients in clinical settings to particular health states. Here, the preference scores can be gathered indirectly by using a health status classification system that comes complete with a preference scoring system. Often the questions are asked on a self-administered interactive computer program which can significantly decrease both respondent and investigator burden.

The time involved in primary collection of preference weights for highly detailed health states might be prohibitive, however, in a CEA that sought to directly assess community preferences within the body of the study. Strategies for gathering community weights can be simplified by measuring preferences using less-time-consuming techniques. These may include direct assignment of preference weights to health scenarios or administration of instruments with fewer domains such as the YHL, the QLHQ, or the EuroQol.

The unsettled nature of the field of preference measurement requires that analysts be sensitive to how their choice of measure will influence study results. Most analyses will not be able to include multiple methods for measuring and valuing outcomes (for purposes of sensitivity analyses), but a great deal more information than is currently available is necessary to understand how, and under what circumstances, the different methods relate to one another. Further research will need to link simpler methods to the more laboratory-derived measurement systems in order to better explore the interval-level qualities of the different approaches. Methods for converting values or riskless measures to risk-based or utility measures also require exploration.

Toward Consistency Across Studies: A National Catalogue of Weights

A number of methods are currently used to collect preference weights for use in CEAs. In some instances investigators have assigned weights to conditions based on the opinion of expert panels (e.g., Stason and Weinstein, 1977; Mandelblatt and Fahs, 1988), while in other instances, weights are collected directly from the patients on whom the CEA is being conducted (Oldridge et al., 1993). In still other studies, weights have been collected from a cross section of the community using one of a number of standardized measurement instruments (Torrance et al., 1982; Boyle et al., 1983; Kaplan et al., 1978). This diversity in how preference weights are gathered markedly constrains the ability to credibly compare analyses where the effectiveness measure is presented in QALYs.

Consider the example of two studies that looked at the cost-effectiveness of screening mammography for breast cancer. Hall et al. (1992) investigated the influence of quality-adjustment on cost-effectiveness ratios for mammography screening using time tradeoff to obtain preference weights for breast cancer. The C/E ratio in this study more than doubled ($7,190 per life year saved versus $16,355 per healthy-years equivalents) for treatment of breast cancer when life years were quality-adjusted by applying the time-tradeoff method to disease-specific states. DeKoning et al. (1991) also looked at the impact of quality adjustment on cost-effectiveness ratios for mammography screening by using a visual analogue scale. In this study, quality adjustment increased the ratio by 5.6% (from $3,825 per life year gained to $4,050 per quality-adjusted life year gained), suggesting that preferences for breast-cancer-related quality of health varied minimally from those for life without breast cancer.

As we have described, differences in approach to measuring and valuing outcomes stem from issues of expediency as well as from disagreements about which is the best measurement strategy. Development and testing of particular measures in order to clarify strengths and weaknesses with respect to theoretical limitations, reliability, validity, responsiveness, performance in different sociodemographic groups, and clinical practicality are ongoing in this technically challenging field.

Our contention has been that a cost-effectiveness analysis should capture all important outcomes of an intervention; not simply the effectiveness of a therapy or program in extending life, but also its ability to improve or maintain the quality of life. However, the lack of a standard measure with which to value outcomes has created significant problems for standardization of CEA across conditions and illnesses.

The differing requirements with respect to source of preferences for a given study suggest the need for an instrument that can be useful in a clinical setting where the preferences of individuals with particular illnesses can be queried—and which can also capture information about community-based preferences for specified health states. In addition, many investigators have limited resources and are unable to collect primary data. A measurement scheme that furnished "off the shelf" weights for health states and illnesses would provide a ready vehicle to aid standardization of analyses.

The ability of CEAs to compare treatments for disparate conditions in a common language would be well served by availability of a standard catalogue of weights that could be used in any CEA without the requirement for collection of primary data. A catalogue of weights would consist of a set of well-described health states, with accompanying scores for each state. Mapping these health states to average weights associated with particular illnesses and/or conditions, as reported for the Beaver Dam population (Fryback et al., 1993), would allow users of secondary data sources with access to information about disease status but not about health states to assign values to particular conditions (Wong et al., 1993). This catalogue could serve as a link across studies that are designed to inform resource allocation.

In conformance with the recommendations in this chapter, and for reasons of practicality, the ideal system for use in a Reference Case analysis should meet the criteria of: (1) derivation from a theory-based method on which empirical data have been collected; (2) availability of weights from a representative, community-based sample of the U.S. population; (3) low burden of administration in clinical and population-based settings; and (4) ability to furnish weights for health states, as well as for illnesses and conditions.

None of the systems presented in Appendix 4.1 meets all of these criteria. In addition, the field of measurement and valuation of outcomes is still a developing one, and premature closure on designating a single system as appropriate for all analyses would be unsatisfactory. However, there may be some use in adapting a strategy where one of the instruments becomes the de facto ''placeholder'' and is used in a sensitivity analysis in all studies that are intended for use in informing resource allocation decisions.

One measurement strategy that may hold promise for placeholding is the instrument developed by the National Center for Health Statistics (as described in Appendix 4.1) in order to track the nation's health status. The Years of Healthy Life (YHL) measure, covering the domains of health perceptions and role function, has been mapped to information collected in the National Health Interview Survey on chronic conditions. Investigators using the YHL have access to weights for health states as well as those associated with particular conditions. The range of scores associated with different conditions can be used in order to model possible gains or decrements associated with improvements in particular conditions. Because the information has been collected on a representative sample of U.S. citizens, adjustments for sociodemographic characteristics are also possible. While the weights for the 30-cell matrix have not been measured directly as yet (failing, therefore, the first criterion listed above), condition scores have shown correlations ranging from 0.77 to 0.83 when compared, respectively, with the QWB and a version of the HUI constructed from the National Health and Nutrition Examination Survey (Gold et al., 1994, 1996.)

Although the use of a placeholder might provide comfort to CEA ''consumers'' with respect to comparability of studies, it is important to note the limitations of such an approach. Each of the measurement systems described in Appendix 4.1 build their health states from differing domains. A system that provides inadequate or absent information regarding a domain that is important to the condition under investigation will be unable to provide sensitive information about changes in that condition; it will not be a valid measure of effect. Comparing that condition to another where change is readily captured on the placeholder system will give misleading information regarding the gains possible from interventions for the different conditions.

On balance, however, the multiplicity of systems currently in use is a significant impediment to comparability of CEAs. While ongoing research may better allow us to understand the relationships of the different measures, thereby permitting appropriate adjustments between analyses that use different valuation techniques, the field is not yet there. With the understanding that there is no consensus on a single measure that will serve all studies equally well, use of the same measurement system in all CEAs

intended to inform resource allocation decisions would be helpful to the ongoing development of the field. Used alongside the measurement strategy selected by an investigator as best suited to a particular analysis, a standard measurement strategy in all
analyses would allow better understanding of the source and magnitude of variation
that stem from different elicitation and scaling techniques.

Recommendations

   1. For a Reference Case analysis, incorporation of morbidity and mortality consequences into a single measure should be accomplished using QALYs.
   2. In general, since lives saved or extended by an intervention will not be in
perfect health, a saved life year will count as less than 1 full QALY.
   3. To satisfy the QALY concept, the quality weights must be preference-based,
interval-scaled, and measured or transformed onto an interval scale where the reference point ''death'' has a score of 0.0 and the reference point ''optimal health''
has a scale of 1.0.
   4. Community preferences for health states are the most appropriate ones for use
in a Reference Case analysis.
   5. When community preferences are used and the program (treatment or prevention) is related to an illness or condition, a sensitivity analysis that furnishes information on the preferences of persons with the condition will provide important ancillary information.
   6. If distinct subgroup preferences are identified that will markedly affect a C/E
ratio, a Reference Case analysis should provide this information and conduct separate
sensitivity analyses that reflect this difference.
   7. The health-related quality of life of those whose lives have been saved or
extended by a health intervention may be influenced by characteristics such as the
age, gender, race, or socioeconomic status of the population involved. This may
affect a Reference Case analysis in ways that are ethically problematic. In these
instances, we recommend that sensitivity analysis be conducted to indicate explicitly
how the analysis is affected by these characteristics.
   8. A CEA should be based on a health-state classification scheme which reflects
domains (attributes) that are important for the particular problem under consideration. If the CEA is intended for use in a Reference Case, the preference measure
used should be a generic one or be capable of being compared to a generic system.
   9. In a Reference Case analysis, health-related quality of life should be captured
by an instrument that, at minimum, implicitly incorporates the effects of morbidity
on productivity and leisure.
   10. Financial consequences related to changes in health status, including the full
value of morbidity time to patients, should be reflected in the denominator of a C/E
ratio through preference weights. Time effects and financial consequences unrelated
to health status should be captured in the numerator.

Research Recommendations

1. Weights should be collected from a representative sample of the U.S. population for preference-based instruments that are candidates for use in a Reference Case analysis.

2. Priority should be assigned to supporting research that assesses the performance of different measurement strategies in relationship to other measures, and with respect to populations with differing social and demographic characteristics.

3. Research is needed on the relationship of community preferences to patient preferences for different health states and conditions.

4. To further the application of cost-effectiveness analysis, comparison of preference results obtained from techniques employing simpler methods (i.e., rating scales and paired comparisons) should be compared to results obtained using the more traditional methods of time tradeoff and standard gamble. Results from self-administered interactive computer approaches should be compared to more traditional interview techniques.

5. A consistent set of community weights for health conditions and health states, used across studies intended to inform resource allocation, would significantly improve the comparability of analyses.

Appendix 4.1:
Generic Preference-Based Measures
for Use in CEA

A number of generic preference-weighted health state classification systems exist that may be used in cost-effectiveness analyses. To help potential users of these systems identify which outcomes are included in these measurement systems, the principal concepts and domains of HRQL contained in these measures are shown in Table 4.3. Narrative accounts of these measures follow; more extensive accounts of these systems are provided in the literature referenced.

Disability/Distress Index

Rosser and colleagues in England (Rosser and Watts, 1972; Rosser and Kind, 1978; Rosser, 1983, 1990) developed an operational definition of health status, originally in an attempt to measure the performance of hospitals. The researchers asked a group of physicians to describe various illnesses. Next the physicians were asked to describe the criteria they used to decide on the severity of a patient's illness, considering only the present state of the patient. Two principal components of severity emerged from these discussions: observed disability (loss of function and mobility) and subjective distress. All other conditions were included within this framework. This classification consists of eight classes of disability and four classes of distress totaling 32 possible cells. One state is the absence of disability and distress. This state is not necessarily equated with perfect health. It distinguishes between the observable state of the patient's disability and his or her subjective feelings of distress. Scores were developed for the 32 cells on a scale where death was 0.0 and no disability and no distress was 1.0. Ratio scaling was used as the measurement approach. In the original scoring a sample of 70 individuals, consisting of both patients and health providers, were used as judges. The original disability/distress states were redefined later as 176 combinations of disability, discomfort, and distress.

EuroQol Instrument

The EuroQol Group, a consortium of investigators in Western Europe, conducted postal surveys in England, the Netherlands, and Sweden using 14 different health states classified using a system with six domains: mobility, self-care, main activity, social relationships, pain, and mood (EuroQol Group, 1990; Brooks et al., 1991; Nord, 1991). The resultant descriptive system defines a theoretical universe of 216 states. The classification system was developed through review of existing classification systems. The descriptive system was also tested against the results of a survey of lay concepts conducted in England (Williams, 1995a).

Recently, the EuroQol has been revised to contain five domains—mobility, self-care, usual activity, pain/discomfort, anxiety/depression—and three levels on each domain— no problem, some problem, major problem (Essink-Bot et al., 1993). The revised system generates a theoretical universe of 243 states, to which have been added (for completeness) "unconscious" and "dead," making 245 in all. The preferences for the health states in the EuroQol system are usually measured using a self-administered visual analogue scale, often by mail, although time-tradeoff measurements have recently been undertaken. These were elicited by household interview from a representative sample of 3,000 members of the adult population of the United Kingdom, using 45 different health states carefully chosen to facilitate the interpolation of values for all 245 states. This work is described in Discussion Paper 136 (Williams, 1995a) and includes the resulting scoring system. Further details are expected to be published during 1996.

15D-Measure of Health-Related Quality of Life

Sintonen and colleagues in Finland have developed a generic 15-dimensional, standardized, self-administered measure of health-related quality of life that can be used as a profile and single index measure (Sintonen, 1981a,b, 1994, 1995; Sintonen and Pekurinen, 1993). Within the two versions of the profile measure, the 15D.1 and 15D.2, the 15 dimensions represent nine basic physiological functions and several aspects of social and psychological function and symptoms. The earlier 15D.1 has four or five levels for each dimension and the 15D.2 five levels for each. As a profile measure the 15D has demonstrated acceptability, reliability, and evidence of content and construct validity (Sintonen, 1994). Preferences for the health states (all five levels plus states described as "being unconscious" and "being dead" on each of the 15 dimensions) have been measured by postal survey of several random samples of the Finnish population using magnitude estimation and direct rating methods. Results of these surveys have demonstrated feasibility, reliability, and convergent evidence of construct validity (Sintonen, 1995). The 15D is being used in evaluation projects in Finland and in several other countries (Sintonen and Pekurinen, 1993).

Health Utilities Index (HUI)

Torrance and colleagues at McMaster University have developed three multi-attribute health status classification systems; HUI:1, HUI:2, and HUI:3. Each system consists of a classification taxonomy and one or more scoring formulae. In all cases the scores are preference-based, interval-scaled, and on the conventional dead–healthy scale where reference-state death has a score of 0.0 and reference-state full health has a score of 1.0. Scores are derived from the preferences of members of the general public. The systems were developed over time, each building in part on the previous one. The systems are designed for use in clinical studies, in program planning and resource allocation (cost-effectiveness studies), and in the measurement and reporting of population health.

HUI:1 was based in part on the QWB system and contains four domains: (1) physical function: mobility and physical activity, (2) role function: self-care and role activity, (3) social-emotional function: emotional well-being and social activity, and (4) health problem. Preference scoring was determined using the visual analogue scale and the time-tradeoff methods. The HUI:1 classification was originally developed for the economic evaluation of neonatal intensive care (Torrance et al., 1982; Boyle et al., 1983) and later modified slightly for use in the general population (Drummond et al., 1987).

The HUI:2 classification system was based on fundamental research to determine the attributes of health status that are considered important by the general public (Cadman et al., 1986). The system was first applied in childhood cancer (Feeny et al., 1992) and has subsequently been slightly modified for general use. The general version contains six attributes—sensation, mobility, emotion, cognition, self-care, and pain—with four to five levels per attribute and with a preference-based, interval-scaled scoring formula. Preference scoring was determined using the visual analogue scale and the standard gamble methods. Accordingly, two scoring formulae are available: a value formula based on the visual analogue results, and a utility formula based on the standard gamble data (Torrance et al., 1992).

The HUI:3 classification system was developed for general use from the start. It is largely based on the Mark II system, and contains eight attributes—vision, hearing, speech, ambulation, dexterity, emotion, cognition, and pain—with five to six levels per attribute. A preference scoring formula based on a random sample of 503 members of the general public is currently under development for the HUI:3 system. The preference measurements for the scoring formulae for the HUI:3 have been taken using the visual analogue scale and the standard gamble instruments, and like the HUI:2, two scoring formulae will be developed. Questionnaires are available in three formats (face-to-face interview, telephone interview, and self-administration) and in two languages (English and French-Canadian) to gather the health status information necessary to classify an individual into either or both the HUI:2 and the HUI:3. The HUI systems are being widely used in clinical studies, cost-effectiveness studies, and, in Canada, in population health surveys (Feeny et al., 1995; Torrance et al., 1995b).

The Quality of Life and Health Questionnaire (QLHQ)

The QLHQ measure (Hadorn and Uebersax, 1995) was designed for use in large-scale observational studies and as a common currency with which to intertranslate more-complex instruments. The QLHQ uses a "graded" paired-comparison technique in preference elicitation (Hadorn et al., 1992). The strength of preference is indicated on an interval-level scale, permitting more straightforward calculation of interval-level scale values from paired comparison data. The QLHQ consists of four questions—one each covering the areas of physical suffering, limits on activities, and outlook on life, and on overall quality of life. The first three questions contain four response levels (corresponding to no, mild, moderate, and severe problems in these areas); the fourth question is answered on a 0–10 rating scale. This configuration of questions was selected based on the results of two pilot studies (Hadorn and Hays, 1991; Hadorn, et al., 1992).

The 16 health states formed by crossing the four levels of physical suffering with the four levels of limits on activities were each rated by 599 subjects of widely diverse backgrounds using direct scaling and paired-comparison methods. No preference subgroups based on demographic or clinical characteristics have been identified.

The values derived from this exercise were used to calibrate the QLHQ for purposes of testing the instrument in a cohort of 400 patients with advanced cancer (Hadorn et al., 1995). Using a multitrait-multimethod validation technique, the investigators demonstrated excellent discriminant and convergent validity for the four basic parameters contained in the QLHQ. The weighted generic health states closely paralleled patients' reports concerning outlook on life and overall HRQL, providing further validation for the generic 16-state framework.

Quality of Well-Being Scale/General Health Policy Model (QWB)

The Quality of Well-Being Scale (Kaplan and Anderson, 1988) classifies patients according to symptoms and distinct levels of functioning. The levels are represented by scales of mobility, physical activity, and social activity. Individuals are also classified by the one symptom or problem that they find to be most undesirable. Symptoms or problems may be severe, such as serious chest pain, or minor, such as taking medication for health reasons. Observable states of health and functioning have been placed onto a 0.0 (death) to 1.0 (full health) scale of preferences using category scaling measurements on a random sample of the general public. The QWB has been used in a wide variety of population studies (Erickson et al., 1989; Anderson et al., 1989). In addition the QWB scale has been used in clinical trials and studies to evaluate therapeutic interventions for a number of medical and surgical conditions (Kaplan, 1993). Specific validity and reliability data are available in each disease area. Further, the QWB was able to track improvements over time in a 2-week intervention for treatment of pulmonary exacerbation with changes in QWB statistically significantly correlated with changes in pulmonary function (Orenstein et al., 1989, 1990).

Years of Healthy Life Measure (YHL)

The National Center for Health Statistics (NCHS), charged with tracking the nation's disease prevention and health objectives for the year 2000, has developed a method for measuring "years of healthy life" using data from the National Health Interview Survey (NHIS), a continuing nationwide survey of households that is conducted annually. The measure of health-related quality of life is built from questions inquiring into the domains of self-perceived health and role function. Role limitation is defined in terms of limitation of major activity as appropriate for a person's age. Six levels are available for assignment. Self-reported health is reported at five levels, ranging from excellent to poor. Both attributes are weighted equally in a multiplicative model developed by Torrance et al. (1995a).

A matrix of 30 health states is defined by perceived health and role limitation. Scores have been assigned by assuming the highest level of function to be 1.0 (not limited, excellent health) and the lowest to be 0.0 (dead). Correspondence analysis was used to quantify the distance between different levels of each of the two health dimensions. The value of the most dysfunctional health state, save death, is assigned a value of 0.1. For purposes of solving the equation for a multiplicative model, one cell (limited role function, excellent health) was mapped to the Health Utility Index Mark I (Drummond et al., 1987). Direct valuation of health states has not yet been accomplished, but the scores have been shown to exhibit convergent validity with other measures (Erickson et al., 1995).

References

Anderson, J.P., R.M. Kaplan, and M. DeBon. 1989. Comparison of responses to similar questions in health surveys. In *Health survey research methods*, ed. F. Fowler, 13–21. Washington, DC: National Center for Health Statistics.

Anderson, N.H. 1979. Algebraic rules in psychological measurement. *American Scientist* 67:555–63.

Balaban, D.J., P.C. Sagi, N.I. Goldfarb, and S. Nettler. 1986. Weights for scoring the quality of well-being instrument among rheumatoid arthritics: A comparison to the general population weights. *Med Care* 24:973–80.

Barry, M.J., A.G. Mulley, J.F. Fowler, and J.W. Wennberg. 1988. Watchful waiting vs. immediate transuretheral resection for symptomatic prostatism: The importance of patients' preferences. *JAMA* 259:3010–17.

Ben-Zion, U., and A. Gafni. 1983. Evaluation of public investment in health care: Is risk irrelevant? *J Health Economics* 2:161–165.

Bergner, M., R.A. Bobbitt, W.B. Carter, and B.S. Gilson. 1981. The sickness impact profile: Development and final revision of a health status measure. *Med Care* 19:787–805.

Boyle, M.H., and G.W. Torrance. 1984. Developing multiattribute health indexes. *Med Care* 22:1045–57.

Boyle, M.H., G. W. Torrance, J.C. Sinclair, and S.P. Horwood. 1983. Economic evaluation of neonatal intensive care of very-low-birth-weight infants. *N Engl J Med* 308:1330–37.

Brooks, R.G., S. Jedteg, B. Lindgren, U. Persson, and S. Bjork. 1991. EuroQol: Health-related quality of life measurement. Results of the Swedish questionnaire exercise. *Health Policy* 18:37–48.

Broome, J. 1993. QALYs. *J Pub Econ* 50:149–67.

Buckingham, K. 1993. A note on HYE (healthy years equivalent). *J Health Economics* 11:301–9.

Cadman, D., C. Goldsmith, G.W. Torrance, Boyle, M., and W. Furlong. 1986. *Development of a health status index for Ontario children*. Final report to the Ontario Ministry of Health on research grant DM648 (00633). Hamilton, Ontario: McMaster University.

Carr-Hill, R.A. 1989. Assumptions of the QALY procedure. *Soc Sci Med* 29:469–477.

Christensen-Szalanski, J.J.J. 1984. Discount functions and the measurement of patients' values: Women's decisions during childbirth. *Med Decis Making* 4:47–58.

Cox, D.R., R. Fitzpatrick, A.E. Fletcher, S.M. Gore, D.J. Spiegelhalter, and D.R. Jones. 1992. Quality-of-life assessment: Can we keep it simple? *J R Statist Soc A* 155: 353–93.

Culyer, A.J., and A. Wagstaff. 1993. QALYs versus HYEs. *J Health Economics* 11:311–23.

Dasbach, E., D.G. Fryback, P.A. Newcomb, R. Klein, and B.E.K. Klein. 1991. Cost effectiveness of strategies for detecting diabetic retinopathy. *Med Care* 29:20–39.

De Koning, H.J., B. M. van Ineveld, G.J. van Oortmarssen, J.C. de Haes, A.J. Collette, J.H. Hendriks, and P.J. van der Maas. 1991. Breast cancer screening and cost-effectiveness: Policy alternatives, quality of life considerations and the possible impact of uncertain factors. *Int J Cancer* 49:531–37.

Donaldson, C., A. Atkinson, J. Bond, and K. Wright. 1988. Should QALYs be programme-specific? *J Health Economics* 7:239–57.

Drummond, M.F., G.L. Stoddart, and G.W. Torrance. 1987. *Methods for the economic evaluation of health care programmes*. New York: Oxford University Press, 1987.

Eddy, D.M. 1991. Screening for cervical cancer. In *Common screening tests*, 255–85. Philadelphia: American College of Physicians.

Eddy, D.M. 1989. Screening for breast cancer. *Ann Intern Med* 111:389–99.

Edelson, J.T., M.C. Weinstein, A.N.A. Tosteson, L. Williams, T.H. Lee, and L. Goldman. 1990. Long-term cost-effectiveness of various initial monotherapies for mild to moderate hypertension. *JAMA* 263:407–413.

Epstein, A.M., J.A. Hall, J. Tognetti, L.H. Son, and L. Conant. 1989. Using proxies to evaluate quality of life. *Med Care* 27:S91–98.

Erickson, P., E.A. Kendall, J.P. Anderson, and R.M. Kaplan. 1989. Using composite health status measures to assess the nation's health. *Med Care* 27(suppl 3):S66–S76.

Erickson, P., R.W. Wilson, and I. Shannon. 1995. *Years of healthy life*. Statistical Note No. 7. Hyattsville, MD: National Center for Health Statistics.

Essink-Bot, M.L., M.E. Stouthard, and G.J. Bonsel. 1993. Generalizability of valuations on health states collected with the EuroQol questionnaire. *Health Econ* 2:237–46.

EuroQol Group. 1990. EuroQol: A new facility for the measurement of health- related quality of life. *Health Policy* 16:199.

Fahs, M., J. Mandelblatt, C. Schecter, and C. Muller. 1992. Cost effectiveness of cervical cancer screening for the elderly. *Ann Intern Med* 117:520–27.

Fanshel, S., and J.W. Bush. 1970. A health-status index and its application to health-services outcomes. *Oper Res* 18:1021–66.

Feeny, D.H., W. Furlong, R.D. Barr, G.W. Torrance, P. Rosenbaum, and S. Weitzman. 1992. A comprehensive multi-attribute system for classifying the health status of survivors of childhood cancer. *J Clin Oncol* 10:923–28.

Feeny, D., W. Furlong, M. Boyle, and G.W. Torrance. 1995. Multi-attribute health status classification systems: Health utilities index. *PharmacoEconomics* 7:490–502.

Froberg, D.G., and R.L. Kane. 1989a. Methodology for measuring health-state preferences. I. Measurement strategies. *J Clin Epidemiol* 42:345–54.

Froberg, D.G., and R.L. Kane. 1989b. Methodology for measuring health-state preferences. II. Scaling Methods. *J Clin Epidemiol* 42:459–71.

Froberg, D.G., and R.L. Kane. 1989c. Methodology for measuring health-state preferences. III. Population and context effects. *J Clin Epidemiol* 42:585–92.

Fryback, D.G. 1993. QALYs, HYEs, and the loss of innocence (editorial). *Med Decis Making* 13:271–72.

Fryback, D.G., E.J. Dasbach, R. Klein, B.E.K. Klein, K. Peterson, and P.A. Martin 1993. The Beaver Dam health outcomes study: Initial catalog of health-state quality factors. *Med Decis Making* 13:89–102.

Gafni, A., and S. Birch. 1995. Preferences for outcomes in economic evaluation: An economic approach to addressing economic problems. *Soc Sci Med* 40:767–76.

Gafni, A., and S. Birch. 1993. Economics, health and health economics: HYEs versus QALYs. *J Health Economics* 11:325–39.

Gold, M.R., P. Franks, and K. McCoy. 1994. Condition weights for chronic diseases from a nationally representative sample. *Med Decis Making* 14:431. (Abstract).

Gold, M.R., P. Franks, and P.A. Erickson. 1996. Assessing the health of the nation: The predictive validity of a preference-based measure and self-rated health. *Med Care* 34:163–77.

Goldman, L., M.C. Weinstein, P.A. Goldman, and L.W. Williams. 1991. Cost-effectiveness of HMG-CoA reductase inhibition for primary and secondary prevention of coronary heart disease. *JAMA* 265:1145–51.

Gottlieb, L.K., B. Schwartz, and S.G. Pauker. 1983. Glaucoma screening: A cost-effectiveness analysis. *Surv Ophthalmol* 28:206–26.

Hadorn, D.C. 1991. The role of public values in setting health care priorities. *Soc Sci Med* 32:773–82.

Hadorn, D.C., and R.D. Hays. 1991. Multitrait-multimethod analysis of health related quality of life measures. *Med Care* 29:829–40.

Hadorn, D.C., R.D. Hays, and T. Hauber. 1992. Improving task comprehension in the measurement of health state preferences. *J Clin Epidemiol* 45:233–43.

Hadorn, D.C., J. Sorenson, and J. Holte. 1995. Large-scale outcome evaluation: How should quality of life be measured? II. Questionnaire validation in a cohort of patients with advanced cancer. *J Clin Epidemiol* 48:619–29.

Hadorn, D.C., and J. Uebersax. 1995. Large-scale outcome evaluation: How should quality of life be measured? I. Calibration of a brief questionnaire and a search for preference subgroups. *J Clin Epidemiol* 48:607–618.

Hall, J., K. Gerard, G. Salkeld, and J. Richardson. 1992. A cost utility analysis of mammography screening in Australia. *Soc Sci Med* 34:993–1004.

Harris, J. 1987. QALYfying the value of life. *J Med Ethics* 13:117–23.

Hatziandreu, E.I., J.P. Koplan, M.C. Weinstein, C.J. Caspersen, and K.E. Warner. 1988. A cost-effectiveness analysis of exercise as a health promotion activity. *Am J Public Health* 78:1417–21.

Hinman, A.R., and J.P. Koplan. 1984. Pertussis and pertussis vaccine: Reanalysis of benefits, risks, and costs. *JAMA* 251:3109–13.

Hornberger, J.C., D.A. Redelmeier, and J. Petersen. 1992. Variability among methods to assess patients' well-being aned consequent effect on a cost-effectiveness analysis. *J Clin Epidemiol* 5:505–12.

Hutchinson, B.G., and G.L. Stoddart. 1988. Cost-effectiveness of primary tetanus vaccination among elderly Canadians. *Can Med Assoc J* 139:1143–51.

Johannesson, M., J.S. Pliskin, and M.C. Weinstein. 1993. Are health-years equivalents an improvement over quality-adjusted life years? *Med Decis Making* 13:281–86.

Johannesson M., J.S. Pliskin, and M.C. Weinstein. 1994. A note on QALYs, time tradeoff, and discounting. *Med Decis Making* 14:188–193.

Kahneman, D., and A. Tversky. 1983. Choices, values, and frames. *Am Psychol* 39:341–50.

Kaplan, R.M. 1993. *Hippocratic predicament: Affordability, access, and accountability in health care.* San Diego: Academic Press.

Kaplan, R.M., and J.P. Anderson. 1988. A general health policy model: Update and applications. *Health Serv Res* Jun 23:203–35.

Kaplan, R.M., J.W. Bush, and C.C. Berry. 1978. The reliability, stability, and generalizability of a health status index. Proceedings, Social Status Section, 704–9. American Statistical Association.

Kaplan, R.M., and J.A. Ernst. 1983. Do category rating scales produce biased preference weights for a health index? *Med Care* 21:193–207.

Koplan, J.P., S.C. Schoenbaum, M.C. Weinstein, and D.W. Fraser. 1979. Pertussis vaccine—an analysis of benefits, risks, and costs. *N Engl J Med* 301:906–11.

Littrup, P.J., A.C. Goodman, C.J. Mettlin. 1993. The benefits and cost of prostate cancer early detection. *CA Cancer J Clin* 43:134–49.

Llewellyn-Thomas, H.A., J.H. Sutherland, and E.C. Thiel. 1993. Do patients' evaluations of a future health state change when they actually enter that state? *Med Care* 31: 1002–12.

Llewellyn-Thomas, H.A., J.H. Sutherland, R. Tibshirani, A. Ciampi, J.E. Till, and N.F. Boyd. 1984. Describing health states: Methodologic issues in obtaining values for health states. *Med Care* 22:543–52.

Llewellyn-Thomas, H.A., J.H. Sutherland, R. Tibshirani, A. Ciampi, J.E. Till, and N.F. Boyd. 1982. The measurement of patients' values in medicine. *Med Decis Making* 2:449–62.

Loomes, G., and L. McKenzie. 1989. The use of QALYs in health care decision making. *Soc Sci Med* 28:299–308.

Mandelblatt, J., and M. Fahs. 1988. Cost-effectiveness of cervical cancer screening for low income elderly women. *JAMA* 259:2409–13.

McDowell, I., and C. Newell. 1987. *Measuring health: A guide to rating scales and questionnaires.* New York: Oxford University Press.

McNeil, B.J., S.G. Pauker, H.C. Sox, Jr., and A. Tversky. 1982. On the elicitation of preferences for alternative therapies. *N Engl J Med* 306:1259–62.

Mehrez, A., and A. Gafni. 1993. Healthy-years equivalents versus quality-adjusted life years: In pursuit of progress. *Med Decis Making* 13:287–92.

Mehrez, A., and A. Gafni. 1989. Quality-adjusted life years, utility theory, and healthy-years equivalents. *Med Decis Making* 9:142–49.

Miller, G.A. 1956. The magical number seven plus or minus two: Some limits on our capacity for processing information. *Psychol Rev* 63:81–97.

Moriyama, I.M. 1968. Problems in the measurement of health status. In *Indicators of Social Change*, ed. E.B. Sheldon and W.E. Moore. New York: Russell Sage Foundation, 573–600.

Najman, J., and S. Levine. 1981. Evaluating the impact of medical care and technologies on the quality of life: A review and critique. *Soc Sci Med* 15F:107–15.

Nease, R.F., Jr., T. Kneeland, G.T. O'Connor, W. Sumner, C. Lumpkins, L. Shaw, D. Pryor, and H.C. Sox. 1995. Variation in patient utilities for outcomes of the management of chronic stable angina: Implications for clinical practice guidelines. Ischemic Health Disease Patient Outcomes Research Team. *JAMA* 273:1185–90.

Nord, E. 1992a. An alternative to QALYs: The saved young life equivalent (SAVE). *BMJ* 305:875–77.

Nord, E. 1992b. Methods for quality adjustment of life years. *Soc Sci Med* 34:559–69.

Nord, E. 1991. EuroQol: Health-related quality of life measurements. Valuation of health states by the general public in Norway. *Health Policy* 18:25–36.

O'Connor, A.M., N. Boyd, and P. Warde. 1987. Eliciting preferences for alternative drug therapies in oncology: Influence of treatment outcome description, elicitation technique and treatment experience on preferences. *J Chronic Dis* 40:811–18.

Office of Technology Assessment (OTA), U.S. Congress. 1992. *Evaluation of the Oregon Medicaid proposal.* OTA-H-531. Washington, DC: U.S. GPO.

Oldridge, N., W. Furlong, D. Feeny, G. Torrance, G. Guyatt, J. Crowe, and N. Jones. 1993. Economic evaluation of cardiac rehabilitation soon after acute myocardial infarction. *Am J Cardiol* 72:154–61.

Orenstein, D.M., P.A. Nixon, E.A. Ross, and R.M. Kaplan. 1989. The quality of well-being in cystic fibrosis. *Chest* 95:344–47.

Orenstein, D.M., E.N. Pattishall, P.A. Nixon, E.A. Ross, and R.M. Kaplan. 1990. Quality of well-being before and after antibiotic treatment of pulmonary exacerbation in patients with cystic fibrosis. *Chest*, 98:1081–84.

Oster, G., D.M. Huse, T.E. Delea, and G.A. Colditz. 1986. Cost-effectiveness of nicotine chewing gum as an adjunct to physician's advice against cigarette smoking. *JAMA* 256:1315–18.

Patrick, D.L. 1976. Constructing social metrics for health status indexes. *Int J Health Services* 6:443–53.

Patrick, D.L., and M. Bergner. 1990. Measurement of health status in the 1990s. *Annu Rev Public Health* 11:165–83.

Patrick, D.L., and R. Deyo. 1989. Generic and disease-specific measures in assessing health status and quality of life. *Med Care* 27:S217–32.

Patrick, D.L., and P. Erickson. 1993. *Health status and health policy: Allocating resources to health care.* New York: Oxford University Press.

Patrick, D.L., and P. Erickson. 1996. Applications of health status assessment to health policy. In *Quality of Life and Pharmacoeconomics,* (2nd edition). ed. B. Spilker, Philadelphia: Lippincott-Raven.

Patrick, D.L., Y. Sittampalam, S. Somerville, W. Carter, and M. Bergner. 1985. A cross-cultural comparison of health status values. *Am J Public Health* 75:1402–7.

Patrick, D.L., H.E. Starks, K.C. Cain, R.F. Uhlmann, and R.A. Pearlman. 1994. Measuring preferences for health states worse than death. *Med Decis Making* 14:9–18.

Read, J.L., R.J. Quinn, D.M. Berwick, H.V. Fineberg, and M.C. Weinstein. 1984. Preferences for health outcomes: Comparisons of assessment methods. *Med Decis Making* 4:315–29.

Richardson, J. 1994. Cost utility analysis: What should be measured? *Soc Sci Med* 39:7–21.

Rosser, R.M. 1990. From health indicators to quality-adjusted life years: Technical and ethical issues. In *Measuring the outcomes of medical care*, ed. A. Hopkins and B. Costain, 1-17. London: Royal College of Physicians.

Rosser, R.M. 1983. Issues of measurement in the design of health indicators: A review. In *Health indicators: An international study for the European Science Foundation*, ed. A.J. Culyer, 34–81. New York: St. Martin's Press.

Rosser, R.M., and P. Kind. 1978. A scale of valuations of states of illness: Is there a social consensus? *Int J Epidemiol* 7:347–58.

Rosser, R.M., and V.C. Watts. 1972. The measurement of hospital output. *Int J Epidemiol* 1:361–68.

Sackett, D.L., and G.W. Torrance. 1978. The utility of different health states as perceived by the general public. *J Chronic Dis* 31:697–704.

Shoemaker, P.J.H. 1982. The expected utility model: Its variants, purposes, evidence and limitations. *J Econ Lit* 20:529–63.

Sintonen, H. 1995. *The 15D-measure of health related quality of life. II. Feasibility, reliability, and validity of its valuation system.* Working Paper 42. Melbourne, Australia: National Centre for Health Program Evaluation.

Sintonen, H. 1994. *The 15D-measure of health related quality of life. I. Reliability, validity of its valuation system.* Working Paper 41. Melbourne, Australia: National Centre for Health Program Evaluation.

Sintonen, H. 1981a. *An approach to economic evaluation of actions for health: A theoretical-methodological study in health economics with special reference to Finnish health policy.* Official Statistics of Finland. Special Social Studies XXXII:74. Helsinki, Finland: Government Printing Centre.

Sintonen, H. 1981b. An approach to measuring and valuing health states. *Soc Sci Med* 15C:55–65.

Sintonen, H., and M. Pekurinen. 1993. A fifteen dimensional measure of health-related quality of life (15D) and its applications. In *Quality of life assessment: Key issues in the 1990s,* ed. S.R. Walker and R.M. Rosser, 185–95, 467–70. Dordrecht, Netherlands: Kluwer Academic Publishers.

Sisk Willems, J., C.R. Sanders, M.A. Riddiough, and J.C. Bell. 1980. Cost-effectiveness of vaccination against pneumococcal pneumonia. *N Engl J Med* 330:553–59.

Slevin, M.L., L. Stubbs, H.J. Plant, P.Wilson, W.M. Gregory, P.J. Armes, and S.M. Downer. 1990. Attitude to chemotherapy: Comparing views of patients with cancer with those of doctors, nurses, and general public. *BMJ* 300:1458–60.

Stason, W.B., and M.C. Weinstein. 1977. Allocation of resources to manage hypertension. *N Engl J Med* 296:732.

Streiner, D.L., and G.R. Norman. 1989. *Health measurement scales. A practical guide to their development and use.* New York: Oxford University Press.

Sutherland, J.H., H. Llewellyn-Thomas, N.F. Boyd, and J.E. Till. 1982. Attitudes towards quality of survival: The concept of "maximal endurable time." *Med Decis Making* 2:299–309.

Taylor, W.C., T.M. Pass, D.S. Shepard, and A.L. Komaroff. 1990. Cost-effectiveness of cholesterol reduction for the primary prevention of coronary heart disease in men. In *Preventing disease: Beyond the rhetoric*, ed. R.B. Goldblum and R.S. Lawrence, 437–41. New York: Springer-Verlag.

Thompson, M.S., J.L. Read, H.C. Hutchings, M. Paterson, and E.D. Harris, Jr. 1988. The cost-effectiveness of auronofin: Results of a randomized clinical trial. *J Rheumatol* 15:35–42.

Thurstone, L.L. 1927. A law of comparative judgment. *Psychol Rev* 34:273–86.

Torrance, G.W. 1987. Utility approach to measuring health-related quality of life. *J Chron Dis* 40:593–600.

Torrance, G.W. 1986. Measurement of health state utilities for economic appraisal. *J Health Economics* 5:1–30.

Torrance, G.W. 1976. Social prefernce for health states: An empirical evaluation of three measurement techniques. *Socio-Economic Planning Sciences* 10:129–36.

Torrance, G.W., M.H. Boyle, and S.P. Horwood. 1982. Application of multi-attribute utility theory to measure social preferences for health states. *Operations Research* 30:1043–69.

Torrance, G.W., P. Erickson, D. Patrick, and J. Feldman. 1995a. Technical Notes. In *Years of healthy life.* Statistical Note No. 7, by P. Erickson, R.W. Wilson, and I. Shannon, 10–14. Hyattsville, MD: National Center for Health Statistics.

Torrance, G.W., W. Furlong, D. Feeny, and M. Boyle. 1995b. Multi-attribute preference functions: Health utilities index. *PharmacoEconomics* 9:503–20.

Torrance, G.W., W.H. Thomas, and D.L. Sacket. 1972. A utility maximization model for evaluation of health care programs. *Health Serv Res* 7:118–33.

Torrance, G.W., Y. Zhang, D. Feeny, W.J. Furlong, and R. Barr. 1992. *Multi-attribute preference functions for a comprehensive health status classification system.* Working Paper No. 92-18. Hamilton, Ontario: McMaster University, Centre for Health Economics and Policy Analysis.

Torrance, G.W., and A. Zipursky. 1984. Cost-effectiveness of antepartum prevention of Rh immunization. *Clin Perinatol* 11:267–81.

Tosteson, A.N.A., D.I. Rosenthal, L.J. Melton, and M.C. Weinstein. 1990. Cost-effectiveness of screening postmenopausal white women for osteoporisis: Bone-densitometry and hormone replacement therapy. *Ann Intern Med* 113:594–603.

von Neumann, J., and O. Morgenstern. 1947. *Theories of games and economic behavior.* Princeton, NJ: Princeton University Press.

Ware, J.E., and D.C. Sherbourne. 1992. The MOS 36-item short-form health survey. *Med Care* 30:473–83.

Weeks, J., J. O'Leary, D. Fairclough, D. Paltiel, and M.C. Weinstein. 1994. The Q-tility Index: A new tool for assessing health-related quality of life and utilties in clinical trials and clinical practice. *Proceedings of the American Society of Clinical Oncology* 13:436 (abstract).

Weinstein, M.C. 1988. A QALY is a QALY is a QALY—or is it? *J Health Economics* 7:289–90.

Weinstein, M.C., and A.N.A. Tosteson. 1990. Cost-effectiveness of hormone replacement. *Ann N Y Acad Sci* 592:162–72.

White, C.C., J.P. Koplan, and W.A. Orenstein. 1985. Benefits, risks, and costs of immunization for measles, mumps, and rubella. *Am J Public Health* 75:739–44.

Williams, A. 1995a. The measurement and valuation of health: A chronicle. Discussion Paper 136. York, Great Britain: Centre for Health Economics, University of York.

Williams, A. 1995b. The role of the EuroQol instrument in QALY calculations. Discussion Paper 130. York, Great Britain: Centre for Health Economics, University of York.

Wong, J.B., D.N. Salem, and S.G. Pauker. 1993. You're never too old. *N Engl J Med* 328:971–975.

5

Assessing the Effectiveness of Health Interventions

J.S. MANDELBLATT, D.G. FRYBACK,
M.C. WEINSTEIN, L.B. RUSSELL, M.R. GOLD, and
D.C. HADORN

Cost-effectiveness analysis (CEA) requires a numerical estimate of the magnitude of the effects of an intervention on health outcomes. The denominator of a cost-effectiveness (C/E) ratio is the difference in effectiveness between an intervention and the alternative to which it is being compared (the net effect), just as the numerator is the difference in cost between the two (the net cost). To estimate the net effect of an intervention, the analyst needs to know the health states that may occur as a consequence of the intervention and the alternative, the probability that each state will occur, when each is likely to occur, and how long each will last. These health states turn on the sequence of events and consequent decisions that take place during or following the intervention and the condition the intervention is intended to treat (or prevent). For example, screening may detect a condition, and treatment may alter it. If the treatment is successful it will alter the condition for the better, but it may also bring undesirable side effects. Screening, treatment, and their immediate and delayed direct effects and side effects comprise a connected chain of events that must be taken into account to assess the overall net effect in this example.

A complete and careful description of the cascade of events emanating from the decision to intervene (or to engage in prevention activities) is fundamental to cost-effectiveness analysis. Appropriate calculation of effectiveness—as well as costs—depends on it. Thus, it is critical that the analysis consider all events that change the health of the patient or that generate costs. Since CEA is a comparative analysis, similar care must be taken to describe the events and health consequences deriving from the alternative to which the intervention or program is being compared.

Because CEA summarizes what happens on average, we are not so much interested in the chain of events that occurs in the unique life of one patient as we are interested in determining how likely different possible sequences of events are in particular populations of patients (or individuals). The process of determining average net effect is devoted to describing and then quantifying the possible sequences of effects, determining the probability of each sequence, and computing average health effects associated with each sequence or pathway following from the intervention and comparator programs.

This chapter reviews the methods commonly used to estimate net effects. Sometimes there exist direct primary data, collected using appropriate and rigorous study designs, that can be used to calculate effectiveness. More typically the CEA requires a synthesis of information from diverse sources of varying quality to make inferences about the likely and/or important sequences of health states in the target population. We will refer to this synthesis process as "modeling."

The primary objective of our discussion is to review the process of estimating effectiveness specifically for CEA, not effectiveness analysis in general. To accomplish this goal, following a general definition and discussion of the terms "effectiveness" and "probability" in the context of CEA, the chapter focuses on methods for determining the probabilities of events and health states, highlighting potential sources of data for determining probabilities. The chapter is organized into two major subsections. The first presents a review of effectiveness information from the perspective of clinical epidemiology, emphasizing issues pertinent to assigning probabilities in a CEA. The second introduces the use of modeling to estimate effectiveness in CEA. A brief summary of the methods for estimating effectiveness in a cost-effectiveness analysis of cholesterol reduction in adults is presented at the end of the chapter to demonstrate how these probabilities, together with the measure of quantity and quality of time spent in each health state, are combined to calculate the net effectiveness estimate for the C/E ratio. The chapter concludes with a summary of recommendations of the panel for estimating effectiveness in CEA.

It should be noted that many of the concepts described in this chapter relate to the numerator of the C/E ratio, net costs, as well as to the denominator. Costs of interventions depend on the probabilities that individuals will experience various morbid events, experience adverse effects of treatment, or utilize health services, and these are often the same kinds of probabilities that go into estimating effectiveness. The difference is that in the numerator, these events are weighted by the costs associated with those events (see Chapter 6), while in the denominator they are weighted by the preference values assigned to health states. (See Chapter 4.)

Assessing the net effectiveness of an intervention for a CEA is detailed, complex, and time-consuming work. The overarching goal of this chapter is not to provide a comprehensive step-by-step guide to this process. Instead, the chapter is designed to give the reader a familiarity with the major concepts and issues and to provide recommendations that can be used as guidelines for gathering data on effectiveness within a CEA.

Definitions

Effectiveness

To approach these tasks, it is first necessary to define what is meant by "effectiveness." Perhaps the simplest definition is that health services are considered to be effective to the extent that they achieve health improvements in real practice settings. Thus, *effectiveness* must be distinguished from two closely related concepts: *efficacy*, which denotes how well the intended objectives are realized in ideal settings—often academic or research environments in which services or treatments are developed and initially tested, and *appropriateness*, which reflects a broader range of issues considered in deciding whether an intervention should or should not be done, including assessments of the extent to which the expected health benefit exceeds the expected negative consequences of the intervention, as well as considerations of acceptability, feasibility, and costs (Park, 1986; Leape, 1990, Leape and Brook, 1990). One role of CEA is to provide guidance in the determination of the appropriateness of an intervention given what is known about its effectiveness and cost.

To illustrate, compliance with a new cholesterol lowering drug which must be taken five times a day will likely be higher in a randomized clinical trial (RCT) than in routine practice. In this situation, the efficacy seen in the RCT for cholesterol reduction will be greater than the effectiveness in general practice. Volunteer effects may also act to inflate the efficacy of interventions observed in RCTs, compared to effects seen in non-RCT settings (Morrison, 1992; Goodwin et al., 1988; Hunter et al., 1987; Mandel et al., 1993). In terms of appropriateness, this new drug, while lowering serum lipid levels, may also have an adverse effect, such as a 50% rate of acute pancreatitis in diabetic patients, rendering it inappropriate therapy for diabetic populations.

The example of cholesterol-lowering treatment also illustrates that effectiveness is often the result of a cascade of effects which lead eventually to changes in health. The initial effect, and that measured by early studies of the intervention, is to lower serum cholesterol. Like effects on tumor progression in cancer or CD4 cell counts in HIV, serum cholesterol is an intermediate outcome which is important for its further health implications. Lowered serum cholesterol is imperfectly associated with the more "distal" and more important effect of decreasing the incidence of coronary heart disease and stroke; this association is imperfect because lowered serum cholesterol may not, in all situations, lower the incidence rates of coronary events such as myocardial infarctions. But the rate at which these incident events occur in the treated versus the untreated groups is still only an intermediate outcome. An even more distal effect is the reduction in deaths and improvement in mobility and pain status associated with coronary heart disease. Finally, the health effect of cholesterol lowering on overall all-cause mortality and health-related quality of life is the ultimate outcome measure of effectiveness of the intervention. It should be noted that, while assessment of intermediate outcomes may be clinically important, the final outcomes of all-cause mortality and health-related quality of life are the most useful for CEA, allowing for comparisons of the costs and effectiveness of interventions for differing health conditions.

The presence of multiple etiologic factors often complicates the task of estimating the effectiveness of an intervention. Ideally the CEA should be derived from research designed in a manner which permits one to isolate the effect of a separable component of the intervention by using appropriate controls. However, even under the most rigorous conditions, it is often not possible to determine the extent to which the intervention is truly responsible for the outcome observed. For example, the observed effect of fecal occult blood testing (FOBT) on colorectal cancer mortality may be due to the increased rate of follow-up colonoscopy in the screened versus the unscreened group, and not due to the FOBT test itself (Lang and Ransohoff, 1994). The more distal the outcome event from the intervention, the more likely it is that the intervention is but one of many potential contributing causes of the outcome, and the more difficult it is to have control over the measurement process.

Measuring the effectiveness of interventions for early detection of disease is plagued by additional problems. Ultimately, effectiveness depends on a finding that the intervention will lead to a better health outcome on average than those seen among individuals whose disease is detected without the intervention. A necessary but not sufficient condition for effectiveness of early detection is that the screening test be sufficiently accurate to detect the target condition earlier than would occur without the test or intervention (USPSTF, 1995). However, it is possible that a screening test can detect disease earlier than would occur in routine practice, but, once detected, there may be no treatment of proven effectiveness available. This is the apparent case, for example, in prostate cancer of high grade (Gleason score 8–10) detected by prostate-specific antigen (PSA) screening (Kramer et al., 1993). In this case, if confirmed by the 15-year National Cancer Institute PLCO (Prostate, Lung, Colorectal, and Ovarian) Cancer Screening Trial, the outcome of the disease for those with some high-grade lesions would not be affected by the screening test. Inherent in isolating the effect of early detection is the dilemma of separating true ''effectiveness'' from the influence of lead time and length biases,[1] both of which are discussed later in the chapter. At this other extreme, screening may uncover disease that poses little or no threat to the host individual, but this fact may be unknown because cases are not left untreated; aggressive treatment of these people may appear very effective under the tacit assumption that the disease is more threatening than is the case. This may be the case with localized prostate cancer in 65–75-year-old men with a Gleason score of 2–4 where long-term survival with conservative treatment appears the same as that of the general population of men this age (Albertsen et al., 1995).

Practically speaking, few primary studies will be able to collect direct data measuring effects along the entire cascade of events from intervention to health outcome. Thus, as discussed in Chapter 3, the analyst must make a judgment about the most reasonable time frame for evaluating the outcomes of interest. Modeling must often be used to combine information from different data sources pertaining to various time horizons in the cascade, using data that span several steps, where possible, to validate model integrity. The time periods over which event probabilities are defined will depend on the nature of the condition. One year is a common time period. The analyst estimates the probabilities that an individual will experience different events each year—for example, the probability that disease will occur, the probabilities the patient will survive if the intervention is used or if the alternative is used, the probabilities that the patient will experience improvements in function or deterioration in function, and so on. As discussed in Chapter 3, the analysis is then carried out over a time horizon of as many years as necessary to capture the main effects and costs of the intervention. For some conditions, however, a year is too long a period. For instance, acute conditions may involve important changes in health states (including death) in just a few days or weeks. For cost-effectiveness analyses of such conditions, the appropriate recurrent time period could be 1 week or 1 month. For other conditions, a mixture of life segments using shorter time periods and others using longer periods may be necessary.

Outcome Probabilities

Probability theory (Colton, 1974) underlies all methods for drawing inferences about outcomes. Clinical epidemiology, for example, is grounded in probability theory as a basis for drawing inferences about clinical outcomes. Probabilities express the degree of certainty that an event will happen on a scale from 0.0 (certainty that the event will not occur) to 1.0 (certainty that the event will occur). Examples of probabilities used in CEA include the following: the probability that a patient has a particular disease (prevalence), the probability that the patient will develop disease (incidence), the probability of a positive test result given a patient's disease status (and the converse of this, the probability that a patient has a disease given a positive test result) (Sox et al., 1988; Weinstein et al., 1980), the probability that a patient will respond to a treatment, the probability that a patient will develop a toxic reaction to a drug, and the probability that a patient will die during a given time interval.

Statistics is the science of drawing inference about probabilities by observing the results of repeated events. According to the "law of large numbers," if the probability of an event is 0.5, then over a large number of trials, the proportion of trials in which the event will occur will probably (but not necessarily) be close to 50%. Thus, for example, if 500 of 1,000 patients respond to a drug, a reasonable inference is that the probability of response is 0.5 (or 50%).

Statistical science provides tools not only for estimating probabilities from data but also for expressing the degree of uncertainty about the estimate itself. For example, we may be interested in the average number of years a person will live (i.e., life expectancy) once diagnosed with a certain condition. Given a set of estimated survival probabilities, it is possible to calculate life expectancy as the area under the survival curve (or, as an approximation, the sum of the annual survival probabilities). Such an estimate of life expectancy is a "point estimate" of the quantity of interest. However, there is generally uncertainty about this estimate because the survival probabilities were estimated from data. This uncertainty can be expressed as a confidence interval around the estimate (Colton, 1974), or Bayesian statistical methods may be used to derive a related, and often similar, interval expressing uncertainty about the point estimate (Eddy et al., 1992; Brophy and Joseph, 1995). We will return to the topic of expressing uncertainty about estimates of effectiveness (and cost-effectiveness) in Chapter 8.

As noted in the Introduction, a major task in assessing effectiveness in CEA is to estimate the appropriate probabilities of health events, or outcomes of interest, from the best available sources. The probabilities (or probability distributions) for each event and population group may be estimated from planned empirical investigations such as randomized controlled trials or observational cohort studies or they may be estimated from other types of empirical observations and expert judgments.

Difficulties in obtaining the proper probabilities with which to estimate effectiveness for use in a CEA include the following:

- Converting probabilities that cumulate hazard over time intervals (e.g., a finding of a 30% difference in cumulative mortality at 12 years after the start of a clinical trial) to annual probabilities (Kuntz and Weinstein, 1995)
- Specializing probabilities estimated from one population in which data were collected, to estimate the probability in a related but not identical population needed for the CEA (e.g., estimating the annual mortality probability for a 70-year-old patient when the original 5-year survival data were collected in a cohort with average age of 50) (Kuntz and Weinstein, 1995)
- Estimating the effect on annual mortality and other event probabilities of multiple risk factors (e.g., they may or may not be independent; they may combine additively or multiplicatively in their effect) (Russell et al., 1995)
- Computing conditional probabilities after multiple tests or prior events when the assumption of conditional independence of those prior tests and events cannot be verified or tested with data (Fryback, 1978)
- Using expert opinion about probabilities when no data are available about critical events for the CEA, recognizing that various biases affect experts' estimates of probabilities (Poses et al., 1988)
- Basing probability estimates on studies that are subject to conventional design flaws, such as bias due to selection factors or uncontrolled confounding

Issues related to the use of modeling are discussed later in this chapter.

Sources of Data for Probability Estimates

In order to calculate the effectiveness of an intervention or diagnostic test, the investigator must model the cascade of events resulting from the intervention or test and compare it to the natural history of the disease or event that the intervention is designed to prevent or treat. Unfortunately, for many conditions the precise natural history is not delineated in sufficient detail for use in a cost-effectiveness analysis. For example, while we know from randomized clinical trials that mammography and clinical breast examination are effective in lowering mortality from breast cancer for women aged 50–74 (Shapiro et al., 1982; Tabar et al., 1985; Andersson et al., 1988), a CEA of a mammography screening program will need to consider a number of specific parameters not directly estimated in the clinical trials. To illustrate, while the induced costs related to diagnosis and treatment of screen-detected in situ lesions can be identified, the effectiveness of screening for in situ lesions is more difficult to evaluate. The probability that a mammographically detected breast carcinoma in situ will progress to invasive cancer is not known, and, if the lesion does progress, the time between preclinical detectability and symptomatic disease (the sojourn time) is also unknown.

For most diseases, determination of the natural history is difficult and must be inferred, since allowing patients to go untreated in order to follow the course of their disease would often be considered unethical. Natural history data may be available from studies predating the availability of treatment. However, comparing a contemporary intervention to such historically untreated groups may overestimate effectiveness, due to improvements in outcomes associated with general improvements in medical care (Cohn et al., 1975). The course of contemporaneous patients refusing treatment can yield some insight into disease progression rates, but this group is not likely to be representative of the general population with the disease. Finally, the natural history of screen-detectable diseases may be estimated from RCTs using data from cases detected in the intervals between screening tests.

As alluded to in the Introduction to this chapter, the quality of the evidence about effectiveness should be considered in selecting the data for use in a CEA (Laupacis et al., 1992). For estimation of effectiveness in a CEA, outcome probability values should be selected from the best designed (and least biased) sources that are relevant to the question and population under study. A greater weight should be given to outcome probability values derived from study designs that are the least prone to bias. The hierarchy of evidence for evaluating the effectiveness of clinical preventive services suggested by the United States Preventive Services Task Force (USPSTF) can be broadly applied to selection of probabilities in a CEA (in decreasing order): RCTs; observational data, including cohort, case-control, and cross-sectional studies; uncontrolled experiments; descriptive series; and expert opinion (USPSTF, 1995). This hierarchy should not, however, be interpreted too rigidly. Qualitative evidence of effectiveness from randomized trials that are too small to provide precise estimates of effect size, which are performed in atypical or insufficiently diverse patient populations, often need to be supplemented by quantitative data from observational studies for use in CEAs. For example, CEAs have built upon the qualitative evidence of the effectiveness of cholesterol lowering from trials such as the Coronary Primary Prevention Trial (Lipid Research Clinics Program, 1984) with quantitative estimates from the Framingham Heart Study on the association between serum cholesterol and coronary heart disease. It should be noted that less-rigorously designed studies, where multiple studies draw similar conclusions, may be the best available source of data for a particular subpopulation or research hypothesis in the absence of other data. Meta-analysis, a synthesis technique which can be applied to all of these types of study designs, may be a useful source of effectiveness data for a CEA, although the quality of the estimates derived from such meta-analyses depend on the quality of the original study data.

Probability data for use in a CEA can be collected as part of a research protocol (primary data) or they can be abstracted or extrapolated from existing published research (secondary data). This section will briefly review each of these potential sources of data and discuss the advantages and disadvantages of each from the perspective of estimating probabilities in cost-effectiveness research. Since most CEAs to date have relied on secondary sources for probability values (and costs), this discussion generally assumes the perspective of secondary data collection. As cost-effectiveness research evolves, more data will be collected as integral elements of primary research designs; the caveats presented here for evaluating secondary data sources should be equally applicable. For further information on effectiveness data and evaluating technology, the reader is referred to other excellent reviews and texts (Mosteller, IOM, 1985; Banta et al., 1981; Banta and Luce, 1993; OTA 1994; 1995).

Randomized Controlled Trials

Randomized controlled trials (RCTs) are generally accepted as the most powerful tool for assessing the effectiveness of interventions, medications, or procedures. By design the blind, random assignment of an adequate number of subjects to study arms and blind assessment of outcomes minimizes bias due to observer bias and confounding due to known and unknown variables. Thus, randomization enhances the comparability of the study and control groups and provides a more valid basis for inferring that the treatment or intervention actually caused the observed outcome. Concurrent control groups avoid problems with the use of historical controls since, as noted previously, trends in treatment and survival which are independent of the study can bias the conclusions.

Use of data from RCTs (or any other source) to estimate outcome probabilities requires that the interventions tested should delineate clear causes and effects and be able to separate the effects of multimodality interventions. For instance, to estimate probabilities associated with the effects of the intervention itself as distinct from the probabilities of nonspecific effects of contact with the medical care system, data from a trial including a nonintervention arm could be useful. As an example of estimating separate effects in a multimodality trial, the recent Canadian National Breast Screening Study was designed so that data could be used to estimate the effects on breast cancer mortality of clinical breast examination (CBE) alone, mammography alone, or CBE and mammography combined (Miller et al., 1992a,b). It should be noted, however, that even this well-conceived RCT has been surrounded by controversy concerning its conduct and results to date (Baines, 1994); a CEA analyst using data from such a source would be well served to be aware of the (potential sources of) threats to validity of the source data and of the possible consequences such issues may have for the effectiveness estimates in the CEA.

The primary disadvantages associated with using estimates of effectiveness and rates of adverse events derived from RCTs include: (1) the select nature of the subjects; (2) the difference between the impact of the intervention under RCT conditions (i.e., efficacy), compared to effects in routine practice; (3) the limited window of opportunity to conduct a RCT prior to widespread dissemination of an intervention into clinical practice (referred to as "contamination" effects); (4) the limited time horizon employed; and (5) the costs of conducting RCTs. We consider these limitations of RCTs in turn.

Patient selection in RCTs

Patient eligibility for RCTs is generally narrowly defined. While this aspect of RCTs allows for specificity of conclusions, the range of patients may not represent those included in a cost-effectiveness analysis. For example, patients eligible for treatment in a clinical trial may have better outcomes than ineligible patients, whether or not they consent to participate; and those consenting to participate and be randomized may also have better health outcomes than the general population (the "healthy volunteer" effect) (Goodwin et al., 1988; Hunter et al., 1987; Mandel, 1993). As an illustration, the authors of an early CEA of coronary artery bypass graft surgery (CABG) noted that survival among patients with single-vessel coronary disease in the control arm of the Veterans Administration trial of CABG was better than that of age-matched persons in the general U.S. population (Weinstein and Stason, 1982). They corrected for this bias by estimating the relative survival benefit of CABG from the RCTs, while relying on observational data to estimate the survival of medically treated CHD patients.

Another problem relating to patient selection in RCTs is underrepresentation of minority groups, the aged, and women (e.g., El Sadr and Capps, 1992). However, these may be the very groups at highest risk for the disease or death from the disease targeted by the intervention. For example, elderly women and African-American women are more likely to have breast cancer diagnosed at advanced stages, and to die with that disease, than younger and nonminority women (Mandelblatt et al., 1991; Wells and Horm, 1992; Hunter et al., 1993; Bassett and Krieger, 1986). Yet, these groups, with few exceptions (Shapiro et al., 1982), have not been included, or have not been included in sufficient numbers, in RCTs evaluating the effectiveness of screening mammography and clinical breast examination.

Such gaps in patient representation in RCTs can have important implications for conducting CEAs and for making policy recommendations. For instance, given the paucity of effectiveness data for women aged 75 or more years, many groups, including the USPSTF, have not made any recommendations about breast cancer screening for this age group. As another example, cardiologists have been reluctant to recommend thrombolysis for elderly patients with acute myocardial infarction, although a CEA based on a meta-analysis of elderly patients included in clinical trials concluded that thrombolysis was indeed likely to be cost-effective in the elderly (Krumholz et al., 1992). In such situations, a cost-effectiveness analyst could use modeling to extrapolate trial (or other) data to subpopulations which were not well represented in the RCT.

Efficacy versus effectiveness in RCTs

Results from a RCT best represent the efficacy of an intervention, not its effectiveness. The RCT generally represents the ideal conditions for implementation of the intervention, conditions which are rarely duplicated in practice settings where the vast majority of care is received. The structure of a trial includes sufficient personnel and attention to follow-up and monitoring to minimize the numbers of patients lost and to maximize the compliance with the research protocol. Few practice settings have such resources. As a consequence results observed in a RCT will likely overestimate the "true" effectiveness of an intervention or test. The recommended practice of analyzing RCT data by "intention to treat," where all patients randomized to an arm are included in analyses of that intervention arm (including patients who drop out, who are lost to follow-up, or who "cross over" to another intervention or treatment), minimizes some of this tendency of an RCT to overestimate effectiveness.

Fully correcting for this bias in CEA is problematic, since ethical concerns preclude performing "effectiveness RCTs" in routine practice settings once an RCT has demonstrated efficacy. Outcomes research based on patient databases and other types of postmarketing surveillance of new technologies may be helpful in this regard, despite problems with achieving adequate controls for confounding factors in observational studies.

Limited window of opportunity for RCTs

For technologies that are introduced rapidly into medical practice it may never be possible to conduct an RCT. For example, the PSA test to screen for cancer has been rapidly incorporated into clinical practice without any systematic assessment of efficacy or effectiveness of screening and treating screen-detected prostate cancers. As a result, any true effect of screening with PSA will be diluted or contaminated, when tested in an RCT, by the high use of the test in the control population (Kramer et al., 1993).

In such a situation, the CEA analyst might rely on data from historical controls predating the use of PSA. In that case, however, as noted above, the PSA group may appear to have better outcomes than the historical control group based solely on general advances in medical care. Alternatively, the analyst could consider using data from a prostate cancer treatment efficacy trial combined with careful studies of the technical characteristics of the screening techniques and studies of stage-specific outcomes associated with prostate cancer treatment (M.L. Brown, personal communication, 1995).

Time horizon limits in RCTs

Another difficulty with using RCT data to estimate the effectiveness of interventions is that the time horizon of the trial is usually limited by practical as well as ethical considerations. Sometimes effectiveness is defined in terms of intermediate end-points, such as changes in clinical markers. It is possible that long-term effectiveness differs from that observed for the intermediate end-point. Even when final outcomes such as mortality are used, trials are usually stopped before it is possible to tell if benefits increase, hold steady, or diminish over time. This problem is of particular concern to analyses of preventive interventions, for which the time interval between the initiation of the intervention and the health outcome is great.

In addition, future adverse effects may not be noted in the course of a trial. Related to this issue is the practice of employing "early stopping" rules in many trials. For example, in the RCTs of aspirin to prevent second myocardial infarcts among men, the benefits of aspirin were considered too great to continue the trials to their conclusion. However, there was also a suggestion of increased risk of hemorrhagic strokes in certain subpopulations of subjects (i.e., hypertensives) (the Steering Committee of the Physicians Health Study Research Group, 1988, 1989). Unfortunately, there were insufficient data at the time of stopping to draw firm conclusions about this risk, and this is likely to remain an unresolved issue. For the analyst assessing the overall cost-effectiveness of this intervention, these data are essential for a complete evaluation of expected outcomes.

Costs of data collection

The intensity of resources needed to conduct an RCT (or large observational study) to assess the effectiveness of a new intervention is considerable. Decisions about resource expenditures for new primary efficacy or effectiveness data collection efforts should consider not only the costs of the undertaking but also the potential benefits of the data. From a policy perspective, new data on an intervention which addresses a condition with a high burden of illness and important resource implications might be a good value (Detsky, 1989).

In summary, well-designed and -conducted RCTs are a preferred source of data for probability values to estimate intervention effectiveness in CEAs owing to the absence of major biases which may affect conclusions. However, such data may be limited in their power and their generalizability to population-based settings and groups that differ from the research subjects and the time horizons of interest. Larger size trials can take some of these considerations, such as healthy volunteer, contamination, and subgroup effects, into account by increasing the power of an RCT to detect clinically important effects, but they are considerably more expensive to conduct. Changing trends in RCT conduct, such as recruitment from practice settings, follow-up observation of ineligible subjects (as a cohort), greater representation of women and minority groups, and inclusion of health-related quality-of-life outcomes, should make RCT data more useful for future CEAs.

As a practical matter, now and in the future, RCT evaluation will not be available for all interventions in all types of patients; even when available, RCT data may be subject to considerable limitations. As a consequence, CEA must also draw on other data sources (as discussed below) and methods of extrapolation, such as modeling.

Epidemiologic (Observational) Studies

Two major types of observational studies, observational cohort and case-control studies, can provide data on the probabilities of particular health outcomes associated with an intervention. Additional study designs, such as cross-sectional studies, case series, and uncontrolled cohort studies, may also provide data for a CEA. These observational studies all differ from RCTs in that the investigators do not have control over which persons receive the intervention.

In *observational cohort studies*, a defined population that is free of the outcome of interest is selected and followed longitudinally (prospectively or retrospectively) to observe the rate of occurrence of the outcome among various subgroups. These subgroups may be defined according to risk factors for disease, according to treatment, or according to exposure to a screening or diagnostic test. The Framingham Heart Study of risk factors for cardiovascular disease is a classic example of an observational cohort study; this study has generated probability data for several cardiovascular health outcomes that could be used to estimate effectiveness in a CEA. (See, for example, Weinstein and Stason, 1976; Goldman et al., 1991.) As another example, the Minnesota Heart Health Program tested a community-level intervention for smoking cessation; the community was then observed for coronary heart disease incidence as an intermediate outcome (Lando et al., 1995).

Observational cohort studies are more prone to bias than RCTs, since interventions may be chosen by patients or physicians on the basis of measurable or unrecognized variables that influence the outcome. Evidence for effectiveness from observational cohort studies which control for relevant confounding variables would have the greatest validity in inferring that the outcomes are attributable to the intervention and not to other extraneous factors. Compared to RCTs, however, observational cohort studies can only control for confounding variables that are known at the time of the study.

An advantage of observational cohort studies is that, compared to RCTs, they are more likely to yield "real-world" effectiveness data. In addition, retrospective observational cohort studies, compared to RCTs, have, by definition, a sufficiently long time period of observation, say until disease development or death, to ascertain most of the pertinent outcomes flowing from the intervention and comparison program that are needed for the CEA. Observational cohorts also have the advantage of generally comprising a broader spectrum of the population of interest than an RCT, although, like RCTs, they may not include sufficient numbers of relevant subpopulations. For example, the Framingham cohort did not include sufficient numbers of Hispanic or African-American residents for meaningful analyses for these groups.

While observational cohort studies can provide valid estimates of effectiveness, like RCTs, they are costly to implement, since they require large samples observed over long periods in order to have sufficient statistical power to measure differences in outcomes. As with all study designs we are discussing, in the situation where an insufficient sample has been observed, a failure to find effectiveness of a new intervention may reflect a true lack of impact, or it may reflect the inability to detect a small, but clinically meaningful difference in outcome. Lastly, as with RCTs, differential rates of loss to follow-up can bias the results of an observational cohort study.

Case-control studies have the advantage of not requiring follow-up, since the study group is selected to have the outcome at the time of study, and exposure to the intervention is assessed retrospectively. Because large numbers of persons with the outcome of interest can be sampled directly, there are rarely problems with sample size.

As in an observational cohort study, however, data from a case-control study are subject to bias from confounding factors. In addition, the retrospective nature of the design introduces the potential for recall bias, with cases more likely to remember a test or exposure than nondiseased controls. Since ascertainment of exposure is occurring after the disease has been diagnosed, measurement of exposure may also be influenced by knowledge of disease status. For example, in a breast cancer study a zealous interviewer may make greater efforts to elicit a positive response to prior use of mammography for controls than for cases, especially if the interviewer is convinced that mammography is effective (observer bias).

The use of case-control studies to evaluate the effectiveness of screening can be further biased by the type of case and/or control group selected (Weiss, 1983; Morrison, 1982; Conner et al., 1991). For example, in evaluating the effectiveness of sigmoidoscopy screening to reduce mortality from colorectal cancer, cases should include all those dying from the disease, and controls should include both those with colorectal cancer who are still alive and those without cancer. Moreover, the definition of cancers in both the case and control groups should include those cancers in reach of the sigmoidoscope and those beyond (Selby, 1992). Such choice of study groups eliminates the lead-time bias that would occur in situations if early stage cases were compared to later-stage cases, where earlier diagnosis resulted in an apparent benefit, even though survival did not actually differ in screened and unscreened groups. Using cases and controls from a large observational cohort study (referred to as cohort case-control or nested case-control designs) can be a practical way to avoid this and other case-control-related biases.

It should also be noted that most case-control studies, by selection of diseased in-dividuals as ''cases,'' will provide CEA data only on intermediate outcomes—unless, as in the colorectal cancer example above, cases are defined as those dying from the disease. As in other settings, however, intermediate outcomes can be extended, using additional data, by modeling.

Other types of observational studies that might provide probability data for a CEA include *cross-sectional studies*, *case series*, and *uncontrolled observational cohort stud-ies*. Examples of cross-sectional data that are often useful in CEA include data from the National Health Interview Survey (NHIS) (Massey et al., 1989) and the National Health and Nutrition Examination Survey (NHANES) (Ezzati et al., 1992). Longitu-dinal follow-up data are sometimes available for such cross-sectional panels (e.g., the NHANES I epidemiologic follow-up cohort, Ingram and Makuc, 1994).

Postmarketing surveillance is a longstanding methodology used to monitor long-term effects of pharmaceuticals. By analogy, data on past use of any technology, such as mammography, could be ascertained and related to current adverse effects, such as rates of false positives, psychological sequelae, or probability of repeat screening. Given the difficulties in separating the impact of confounding variables and chance from the true effect of the intervention, such results need to be interpreted with caution. However, in some situations, these may the only available estimates of effect for particular sub-populations.

Disease registries and *administrative databases* can also be used as sources of in-formation for estimating outcome probabilities for a CEA. For example, databases such as the National Cancer Institute's Surveillance, Epidemiology, and End-Results (SEER) registry[2], together with data on screening use (the NCI Breast Cancer Database Project, linking radiology records to SEER data), could be used to assess the impact of breast cancer screening technologies on disease mortality. The advantage of a database such as SEER is that it is population based (minimizing selection bias), has high rates of ascertainment, and includes a large-enough population over a long-enough time period to evaluate effectiveness among different age- or race-specific population subgroups.

Administrative databases, such as the Medicare Provider Analysis and Review (MEDPAR) files (Office of Statistics and Data Management, 1995), may be useful for calculating probabilities of particular health events among the beneficiary population. In general, these types of data sources may be limited by the type and completeness of data collected, the ability to retrieve records, the need for protection of confidentiality, and the inability to control for potential selection biases or other confounding variables.

Synthesis Methods

When there are insufficient data from any one source or when studies conflict, infor-mation from many good quality studies can be combined to provide probability values for estimating effectiveness. The two major approaches that will be discussed here are meta-analysis and Bayesian methods; expert opinion and consensus panels will be mentioned briefly. For further information on the use of synthesis methods in CEA, the reader is referred to additional sources (Schultz, 1995; Hasselblad and McCrory, 1995; Petitti, 1994; Eddy et al., 1990).

Meta-analysis is a tool for combining and integrating the results of independent studies of an intervention effect (Fleiss and Gross, 1991; Dickersin and Berlin, 1992; Hasselblad and McCrory, 1995). Combining data from a variety of studies can increase the power to detect effects, improve the precision of the estimate of effect size, or address a question not previously posed by the original investigations. To maximize the validity of the results of a meta-analysis, it is suggested that several criteria be fulfilled: (1) All relevant reports should be identified in an exhaustive search of multiple sources; (2) the studies included in the summary should be of good quality, the patient populations similar, the interventions similar, and the outcomes measured in the same manner; (3) homogeneity of effects across studies should be evaluated statistically (Mantel, 1977; Mantel et al., 1977; DerSimonian and Laird, 1986); (4) bias in the selection of studies for inclusion should be controlled; and (5) analyses should be done to evaluate the impact of including or excluding certain studies (Sacks et al., 1987; L'Abbe et al., 1987; Schultz, 1995).

When effect size is not homogeneous across studies, methods that assign weights to studies in less than direct proportion to their sample size should be used. These methods (Dersimonian and Laird, 1986), which are based on the assumption that different studies represent different subpopulations within the population at large, are related to the more general class of methods known under the rubric of *hierarchical models*. These methods recognize that large numbers of small studies contain information about the larger population that is not available from one or two large studies drawn from particular subpopulations.

When results of individual studies are inconclusive, or where large samples are required to demonstrate an effect, meta-analysis can be a useful technique. For example, recent meta-analyses of the effectiveness of breast cancer screening, including analyses for women 40–49 years old, have contributed to changes in practice recommendations (Kerlikowske, 1995; Eddy et al., 1990). It has been demonstrated that, if meta-analysis had been used sooner, the evidence of effectiveness of such interventions as beta blockade after acute myocardial infarction might have been available sooner (Lau et al., 1992).

Meta-analysis is prone to many of the same pitfalls that apply to the study designs described previously. For instance, a meta-analysis of breast self-examination (BSE) in relation to extent of disease at diagnosis found significant improvements in outcome (as measured by tumor size and lymph node metastases) in women practicing BSE compared to those not performing BSE (Hill et al., 1988). Unfortunately, it is not clear from this analysis whether BSE is effective in reducing mortality from breast cancer, since tumor size, and not death, was the outcome, and lead time bias was not examined. (See the section on modeling, below, for further discussion of lead-time bias.)

There is some disagreement about whether unpublished data should be included in a meta-analysis. Negative studies are more likely to be unpublished than positive ones, so meta-analyses relying on published studies could overestimate effectiveness (''publication bias''); however, reasons for excluding unpublished data, such as lack of peer review, are equally valid (Cook, 1993). Meta-analysis is traditionally applied to RCT data; data from observational studies can also be analyzed in this manner if attention is paid to the quality of the studies, particularly their control of confounding (Fleiss and Gross, 1991; Spitzer, 1991). Limitations of the technique include, as noted above, the potential to overestimate effectiveness due to publication bias and biased estimation as a result of poor inclusion/exclusion criteria. These limitations are not confined to meta-analysis: For instance, published reports of primary data, such as RCTs, may overestimate effectiveness as a result of publication bias as well.

Bayesian methods describe the class of meta-analytic techniques that combine empiric data with an explicit use of subjective probability. The confidence profile method (Eddy et al., 1992) is one such method that can be used to estimate a probability distribution of a parameter (or a joint distribution of multiple parameters). Here Bayes' rule is applied to revise prior (subjective) probability distributions for unknown parameters—using the likelihood functions associated with observed data from clinical studies. Both of these components—prior distributions of unknown parameters and likelihood functions for observed data—require subjective judgment on the part of the analyst. Specifically, the analyst is required to assess a prior distribution for each estimated parameter as well as estimates of the probability distributions of the magnitude of bias from each type of study data. For this reason, the end result of a confidence profile analysis may not correspond to the result that would be obtained from a decision maker with different prior judgments. This limitation is also an advantage, however, in that it permits synthesis of a broader range of studies. An example of a Bayesian analysis to express uncertainty about a point estimate of critical outcomes from clinical trial data is found in a recent reanalysis of the results of the Global Utilization of Streptokinase and Tissue Plasminogen Activator in Occluded Arteries (GUSTO) trial (Brophy and Joseph, 1995).

Expert opinion and *consensus panels* are additional synthesis techniques often used to estimate effectiveness, although the process for combining information is left implicitly to the judgment of the expert or panelist. For example, the original Oregon priority list relied upon educated guesses of experts who estimated the ability of particular technologies and practices to improve survival (Klevit et al., 1991). Several parameters in the colon screening model discussed below were estimated using expert clinical opinions (Eddy, 1990b).

Expert judgment should be used sparingly as the basis for probability assessments in CEAs; it should be primarily relegated to situations where no other data sources are available or to variables of secondary importance in the analysis. When expert judgment is used as a data source for effectiveness estimation in a CEA, it should be elicited in a structured way, such as via the Delphi method or other methods for structured elicitation of group judgments (Gustafson et al., 1986) or individual judgments (Poses et al., 1988). Any variables based on expert judgment should be subjected to sensitivity analyses within the CEA. (See Chapter 9 for additional discussion of sensitivity analysis.)

Modeling to Estimate Effectiveness in a CEA

As we have noted previously (Chapter 3), data from the above types of studies will inevitably be incomplete, and the analyst must rely on methods of extrapolation and imputation to estimate the magnitude of health effectiveness in terms useful for CEA. When direct primary or secondary empriical evaluation of effectiveness is not possible, the use of modeling to estimate effectiveness is a valid form of scientific inquiry. Mathematical models developed in order to piece together the aggregate implications of diverse pieces of evidence from multiple epidemiologic sources are tools with which to accomplish these tasks. Models can be used to combine available probability estimates and, when complete data are not available, can be of use in addressing the question of what the data parameters would need to be in order for an intervention to be considered cost-effective.

Types of Models

Models for estimating health-effectiveness may be characterized in terms of several nonmutually exclusive characteristics. First, models must employ an analytic methodology to account for events that occur over time. As discussed below, decision tree models, state-transition models, and other types of dynamic models are different but related mathematical methods that represent the unfolding of a process over time. Second, models may apply to cohorts longitudinally or to populations cross-sectionally. Third, models can be either *deterministic or stochastic* (probablistic); in the former case, the average number of events per population is used, while in the latter case, randomization is used to simulate the probability distributions of events that may occur.

It should be noted that models are often used in drawing inferences from data to address a research question. The data may be drawn from any of the primary or secondary data sources previously discussed. Applying statistical models requires assumptions about the data—for example, that a treatment effect is additive or multiplicative, independent of, or interactive with, confounding variables, constant or variable over time, distributed according to a normal, lognormal, or other distribution, and so forth. Assumptions are made regarding the statistical sampling distributions in clinical studies and the homogeneity of the populations studied. The assumptions made in modeling for cost-effectiveness analysis are made for the same purpose: to simplify the representation of reality to a level which permits insightful analysis useful for decision making.

No model is a perfect representation of reality; its validity rests on whether its assumptions are reasonable in light of the needs and purposes of the decision maker and, importantly, in light of whether, after close examination, its implications make sense.

Analytic methodology

Decision tree models represent the sequence of chance events and decisions over time (Raiffa, 1968; Weinstein et al., 1980; Sox et al., 1988). Each chance event is assigned a probability, often estimated from data in clinical studies. Each path through the decision tree represents one possible sequence of chance and decision events, and is associated with a consequence, which is valued in terms of a utility. Alternative decision strategies, such as screening versus not screening for breast cancer, are evaluated by calculating their average, or *expected utility*. When utility is defined in terms of the number of quality-adjusted life years associated with a consequence, the measure of effectiveness is the *quality-adjusted life expectancy* associated with the strategy. Decision analysis models have been used extensively in the medical literature—for example, to estimate gains in life expectancy from vaccines (Lieu et al., 1994; Willems et al., 1980; Riddiough et al., 1983) and from screening elderly women for breast cancer (Mandelblatt et al., 1992).

One limitation of decision tree models is that they are not well suited to representing recurrent events that repeat over time. In chronic diseases, events such as complications of the chronic disease or its treatment, recurrence of disease, and mortality, are confronted repeatedly during a lifetime, albeit with probabilities that change with time, age, and health status. Rather than model each event as a separate branch of a complex decision tree, modelers rely on more efficient mathematical representations of such events.

State-transition models are one such tool. State-transition models allocate, and subsequently reallocate, members of a population into one of several categories, or *health states*. Health states may be defined according to disease stage, treatment status, or a combination of the two. Transitions occur from one state to another at defined recurring time intervals (usually 1 year, but sometimes 3 months or 1 month for rapidly progressive diseases) according to *transition probabilities*. For example, mortality is represented by the transition probabilities from each other possible state into the state "dead." Transition probabilities can be made dependent on population characteristics, such as age, by specifying the probabilities as functions of these characteristics. Through simulation, or mathematical calculation, the number of members of the population passing through each state at each point in time can be estimated. State-transition models can be used to calculate life expectancy or quality-adjusted life expectancy, depending on whether all states are weighted at 1.0 or according to preference weights. A special type of state-transition model in which the transition probabilities depend only on the current state (and not, for example, on the previous states or the path by which the state was entered) is called a *Markov model* (Beck and Pauker, 1983). State-transition models have been used to estimate outcomes in a large number of cost-effectiveness studies, including coronary heart disease prevention (Weinstein et al., 1987), breast cancer screening (Eddy, 1987a, 1989), cervical cancer screening in the elderly (Fahs et al., 1992), prostate cancer screening (Krahn et al., 1994), hormone replacement therapy (Tosteson et al., 1990), abdominal aneurysm screening (Frame et al., 1993), and osteo-porosis screening (Tosteson et al., 1990). Decision tree models have been augmented in the past decade to include *Markov nodes*—or branching points within the tree that lead into a Markov process—thereby incorporating the capabilities of both decision tree and Markov models (Sonnenberg and Beck 1993). Several computer programs, such as SMLTREE (copyright 1989, J. Hollenberg), DATA (copyright 1994, TreeAge Software, Inc.), and Decision Maker (copyright 1980; 1993, S.G. Pauker, F.A. Son-nenberg, and B. Wong, New England Medical Center, Boston, MA) can be used to construct such models.

Other types of dynamic models are also used to project outcomes. *Difference equa-tions*, for example, are used in epidemic models in which the numbers of susceptible, immune, and infected persons in a population are modified each time period according to an equation that relates the change in the number of persons in each category to the numbers of persons in each category in the preceding time period as well as to variables that may be modified by intervention, such as contact rates and infectivity rates. The effectiveness of AIDS prevention programs has been assessed using difference equation models (Paltiel and Kaplan, 1991).

Longitudinal and cross-sectional models

Longitudinal cohort models estimate effectiveness by calculating expected outcomes for homogeneous cohorts longitudinally through time under alternative programs. This is typically the approach in models based on decision analysis, for which decisions and outcomes for "typical" patients are represented in a decision tree. This is also the approach in models appended to data from clinical trials, where the follow-up period for the arms of the trial are synthetically extended in time until death. The measure of effectiveness in longitudinal models is usually the gain in life expectancy, quality-adjusted life expectancy, or other lifetime measure of health for persons with the char-acteristics specified for the modeled cohort.

Cross-sectional population models track outcomes in a population over time. Often, as in the Coronary Heart Disease (CHD) Policy Model (Weinstein et al., 1987), the population is that of the United States within a specified age range, 35–84 in the case of the CHD Policy Model. The model tracks the health status in the population in each time period, then sums across time to estimate an aggregate measure of health status, such as quality-adjusted person years. The difference between the aggregate health status of the population under alternative programs is the measure of effectiveness.

CAN*TROL is another example of a cross-sectional population model (Eddy, 1986). This deterministic model, designed to evaluate cancer screening programs, requires that the user specify the key information to estimate effectiveness, such as expected stage shifts or improvement in survival curves. The model then computes cancer cases and deaths that would be expected for the specified level of effectiveness. Revisions of this model are in progress (M.L. Brown and A. Potosky, personal communication, 1995).

Population models are best suited to modeling heterogeneous populations, possibly disaggregated by subgroup within the model. They are also useful when measures of aggregate effectiveness or cost are desired, as opposed to effectiveness or cost per person.

Deterministic and stochastic models.

Deterministic models assume certainty about the numbers of health events, while stochastic models use uncertainty explicitly as part of the calculation. For example, suppose that we are interested in the number of people in a cohort of 10,000 that will be dead in 10 years from a particular disease, and suppose further that we know that the annual disease-specific mortality rate is 10% and that the average annual other-cause mortality rate is 1%. We could compute the number that will be dead from the disease directly by multiplying the survival percentages by the number of survivors in each of the 10 years. This is a *deterministic* computation, because the proportion dying in each year is treated as certain. Not only do we assume that the 10% is known to be the mortality rate, but we assume that exactly 10% of persons in the cohort will die of the disease in each year. With more work and the analytic machinery (statistical models) of survival analysis we can compute other summary statistics that might be used as outcomes in a cost-effectiveness analysis (e.g., average number of life years accrued by the cohort over the next 10 years). Decision trees that do not have Markov nodes are generally deterministic models. Some state-transition models may use deterministic computations (e.g., Weinstein et al., 1987; Frame et al., 1993).

Stochastic models, also known as *discrete event simulations*, approach the same calculations differently. In a *first-order* simulation, the individual history of each individual in the cohort is simulated using random numbers to represent chance events. To simulate a 5% chance of death in a given year, the computer is directed to generate a random integer between 1 and 100, and if that integer is 5 or less the computer program tallies the simulated person as dying in that year. Each possible event that affects health outcomes is simulated for each simulated person in this fashion, and summary statistics are computed by cumulating counts of these events over the simulated time span as if there were an omniscient observer recording the cohort results across that time. The number of people in the cohort who are "observed" to live the full 10 years in the simulation is used as an estimate of the number that would be observed were a real study done under conditions of the simulation. Because this represents one possible experimental observation, the entire simulation is repeated many times (usually several thousand) and the counts are averaged across simulation runs. As the number of runs grows large—often into the thousands—these averages approach the values that would be computed by deterministic calculations.

In Chapter 8, we also discuss the role of *second-order* stochastic simulations in performing sensitivity analyses. In second-order simulations, the probabilities them-selves are regarded as uncertain; for example, the 10% mortality rate might actually be the mean of a probability distribution in the range from 0% mortality to 100% mortality. Each replication would represent a random "draw" from the distribution of possible parameter values.

Deterministic calculations have the advantage of being exact. However, if a model is complex, involving many possible events and intervening decisions based on those events, deterministic computations must exhaustively calculate the probability of every possible combination of events and decisions; in problems of even moderate complexity this may involve millions of combinations. Stochastic models are in essence empirical samplings from these combinations, so each combination appears in the final counts in proportion to its likelihood. Further, a deterministic computation may be made hope-lessly complex if it attempts to incorporate characteristics of the individuals being simulated in any detail.

In addition to greater ease of complex simulation, stochastic models have the addi-tional advantage of yielding not only average effects but also measures of the uncer-tainty around the average. For example, the modeler can keep counts of how long each simulated individual survives; from these simulated data, it is then possible to compute not only average life span (i.e., life expectancy) but also a variance for that average or an estimate of the entire distribution of life spans.

The practical disadvantage of stochastic models is computing time; since tens or hundreds of thousands of replications are often needed in order to obtain stable estimates of event probabilities, especially in the presence of infrequent events (e.g., mortality from diagnostic tests or fatal vaccine reactions), even modern computers can be taxed. As electronic technology advances, this latter limitation of stochastic modeling will become less salient, and stochastic simulation models may become more prevalent.

A less obvious limitation of stochastic models is that complex simulations require intricate knowledge in order to estimate the parameters of the simulation, or even to specify the functional forms of the relationships among variables. The most obvious manifestation of this limitation is that we must often assume that two or more events are statistically independent in the simulation, when in real life they may have complex dependencies. For example, the sensitivity of screening mammography (the ability of the examination to pick up true disease) depends on the size of the tumor. Sensitivity is less for in situ cancer than for tumors that are 2 cm in diameter. But it is very difficult to find reliable data from which to estimate sensitivity as a function of tumor size and nature. The modeler may choose to treat sensitivity as a constant or, if not, then must make "ballpark" estimates about this function to use in a discrete event simulation of a mammography screening program that incorporates tumor inception and growth over time. Although stochastic modeling allows incorporation of this complexity, lack of quantitative data on which to build the model may considerably blunt this advantage of the modeling technique. In deterministic modeling this lack of knowledge may be addressed through sensitivity analyses—varying the model parameters through reasonable ranges to observe the effect on the computational results. In stochastic modeling, sensitivity analyses are also used, but performing extensive sensitivity analyses considerably increases the computational time burden.

Choice of modeling technique

As implied above, choice of modeling approach involves a balance of many considerations. Generally it is desirable to use the simplest model possible that captures the level of complexity that is absolutely necessary and for which data are available for describing the model parameters.

To make relatively broad estimates of cost-effectiveness where there exist data from RCTs or observational cohorts linking initial conditions (e.g., a particular screening protocol) to final outcomes of interest, simple deterministic computations may suffice. This may or may not involve a decision tree. For example, Eddy (1989) used deterministic calculations for evaluation of the cost-effectiveness of breast cancer screening; and Grady and colleagues (Grady et al., 1992) used a decision tree model and made deterministic computations. For problems of limited complexity, in which not a great deal of individual differentiation of patients is required, but in which we wish to study an intervention process over time (e.g., where mortality from a disease being screened for is contrasted to other-cause mortality) a deterministically calculated state-transition model may well be used (e.g., Frame et al., 1993).

If we wish to tailor the results more by individual characteristics or to take more complex and numerous events into account, then there may be little option but to use a stochastic approach. Generally the more the modeler wishes to have a ''high fidelity'' representation of a complex process that unfolds over time, the greater the need to use a stochastic approach. However, this must be balanced against availability of data from which to develop critical structures and parameters in the model.

As noted at the beginning of this section, when data are not available, models may still be developed that are useful to address questions concerning what the data parameters would need to be in order for an intervention to be considered cost-effective. (See, for example, Schulman et al., 1991).

Choice of the level of complexity to incorporate (and thus the modeling approach dictated) is at present an art with no hard-and-fast rules. A model is not the real problem; it is an abstract representation of the problem. It must be sufficiently faithful to the problem to be useful, yet not so complex that it goes beyond the data or that it becomes entirely a ''black box'' for intended users (and peer reviewers) who must evaluate how much credence to put in the analytic results. For instance, a model produced using a generic software package such as SMLTREE (copyright 1989, James Hollenberg) may be more readily transparent and reproducible by others than a model developed using the CAN*TROL package (copyright, Eddy, 1986, NCI). However, dedicated models that are well documented may lend themselves more readily to replication, provided that full disclosure of parameter values is available.

Other Issues in Modeling to Estimate Effectiveness in CEA

Several issues that are germane to modeling will be briefly reviewed in this section, including specification of survival parameters, use of disease-specific or total mortality data, modeling patient characteristics, using models to improve program performance, using models to "correct" for lead time and length biases, verification of models, and, finally, peer review of models. Much of this discussion is equally applicable to estimation of effectiveness in CEAs that do not rely primarily on modeling.

Specification of survival parameters

In cost-effectiveness analysis, the effectiveness measure is often life expectancy or some other statistic derived from life tables. In order to calculate life expectancy under a health program, probabilities of survival must be estimated starting at the age of initiation of the program and continuing until death or some arbitrary age horizon. Clinical trials and observational studies typically provide estimates of risk reduction or relative risk during the course of the follow-up period, but they give little indication how to estimate the survival curve for individuals at later ages. Moreover, a clinical trial restricted to a particular demographic or clinical group begs the question of what the effect might be in persons of younger or older ages, in persons of the opposite sex, or in persons with comorbidities that raise their baseline mortality rates (or hazard functions). Thus, the analyst must make assumptions regarding the appropriate basis for extrapolation to populations with varying survival curves. For example, in a recent CEA comparing two thrombolytic therapies for acute myocardial infarction, the analysts used primary data from an RCT (GUSTO) to estimate 1-year survival, but they extended the observation period to 15 years by modeling survival based on a database of CHD patients (Mark et al., 1995).

The simplest assumption to make is that the age-sex-specific hazard function (i.e., the age-sex-specific instantaneous probability of mortality at any point in time) for the affected population is modified by (1) the disease in question, (2) the intervention being evaluated, and (3) any comorbidities that increase or decrease survival relative to the general population. The key choice is often whether these three effects are additive or multiplicative. For example, does coronary heart disease multiply the age-sex-specific mortality rates by a constant amount or does it add a constant amount to the mortality rate? Similarly, does cholesterol reduction reduce the mortality rate proportionally, or does it subtract a constant from it? Sometimes, empirical data can shed light on these questions—for example, if clinical studies have been conducted in different age groups. Often, however, there is insufficient power in clinical studies to infer age-specific effects, so these relationships must be assumed by the analyst in absence of data.

The implications of the choice of an additive versus a multiplicative functional form can be striking (Kuntz and Weinstein, 1995). Additive hazard functions tend to ascribe greater benefit to interventions at younger ages than do multiplicative functions, while the reverse is true for interventions at older ages or in high-risk populations. The reason is that the higher baseline hazard functions in the latter populations are affected more by a multiplicative effect. For example, suppose a clinical trial finds that mortality from a disease in 50-year-old women can be reduced from 0.004 to 0.003 with an intervention. Suppose the baseline mortality at an older age is 0.010. Under the additive assumption, this would be reduced by 0.001 with the intervention, to 0.009. Under the multiplicative assumption, the mortality rate would be reduced by 0.0025 to 0.0075.

Both additive and multiplicative functional forms are widely used. The Cox proportional hazards model of the effects of treatments and other covariates is essentially multiplicative. So is the logistic regression model of the effects of risk factors on mortality and morbidity, as frequently used with data from the Framingham Heart Study in models of cardiovascular interventions (e.g., Weinstein et al., 1987; Goldman et al., 1991; Oster and Epstein, 1987; Weinstein and Stason, 1976; Russell et al., 1995). Psaty and colleagues examined risk factors for cardiovascular disease in the elderly and concluded that some relationships are linear with respect to disease risk, while others are multiplicative (Psaty et al., 1990). The declining exponential approximation to life expectancy model (DEALE) is essentially additive (Beck et al., 1982; Keeler and Bell, 1992).

In cost-effectiveness analyses of prevention, where effects continue over long periods of life, the choice of functional form can be critical and can lead to widely varying results. Therefore, where practical, and where extrapolations to widely varying age and risk groups are made based on point estimates of relative risk, sensitivity analysis with respect to the specification of the model is desirable. This discussion is revisited in Chapter 8.

Disease-specific and all-cause mortality

Estimating length of life is a central problem in CEA. Analysts must use evidence about survival and mortality from many sources. This section discusses the impact of the data that might be used to estimate survival in CEA. The main end-point in many trials is disease-specific mortality—that is, mortality due to the disease addressed by the trial. Analysts rely on these data to calculate differences in life expectancy due to the intervention being studied by the CEA. However, the disease-specific mortality may be only part of the problem. For example, in estimating the effectiveness of cholesterol-lowering drugs in reducing deaths from cardiovascular disease, use of cardiovascular disease-specific mortality will overstate effectiveness compared to the use of all-cause mortality if in fact the intervention also leads to a higher rate of death from other causes (Muldoon et al., 1990; Expert Panel on Detection, Evaluation, and Treatment of High Blood Cholesterol in Adults, 1993).

An additional caveat regarding the use of disease-specific mortality to estimate effectiveness in a CEA concerns misclassification (Brown et al., 1993). In carefully controlled RCTs, where the investigators have drawn careful protocols for attribution of cause of death and can make this determination in follow-up of study participants, the attributed disease-specific mortality rates may be useful inputs to the CEA modeling process. However, in less-controlled studies the recorded cause of death is nonspecific, resulting in an underreporting of disease-specific causes.

The opposite can happen as well. For example, men with known prostate cancer who in fact die of unrelated or distantly related causes may be likely to have the cancer listed as a "contributing cause" on a death certificate simply because they are known to have the disease. If screened men were more likely to have cancer listed as the cause of death than unscreened men, then screening effectiveness would be underestimated in models using disease-specific mortality data.

Thus, in general, it is suggested that all-cause mortality be used as the basis for estimating life-expectancy gains in CEA, especially if source data are from population surveys, cancer registries, and observational studies where rigidly followed detailed protocols for attribution of cause of death are not used. When using trial data where only cause-specific mortality is reported, modeling should be used to take competing causes of mortality into account.

Modeling patient characteristics

Besides survival, other event probabilities in CEA models are often represented as conditional upon patient characteristics, including age, gender, risk factors, stage of disease, and prior morbid events (e.g., Kaplan and Feinstein, 1974; Charlson et al., 1987; Greenfield et al., 1987, 1988, 1993). These probabilities can be estimated separately for relevant subpopulations when data permit, but more often they are specified by an equation derived by assuming a statistical relationship between event probabilities and patient characteristics.

Derivation, or modeling, of subpopulation-specific probabilities presents the analyst with many choices. The predictive equations can be derived using logistic regression, Poisson regression, proportional hazards models, or Bayesian analysis, to name a few techniques. These analyses can assume independence among the characteristics, or they may allow for interactions (e.g., effect modification). They can be additive or multiplicative. The dependent variable can be modeled as the instantaneous or annual event rate, the cumulative event rate over a specified time interval, or the time until occurrence of an event. All of these model specifications have their roles and have been used in cost-effectiveness models.

Using models to vary program parameters

Models have the advantage of providing the user with a number of "dials" and "levers" to manipulate an intervention program in ways that are not possible in real-time experiments with human subjects. Models allow simulation of the effect of starting an intervention, such as breast cancer or cervical cancer screening or cholesterol reduction, at different ages. They enable exploration of the implications of different screening intervals, such as annual, biannual, or triennial cervical screening. They allow simulation of the effects and costs of ending a screening program or chemoprevention program at a given age, such as whether to continue cervical screening or hormone replacement into the ninth decade of life. Models allow examination of the implications of using different cutoff points for screening tests, such as the cholesterol level chosen for initiating dietary or pharmacologic intervention, or the bone mineral density level chosen for initiating treatment for osteoporosis.

Clinical trials cannot possibly compare all important alternative program designs, and yet the critical data obtained from trials must be combined with other evidence in order to optimize a program. Clearly there is a tradeoff between obtaining direct evidence of effects of different program designs and the cost of obtaining such evidence. Models can facilitate the process of squeezing as much information as possible from data in clinical studies.

An example of a situation where a model could be valuable is the case of fecal occult blood test (FOBT) screening for colon cancer. Recently, a 13-year RCT compared a program of annual screening using rehydrated FOBT slides with colonoscopic follow-up of positive tests to a control group without a systematic screening program. The trial demonstrated a statistically significant reduction in colon cancer mortality from 8.8 deaths per 1,000 persons in the nonscreened group to 5.9 deaths per 1,000 persons in the group screened annually. There was no statistically significant reduction in colon cancer mortality at 13 years in persons screened biennially compared to the control group, although trends in the data suggest there may have been a reduction in mortality for the biennial group if the trial were carried farther into the future (Mandel et al., 1993). In order to perform a complete cost-effectiveness analysis of all realistic options, it would be important to compare annual FOBT to biennial screening and to compare FOBT to various endoscopic and radiologic approaches to screening. Furthermore, it would be useful to compare effects in FOBT screening programs that rehydrate slides to effects in programs that do not rehydrate the slides. It is a certainty that trials of all possible protocols will not be conducted; in this setting modeling must be used to simulate alternative protocols if CEAs are to be done for them.

Use of modeling to address lead-time and length biases
Two related types of bias—lead time and length—make it difficult to determine with certainty if a screening intervention is effective in improving outcomes (USPSTF, 1995; Prorok et al., 1981). This section describes these biases and discusses the use of modeling to "correct" estimates of effectiveness for lead-time and length biases.

Lead time in a screening program is the time, in the normal course of disease, between the average time of early diagnosis by screening or case finding, and the average time of diagnosis in the absence of screening. Lead-time bias is an overestimate of the increased survival associated with screening, owing to the fact that the disease is diagnosed earlier in its natural history. In extreme cases, all of the observed increase in survival with screening may be attributable to lead-time bias, and there may be no actual prolongation of life (Morrison, 1992; Black and Welch, 1993).

Lead time may have another consequence that is important for effectiveness estimation: Earlier diagnosis and treatment afforded by screening may result in the patient being exposed to a longer period of adverse treatment effects than would occur in the absence of screening. This result, which is germane, for instance, to cancer screening and treatment, is often not considered in CEAs.

Length bias, another unique problem in assessing prevention interventions, is related to disease biology.[3] Length bias refers to the tendency for slower-growing, less-virulent disease to be detected in a screening program more often than more aggressive disease. This is a consequence of the fact that there is a longer preclinical detectable time (sojourn time) for the less-aggressive disease than for the more virulent form of the disease, providing greater opportunities for the former to be detected in a screening program compared to the latter. As a result, those with aggressive disease are under-represented in screened populations, and patients detected by screening may do better than unscreened patients, regardless of whether screening actually influences outcome. Thus, this bias can also lead to an overestimation of screening effectiveness (USPSTF, 1995; Morrison, 1992).

Models can be used by the analyst to address these biases by modeling the disease process directly. These models generally require more detailed assumptions and estimates of such variables as tumor progression, stage-specific screening sensitivity, and stage-specific treatment response than are directly available from primary data. One simulation model that incorporates disease process modeling to avoid lead time and length biases to the extent possible is the MISCAN model (Habbema, 1984). For examples of this, and other approaches, the reader is referred to other sources (Feuer and Wun, 1992; Chang, 1993; Eddy, 1980, 1989, 1990a,b; Shwartz, 1978, 1981, van Oortmarssen, 1990).

Model Validation

Models are only as good as their ability to represent reality at the level needed to draw useful conclusions; this, in turn, depends on their structure and on the assumptions that go into the models. Models often cannot be validated directly; indeed, if credible data regarding all of a model's outputs of interest were available, there might not be a reason to use the model in the first place.

The results of a model should, therefore, be accompanied by a range of *sensitivity analyses*, as discussed in Chapter 8. The report of the sensitivity analyses should identify which model inputs and parameters exert the most leverage on model outputs. However, some aspects of models, such as which variables are included in the model inputs and their qualitative relationships in the model's structure, are not easily amenable to sensitivity analysis.

Thus, *face validation* of a model may have to rest solely on evaluating the inherent reasonableness of model assumptions as a representation of reality. Ultimately, the users of the model must decide whether the cumulative evidence relevant to judging the model's validity is sufficient to justify its use for the decision makers' purposes. In this regard, users must decide whether the model is sufficiently detailed to capture the important features of the problem. However, complex models for which few or no data exist may have high face validity because they appear to incorporate the complexities of the real problem, but they may be difficult to test for technical accuracy.

The technical accuracy of models must be verified to ensure that the model performs the calculations correctly as claimed. Computer programming errors, data entry errors, and logical inconsistencies in model specification can all lead to errors that should be detected in the verification process. Verification can be accomplished by testing the model under hypothetical conditions in which the results should be obvious and predictable. Examples include extreme assumptions that a treatment has 100% mortality, 0% effectiveness, or 100% effectiveness, or that a screening test has 100% sensitivity. Also, intermediate outputs can be examined to ensure that they are consistent with the data entered. Reports based on models should contain assurances that the model has been verified in this manner.

The *predictive validity* of a model should also be evaluated when data are available to validate intermediate or final numerical predictions. For instance, predictions of cancer models can be compared with data on observed patterns in cancer incidence, staging, and mortality (e.g., Eddy, 1987b). As another example, the Coronary Heart Disease Policy Model (Weinstein et al., 1987) was validated by comparing the model's predictions of coronary heart disease mortality in 1990 with actual mortality data. In doing so, the assumptions in the model, regarding risk factors in the population and the effectiveness of treatments, had to be changed to incorporate new data obtained during the intervening decade since the model was developed. After all, the model cannot be expected to predict future changes in its inputs, only to reflect accurately the relation between its inputs and outputs.

Peer Review of Models

Models are black boxes to those who cannot or choose not to view their inner workings. It is incumbent upon the modeler therefore, to provide for the possibility of peer review and replication by colleagues who are able to examine the inner workings of the model. We return to this discussion in Chapter 9.

For most models, providing the detailed structural assumptions and data for a model is sufficient to permit peer review. Development of structured formats for presenting information about models, including analytic structure, definitions of variables, equations relating variables to one another, and specific data, might be useful as part of a future CEA research agenda.

Occasionally, it may be desirable for electronic copies of the model to be released to peer reviewers. In economics research there is precedent for this type of review, such as the economic modeling replication project conducted by the *Journal of Money and*

Banking, where third parties attempted to replicate the results of previously published articles (DeWald et al., 1986).

Ultimately, the reputation and assurances of the modeler must carry weight to minimize the burden on peer reviewers. Just as the possibility of auditing clinical trial data protects the integrity of clinical investigation, at a minimum, a willingness to release model software and data for peer review under appropriate protection must exist on the part of CEA investigators in order to guarantee the integrity of modeling.

Calculation of Net Effectiveness

The process of calculating the denominator for the C/E requires computation of the net effectiveness of the intervention where net effect is defined as the *magnitude* of the difference in outcome between persons who are subjected to the intervention and persons experiencing the alternative(s) to which the intervention is being compared. This calculation requires the synthesis of the diverse data described here and in Chapter 4 in order to represent the full cascade of events occurring along the continuum from the intervention to the final health outcome observed (usually death). This synthesis involves estimating the probabilities of each health-state outcome and multiplying these probabilities by the values for the health states and the quantity of time spent in the health states in order to yield a summary measure such as QALYs.

In addition, the evaluation of *net* effectiveness of an intervention should consider important potential adverse effects. For instance, thalidomide was effective in reducing emesis in pregnancy but resulted in catastrophic unanticipated abnormalities in offspring. Another example, often overlooked, are the adverse psychological and time costs of false-positive diagnoses in screening programs. In this latter example, however, decrements in utility associated with health states which may be relatively short-lived are less likely to have a major impact on CEA results.

To illustrate the general process of completing this final step to calculate the denominator of the C/E ratio, this section presents a summary of the methods used to estimate effectiveness in a CEA of interventions intended to lower serum cholesterol in adults. An in-depth presentation of the analysis is contained in Appendix C. Briefly, the analysis compares several strategies to reduce cholesterol—involving diet, niacin, and lovastatin—in various subgroups defined by serum lipid levels, prior history of coronary heart disease (CHD), other coronary risk factors, age, and sex. As an additional comparator strategy, a status quo alternative was based on the assumption that existing patterns of serum cholesterol would continue. The analysis uses secondary data to model the impact of these alternative cholesterol-lowering strategies on quality-adjusted all-cause mortality among different age, sex, and risk groups in the U.S. population. This approach was selected since the large sample and long period of observation that would be required for a primary cost-effectiveness trial make such a trial highly unlikely.

The analysis defines and follows a cascade of effects: (1) from intervention to cholesterol changes; (2) from cholesterol changes to changes in CHD incidence; (3) from CHD incidence to mortality and morbidity; and (4) from changes in mortality and morbidity to changes in (a) life years lived, (b) health-related quality of life, and (c) cost.

1. *From intervention to cholesterol changes.* The proximal effects of interventions were measured in terms of changes in serum low-density lipoprotein cholesterol (LDL) and serum high-density lipoprotein cholesterol (HDL). Except for the estimation of effects of lovastatin from one RCT (Bradford et al., 1991), no one study was sufficiently powered to estimate effects of other strategies for all age, risk, and/or gender groups. Thus, percent changes in HDL and LDL associated with the use of diet and niacin were estimated by performing a meta-analysis of published clinical studies. Guided by the criteria described earlier in the chapter for considering the quality of the evidence of effectiveness for use in a CEA, the general approach included the identification and selection of the best available data that were relevant to the populations of interest. For instance, studies included in the estimation of the effectiveness of diet were limited to those conducted with community populations consuming routine step 1 diets (i.e., not patients on metabolic wards, or persons using special prepared foods). However, in assessing the effects of niacin, since few studies presented data for the unique effects of niacin (i.e., absent other antihyperlipemic medication) on LDL, HDL, and total cholesterol (TC), all possible data were considered for inclusion.

   Treatment failures, compliance, and treatment crossovers are included in the analysis by estimating cholesterol changes on an intention to treat basis. In other words, the cholesterol change associated with a treatment strategy is based on the mean change resulting from a range of possible treatment changes and discontinuations. For example, a certain proportion of persons started on niacin are assumed to experience intolerable side effects, such as flushing, and to either switch to lovastatin or discontinue medication. The probabilities of these events, and all other events, were estimated by reviewing the best quality data available for each treatment regimen. The cholesterol changes associated with the niacin strategy were then estimated as the weighted average (i.e., a product of the probabilities) of the changes associated with each pattern of treatment (continuation on niacin, switch to lovastatin, or discontinue medication).

2. *From cholesterol changes to CHD incidence.* The changes in LDL and HDL were then used as inputs into the Coronary Heart Disease Policy Model, a deterministic, state-transition model of CHD in the U.S. adult population (Weinstein et al., 1987). State-transition probabilities were again estimated using the best data available in the literature. The model uses

logistic regression equations to predict age-sex-specific rates of CHD incidence, conditional upon LDL, HDL, and other risk factors, in persons previously free of CHD. (Persons with previous CHD are handled separately, as described below.) The logistic regression equations are based largely on data from the Framingham Heart Study and are calibrated to match national CHD incidence rates. In each simulated calendar year, a certain number of persons within each risk-factor stratum are estimated to develop CHD. Thus, these regressions are used to combine data to estimate probabilities needed for the model.

3. *From CHD incidence to mortality and morbidity.* Conditional on a new CHD event, the model first allocates patients to various presenting CHD events, including cardiac arrest, myocardial infarction, and angina pectoris, based on data from the clinical literature. Cardiac arrests and myocardial infarctions, also estimated from the literature, are each associated in the model with 30-day mortality rates. Then a part of the model called the Disease History submodel assigns patients with various CHD histories to new events in each calendar year, including subsequent cardiac arrests, myocardial infarctions, and coronary revascularization procedures (bypass surgery and angioplasty). Each of these events, in turn, has an associated case-fatality rate and has implications for future event rates. Thus, in each calendar year, the model keeps a tally of the numbers of persons experiencing each type of cardiac event, the numbers of persons dying of CHD, as well as the numbers of persons with each possible history of cardiac events.

In addition to counting CHD deaths secondary to CHD events and chronic CHD states, the model also counts non-CHD deaths associated with age and sex. In the Reference Case analysis example, presented in Appendix C, the effect of cholesterol change was assumed to be limited to CHD incidence, and resulting CHD mortality, with no direct effect on non-CHD mortality (except by the process of competing risks). The effect on non-CHD mortality was assumed to be zero based on results from published research (Scandinavian Simvastatin Survival Study Group, 1994; Gould et al., 1995). However, due to lingering controversy over the possible adverse effects of lower total cholesterol on non-CHD mortality (Jacobs et al., 1992; Expert Panel on Detection, Evaluation, and Treatment of High Blood Cholesterol in Adults, 1993), a sensitivity analysis examined the possibility of a direct link between total cholesterol change and non-CHD mortality.

Persons with previous CHD events are modeled entirely within the Disease History submodel. The effect of cholesterol reduction in such persons is modeled by assuming the same percent change in CHD events that is implied by the logistic regression equations.

4(a). *From mortality to life years.* As described above, the model counts the numbers of CHD deaths and non-CHD deaths, by age and sex, in each calendar year following the initiation of each preventive intervention strategy (including the "status quo" strategy). The model thus calculates the number of person years lived by each population subgroup under each treatment strategy. However, before these life years can be used in the denominator of the C/E ratio to make comparisons between the differing strategies, each person year in the model is quality-adjusted, as described below.

4(b). *From morbidity and disease history to health-related quality of life.* The Disease History submodel of the CHD Policy Model consists of a large number of "states"—defined according to age, sex, and CHD history— and "events" which may occur in any year, including cardiac arrest, myocardial infarction, and coronary revascularization. CHD history, in turn, is defined by the presence or absence of a prior cardiac arrest, myocardial infarction, or coronary revascularization.

Every person year is assigned a health-related quality of life (HRQL) weight associated with the state in which it is spent, but averaged together with the (lower) short-term HRQL weight associated with the short-term event during that year. Thus, for example, a year of life experienced by a person with a history of angina only (no prior myocardial infarction, cardiac arrest, or revascularization), but who undergoes a coronary bypass procedure during a given year, would be assigned a weight corresponding to the state "angina," averaged together with the short-term weight associated with the event "coronary bypass surgery," where the averaging reflects an estimate of the mean duration of the short-term event and its recovery as a fraction of 1 year.

Since the "states" and "events" in the model do not correspond to classification systems for which HRQL weights are available, it was necessary to "map" the set of CHD states in the model to a standard system of health states. This was done by means of a two-stage procedure. In the first stage, data from the Framingham Heart study were used to estimate the proportions of persons in each model "state" who were experiencing angina pectoris and/or congestive heart failure (CHF). These two conditions were singled out because they were judged to be the chronic CHD-related conditions that most affect HRQL.

In the second stage, weights (from zero to one) were assigned to time spent with angina and CHF. For this example, these weights were based on pooling time-tradeoff utilities from two surveys of CHD patients (Ed Guadnagoli and Paul Cleary, personal communication, 1995; Fryback et al., 1993), stratified according to whether they were experiencing angina and/ or CHF; persons not experiencing angina or CHF are assumed to have the average utility of persons without these conditions (i.e., a utility less than

    1). For sensitivity analyses, several approaches are considered. They are discussed more fully in Appendix C.

4(c). *From morbidity to treatment cost.* Each "event" in the CHD Policy Model is assigned a unit cost, based largely, but not exclusively, on Medicare data. In addition, each person year spent in a CHD "state" is assigned an annual cost estimated from similar data. Since the model counts numbers of person years in each CHD state, as well as numbers of CHD events in each calendar year, it is able to calculate the total CHD-related cost, over time, in each subpopulation and under each treatment strategy. Age-specific estimates of non-CHD costs are also used to estimate "unrelated health care costs" for all persons in the model. All of these cost streams are then combined with the cost of the cholesterol-lowering intervention in each group to estimate total cost. Thus, the calculation of expected costs for each intervention is linked to the intermediate clinical events predicted by the model.

Conclusion

This chapter began by noting that a calculation of net effectiveness for the denominator of the C/E ratio involves accounting for the many events that follow from the decision to intervene with patients or populations. These events link in a chain that eventually influences health outcomes. As can be seen in the above overview example (and in more depth in Appendix C), estimates of net effectiveness will rarely be based on the direct empirical results from a single well-designed study that collects all of the outcomes of interest for the alternatives to be analyzed. Much more frequently, the process of estimating effectiveness will be one of constructing models that combine diverse information from across the medical literature. To estimate the cost-effectiveness of several strategies intended to lower cholesterol, the example here combines data on effectiveness, event probability, patient (and population) utilities for the observed outcomes, and costs from a variety of sources, including prospective randomized studies, longitudinal cohort studies, cross-sectional surveys, published vital statistics, and expert clinical opinion. To compute net effectiveness, these data elements were linked using a complex deterministic state-transition model as the "engine" to simulate various cholesterol lowering strategies.

    Our purpose in reviewing not only experimental and nonexperimental designs, but also in spending a good deal of time reviewing modeling methods for this chapter, was to draw attention to the fact that much of the contemporary CEA process relies on modeling. While in the future we may see more studies that are designed specifically to collect some or all of the primary data needed for a CEA (Revicki and Luce, 1995), we are likely to continue to rely on approaches that combine primary and secondary data in mathematical models.

    Computing net effectiveness is becoming an increasingly sophisticated and complex process. We have tried here to provide some initial insights into the scope, complexity, and common pitfalls of estimating effectiveness for use in CEA.

Recommendations

The following are the summary recommendations of the panel for evaluating and estimating the effectiveness of health care interventions in CEAs:

1. When designing primary data collection efforts, or deriving the necessary probability estimates from secondary data sources for estimation of effectiveness in a CEA, outcome probability values should be selected from the best designed (and least biased) sources that *are relevant to the question and population under study.*
2. Evidence for effectiveness may be obtained from RCTs, observational data, uncontrolled experiments, descriptive series, and expert opinion.
2.1. Good-quality meta-analysis and other synthesis methods can be used to estimate effectiveness where any one study has insufficient power to detect effects or where results conflict.
2.2. Expert judgment should only be used to fill in values where no adequate data sources exist or when the parameter is of secondary importance in the analysis.
3. Where direct primary or secondary empirical evaluation of effectiveness is not possible (for example, in important subpopulations or in differing time frames), the use of modeling to estimate effectiveness is a valid mode of scientific inquiry.
4. Evaluation of effectiveness should incorporate both benefits and harms of alternative interventions.

Research Recommendation

1. If an intervention is deemed of sufficient importance because it addresses a condition with a high burden of illness, or because of its high cost, and where sufficient good-quality data do not exist, additional RCTs or large-scale observational studies should be supported.

Notes

Acknowledgments: Dr. Mandelblatt's work on this chapter was supported, in part, by grant #RO1 HS08395, "Care, Costs, and Outcomes of Breast Cancer in the Elderly," from the Agency for Health Care Policy and Research.

1. Lead-time bias refers to the erroneous finding of improved survival after detection, which is the result of an earlier diagnosis rather than a true prolongation of life. Length bias refers to

the tendency for slower growing, less virulent disease to be detected more often by screening than aggressive disease.

2. The Surveillance, Epidemiology and End-Results (SEER) Registry is maintained by the Division of Cancer Prevention and Control of the National Cancer Institute, National Institutes of Health, Public Health Service, U.S. Department of Health and Human Services.

3. Overdetection (or overdiagnosis) bias is a special type of length bias. Overdetection bias occurs when persons with a disease or condition that is likely to ordinarily escape medical attention (e.g., one which is mild or asymptomatic) are under more frequent medical surveillance than persons without the condition.

References

Albertsen, P.C., D.G. Fryback, B.E. Storer, T.F. Kolon, and J. Fine. 1995. Long-term survival among men with conservatively treated localized prostate cancer. *JAMA* 274(8):626–631.

Andersson, I., K. Aspegren, L. Janzon, T. Landberg, K. Lindholm, F. Linell, O. Lungberg, J. Ranstam, and B. Sigfússon. 1988. Mammographic screening and mortality from breast cancer: The Malmö mammographic screening trial. *BMJ* 297:943–48.

Baines, C.J. 1994. The Canadian national breast screening study: A perspective on criticisms. *Ann Intern Med* 120:326–34.

Banta, H.D., C.J. Behney, and J.S. Willems. 1981. *Toward rational technology in medicine*. Vol 5. New York: Springer Publishing.

Banta, H.D., and B.R. Luce. 1993. *Health care technology and its assessment*. Oxford: Oxford Medical Publications.

Bassett, T., and N. Krieger. 1986. Social class and black-white differences in breast cancer survival. *Am J Public Health* 76:1400–1403.

Beck, J.R., and S.G. Pauker. 1983. The Markov process in medical prognosis. *Med Decis Making* 3:419–58.

Beck, J.R., S.G. Pauker, J.E. Gottlieb, K. Klein, and J.P. Kassirer. 1982. A convenient approximation of life expectancy (the ''DEALE''). II. Use in medical decision-making. *Am J Med* 73:889–97.

Black, W.C., and H.G. Welch. 1993. Advances in diagnostic imaging and overestimations of disease prevalence and the benefits of therapy. *N Engl J Med* 328:1237–43.

Bradford, R.H., C.L. Shear, A.N. Chremos, C. Dujovne, M. Downtown, F.A. Franklin, A.L. Gould, M. Hesney, J. Higgins, D.P. Hurley, A. Langendorfer, D.T. Nash, J.L. Pool and H. Schnaper. 1991. Expanded clinical evaluation of Lovastatin (EXCEL) study results: I. Efficacy in modifying plasma lipoproteins and adverse event profile in 8245 patients with moderate hypercholesterolemia. *Arch Intern Med* 151:43–9.

Brophy, J.M., and L. Joseph. 1995. Placing trials in context using Bayesian analysis. GUSTO revisited by Reverend Bayes. *JAMA* 273:871–75.

Brown, M.L. National Cancer Institute. Electronic mail exchange, February 1995.

Brown, M.L. and A. Potosky. National Cancer Institute, Electronic mail exchange, February 1995.

Brown, M.L., C. Brauner, and M.C. Minnotte. 1993. Noncancer deaths in white adult cancer patients. *J Natl Cancer Inst* 85:979–87.

Chang, P. 1993. A simulation study of breast cancer epidemiology and detection since 1982: The case for limited malignant potential lesions. Ph.D. diss., Department of Industrial Engineering, University of Wisconsin–Madison.

Charlson, M.E., P. Pompei, K.L. Ales, and C.R. MacKenzie. 1987. A new method of classifying prognostic comorbidity in longitudinal studies: development and validation. *J Chron Dis* 40:373–83.

Cohn, L.H., C.M. Boyden, and J.J. Collins. 1975. Improved long-term survival after aortocoronary artery disease. *Am J Surg* 129:380–85.

Colton, T. 1974. *Statistics in medicine.* Boston: Little, Brown.

Conner, R.J., P.C. Prorok, and D.L. Weed. 1991. The case-control design and the assessment of the efficacy of cancer screening. *J Clin Epidemiol* 44:1215–21.

Cook, D.J., G.H. Guyatt, G. Ryan, J. Clifton, L. Buckingham, A. Willan, W. McIlroy, and A.D. Oxman. 1993. Should unpublished data be included in meta-analyses? *JAMA* 269:2749–53.

DerSimonian, R., and N. Laird. 1986. Meta-analysis in clinical trials. *Control Clin Trials* 7:177–89.

Detsky, A.S. 1989. Are clinical trials a cost-effective intervention? *JAMA* 262:1795–1800.

DeWald, W.G., J.G. Thursby, and R.G. Anderson. 1986. Replication in empirical economics: The journal of money, credit and banking project. *American Economic Review* 76:587–603.

Dickersin, K., and J.A. Berlin. 1992. Meta-analysis: State-of-the-science. *Epidemiol Rev* 14:154–76.

Eddy, D.M. 1990a. Screening for cervical cancer. *Ann Intern Med* 113:214–16.

Eddy, D.M. 1990b. Screening for colorectal cancer. *Ann Intern Med* 113:373–84.

Eddy, D.M. 1989. Screening for breast cancer. *Ann Intern Med* 111:389–99.

Eddy, D.M. 1987a. *Breast cancer screening for Medicare beneficiaries: Effectiveness, costs to Medicare and medical resources required.* Washington, DC: U.S. Congress, Office of Technology Assessment Health Program.

Eddy, D.M. 1987b. The frequency of cervical cancer screening. Comparison of a mathematical model with empirical data. *Cancer* 60:1117–22.

Eddy, D. 1986. A computer-based model for designing cancer control strategies. In *Cancer control objectives for the nation: 1985–2000,* ed. P.G. Greenwald and E.J. Sondik. NIH Publication No. 86-2880, Number 2.

Eddy, D.M. 1980. *Screening for cancer: Theory, analysis and design.* Englewood Cliffs, NJ: Prentice-Hall.

Eddy, D.M., V. Hasselblad, and R. Schachter. 1992. *Meta-analysis by the confidence profile method: The statistical synthesis of evidence.* Boston: Academic Press.

Eddy, D.M., V. Hasselblad, and R. Schachter. 1990. A Bayesian method for synthesizing evidence: The confidence profile method. *Int J Technol Assess Health Care* 6:31–55.

El-Sadr, W. and L. Capps. 1992. The challenge of minority recruitment in clinical trials for AIDS. *JAMA* 267:954–57.

Expert Panel on Detection, Evaluation, and Treatment of High Blood Cholesterol in Adults. 1993. Summary of the second report of the National Cholesterol Education Program (NCEP) expert panel on detection, evaluation, and treatment of high blood cholesterol in adults (Adult Treatment Panel II). *JAMA* 269:3015–23.

Ezzati, T.M., J.T. Massey, J. Waksberg, A. Chu, and K.R. Maurer. 1992. Sample design: Third National Health and Nutrition Examination Survey. *Vital Health Stat 2* 113:1–35.

Fahs, M., J. Mandelblatt, C. Schechter, and C. Muller. 1992. The costs and effectiveness of cervical cancer screening in the elderly. *Ann Intern Med* 117:520–27.

Feuer, E.J., and L.M. Wun. 1992. How much of the recent rise in breast cancer incidence can be explained by increases in mammography utilization? A dynamic population model approach. *Am J Epidemiol* 136:1423–36.

Fleiss, J.L., and A.J. Gross. 1991. Meta-analysis in epidemiology, with special reference to studies of the association between exposure to environmental tobacco smoke and lung cancer: A critique. *J Clin Epidemiol* 44:127–39.

Frame, P.S., D.G. Fryback, and C. Patterson. 1993. Screening for abdominal aortic aneurysm in men ages 60 to 80 years. A cost-effectiveness analysis. *Ann Intern Med* 119:411–16.

Fryback, D.G. 1978. Bayes' theorem and conditional non-independence of data in medical diagnosis. *Comput Biomed Res* 11:423–34.

Fryback, D.G., E.J. Dasbach, R. Klein, B.E.K. Klein, N. Dorn, K. Peterson, and P.A. Martin. 1993. The Beaver Dam health outcomes study: Initial catalog of health-state quality factors. *Med Decis Making* 13:89–102.

Goldman, L., M.C. Weinstein, P.A. Goldman, and L.W. Williams. 1991. Cost-effectiveness of HMG-CoA reductase inhibition for primary and secondary prevention of coronary heart disease. *JAMA* 265:1145–51.

Goodwin, J.S., W.C. Hunt, C.G. Humble, C.R. Key, and J.M. Samet. 1988. Cancer treatment protocols. Who gets chosen? *Arch Intern Med* 148:2258–60.

Gould, A.L., J.E. Rossouw, N.C. Santanello, J.F. Heyse, and C.D. Furberg. 1995. Cholesterol reduction yields clinical benefit: A new look at old data. *Circulation* 91:2274–82.

Grady, D., S.M. Rubin, D.B. Petitti, C.S. Fox, D. Black, B. Ettinger, V.L. Ernster, and S.R. Cummings. 1992. Hormone therapy to prevent disease and prolong life in postmenopausal women. *Ann Intern Med* 117:1016–37.

Greenfield, S., G. Apolone, B.J. McNeil, and P.D. Cleary. 1993. The importance of co-existent disease in the occurrence of postoperative complications and one-year recovery in patients undergoing total hip replacement. *Med Care* 31:141–54.

Greenfield, S., H.U. Aronow, R.M. Elashoff, and D. Watanabe. 1988. Flaws in mortality data. The hazards of ignoring co-morbid disease. *JAMA* 260:2253–5.

Greenfield, S., D.M. Blanco, R.M. Elashoff, and P.A. Ganz. 1987. Patterns of care related to age of breast cancer patients. *JAMA* 257:2766–70.

Guadnagoli, E. and P. Cleary. Principal Investigators, Acute Myocardial Infarction Patient Outcomes Research Team. Telephone conversation, July 1995.

Gustafson, D.H., D.G. Fryback, J.H. Rose, V. Yick, C.T. Prokop, D.E. Detmer, and J. Moore. 1986. A decision theoretic methodology for severity index development. *Med Decis Making* 6(1):27–35.

Habbema, J.D.F., G.J. van Oortmarssen, J.T.H.N. Lubbe, and P.J. van der Maas. 1984. The MISCAN simulation program for the evaluation of screening for disease. *Comput Methods Programs Biomed* 20:79–93.

Hasselblad, V., and D.C. McCrory. 1995. Meta-analytic tools for medical decision making: A practical guide. *Med Decis Making* 15:81–96.

Hill, D., V. White, D. Jolley, and K. Mapperson. 1988. Self examination of the breast: Is it beneficial? Meta-analysis of studies investigating breast self examination and extent of disease in patients with breast cancer. *BMJ* 207:271–5.

Hunter, C.P., R.W. Frelick, A.R. Feldman, A.R. Bavier, W.H. Dunlap, L. Ford, D. Henson, D. MacFarlane, C.R. Smart, R. Yancik, and J.W. Yates, 1987. Selection factors in clinicial trials: Results from the community clinical oncology program physician's patient log. *Cancer Treat Rep* 71:559–65.

Hunter, C.P., C.K. Redmond, V.W. Chen, D.F. Austin, R.R. Greenberg, P. Correa, H.B. Muss, M.R. Forman, M.N. Wesley, R.S. Blacklow, R.J. Kurman, J.J. Dignam, B.K. Edwards, S. Shapiro, and other members of the Black/White Cancer Survival Group. 1993. Breast cancer: Factors associated with stage at diagnosis in black and white women. *J Natl Cancer Inst* 85:1129–37.

Ingram, D.D., and D.M. Makuc. 1994. Statistical issues in analyzing the NHANES I epidemiologic followup study. *Vital Health Stat 2* 121:1–30.

Jacobs, D., H. Blackburn, M. Higgins, D. Reed, H. Iso, G. McMillan, J. Neaton, J. Nelson, J. Potter, and B. Rifkind. 1992. Report of the conference on low blood cholesterol: Mortality associations. *Circulation* 86:1046–60.

Kaplan, M.H., and A.R. Feinstein. 1974. The importance of classifying initial co-morbidity in evaluating the outcome of diabetes mellitus. *J Chron Dis* ;27:387–404.

Keeler, E., and R. Bell. 1992. New DEALEs: Other approximations of life expectancy. *Med Decis Making* 12:307–11.

Kerlikowske, K., D. Grady, S.M. Rubin, C. Sandrock, and V.L. Ernester. 1995. Efficacy of screening mammography. A meta-analysis. *JAMA* 273:149–54.

Klevit, H.D., A.C. Bates, T. Castanares, E.P. Kirk, P.R. Sipes-Metzler, and R. Wopat. 1991. Prioritization of health care services. A progress report by the Oregon Health Services Commission. *Arch Intern Med* 151:912–6.

Krahn, M.D., J.E. Mahoney, M.H. Eckman, J. Trachtenberg, S.G. Pauker, and A.S. Detsky. 1994. Screening for prostate cancer. A decision analytic view. *JAMA* 272:773–80.

Kramer, B.S., M.L. Brown, P.C. Prorok, A.L. Potosky, and J.K. Gohagan. 1993. Prostate cancer screening: What we know and what we need to know. *Ann Intern Med* 119:914–23.

Krumholz, H., R.C. Pasternak, M.C. Weinstein, G.C. Friesinger, P.M. Ridker, A.N. Tosteson, and L. Goldman. 1992. Cost effectiveness of thrombolytic therapy with streptokinase in elderly patients with suspected acute myocardial infarction. *N Engl J Med* 327:7–13.

Kuntz, K.M. and M.C. Weinstein. 1995. Life expectancy biases in clinical decision modeling. *Med Decis Making* 15:158–169.

L'Abbé, K.A., A.S. Detsky, and K. O'Rourke. 1987. Meta-analysis in clinical research. *Ann Intern Med* 107:224–33.

Lando, H.A., T.F. Pechacek, P.L. Pirie, D.M. Murray, M.B. Mittelmark, E. Lichtenstein, F. Nothwehrs, and C. Gray. 1995. Changes in adult cigarette smoking in the Minnesota Heart Health Program. *AJPH* 85:201–8.

Lang, C.A., and D.F. Ransohoff. 1994. Fecal occult blood screening for colorectal cancer. Is mortality reduced by chance selection for screening colonoscopy? *JAMA* 271:1011–13.

Lau, J., E.M. Antman, J. Jimenez-Silva, B. Kupelnick, F. Mosteller, and T.C. Chalmers. 1992. Cumulative meta-analysis of therapeutic trials for myocardial infarction. *N Engl J Med* 327:248–54.

Laupacis, A., D. Feeny, A.S. Detsky, and P.X. Tugwell. 1992. How attractive does a new technology have to be to warrent adoption and utilization? Tentative guidelines for using clinical and economic evaluations. *Can Med Assoc J* 146:473–81.

Leape, L.L. 1990. Practice guidelines and standards: An overview. *Quality Review Bulletin* 16(2):42–49.

Leape, L.L. and R.H. Brook. 1990. *RAND Corporation Appropriateness Rating Program: Context and purpose.* Paper presented at Workshop to Improve Group Judgement for Medical Practice and Techology Assessment sponsored by the Council of Health Care Techology, Division of Health Care Services, Institute of Medicine, 15–16 May, Washington, DC.

Lieu, T.A., S.L. Cochi, S.B. Black, M.E. Halloran, H.R. Shinefield, S.J. Holmes, M. Wharton, and A.E. Washington. 1994. Cost-effectiveness of a routine varicella vaccination program for US children. *JAMA* 271:375–81.

Lipid Research Clinics Program. 1984. The Lipid Research Clinics Coronary Primary Prevention Trials results, I. Reduction in incidence of coronary heart disease. *JAMA* 251:251–64.

Mandel, J.S., J.H. Bond, T.R. Church, D.C. Snover, G.M. Bradely, L.M. Schuman, and F. Ederer.

1993. Reducing mortality from colorectal cancer by screening for fecal occult blood. Minnesota Colon Cancer Control Study. *N Engl J Med* 328:1365–71.

Mandelblatt, J., H. Andrew, J. Kerner, A. Zauber, and W. Burnett. 1991. Determinants of late stage diagnosis of breast and cervical cancer: The impact of age, race, social class, and hospital type. *Am J Public Health* 81:646–49.

Mandelblatt, J.S., M.E. Wheat, M. Monane, R. Moshief, J. Hollenberg, and J. Tang. 1992. Breast cancer screening for elderly women with and without co-morbid conditions: A decision model. *Ann Intern Med* 116:722–30.

Mantel, N. 1977. Tests and limits for the common odds ratio of several 2 x 2 contingency tables: Methods in analogy to the Mantel-Haenszel procedure. *J Stat Plann Inf* 1:179–89.

Mantel, N., C. Brown, and D.P. Byar. 1977. Tests for homogeneity of effect in an epidemiologic investigation. *Am J Epidemiol* 106:125–29.

Mark, D.B., M.A. Hlatky, R.M. Califf, C.D. Naylor, D. Phil, K.L. Lee, P.W. Armstrong, G. Barbash, H. White, M.L. Simoons, C.L. Nelson, N. Clapp-Channing, J.P. Knight, F.E. Horrell, J. Simes, and E.J. Topol. 1995. Cost effectiveness of thrombolytic therapy with tissue plasminogen activator as compared with streptokinase for acute myocardial infarction. *N Engl J Med* 332:1418–24.

Massey, J.T., T.F. Moore, V.L. Parsons, and W. Tadros. 1989. Design and estimation for the National Health Interview Survey, 1985–94. *Vital Health Stat 2* 110

Miller, A.B., C.J. Baines, T. To, and C. Wall. 1992a. Canadian National Breast Screening Study: 1. Breast cancer detection and death rates among women aged 40 to 49 years. *Can Med Assoc J* 147:1459–76.

Miller, A.B., C.J. Baines, T. To, and C. Wall. 1992b. Canadian National Breast Screening Study: 2. Breast cancer detection and death rates among women aged 50 to 59 years. *Can Med Assoc J* 147:1477–88.

Morrison, A.S. 1992. *Screening in chronic disease.* 2d ed. New York: Oxford University Press.

Morrison, A.S. 1982. Case definition in case-control studies of the efficacy of screening. *Am J Epidemiol* 115:6–8.

Mosteller, F. 1985. *Assessing medical technologies.* Institute of Medicine, Committee for Evaluating Medical Technologies in Clinical Use. Washington, DC: National Academy Press.

Muldoon, M.F., S.B. Manuck, and K.A. Matthews. 1990. Lowering cholesterol concentrations and mortality: A quantitative review of primary prevention trials. *BMJ* 301:309–14.

Office of Statistics and Data Management, Bureau of Data Management and Strategy. 1995. *Public Use Files Catalog.* Baltimore, MD. Health Care Financing Administration.

Office of Technology Assessment (OTA), U.S. Congress. 1995. *Identifying health technologies that work: Five background papers.* BP-H-142. Washington, DC: U.S. GPO.

Office of Technology Assessment (OTA), U.S. Congress. 1994. *Identifying health technologies that work: Searching for evidence.* OTA-H-608 Washington, DC: U.S. GPO.

Oster, G., and A.M. Epstein. 1987. Cost-effectiveness of antihyperlipemic therapy in the prevention of coronary heart disease. *JAMA* 258:2381–7.

Paltiel, A.D., and E.H. Kaplan. 1991. Modeling zidovudine therapy: a cost-effectiveness analysis. *J Acquir Immune Defic Syndr* 4:795–804.

Park, R.E., A. Fink, R.H. Brook, M.R. Chassin, K.L. Kahn, N.J. Mernck, J. Kosecoff, and D.H. Solomon. 1986. Physician ratings of appropriate indicators for six medical and surgical procedures. *Am J Pub Health* 76:766–72.

Petitti, D.B. 1994. *Meta-analysis, decision analysis, and cost-effectiveness analysis: Methods for quantitative synthesis in medicine.* Oxford: Oxford University Press.

Poses, R.M., R.D. Cebul, and R.M. Centor. 1988. Evaluating physicians' probabilistic judgments. *Med Decis Making* 8:233–40.

Prorok, P.C., B.F. Hankey, and B.N. Bundy. 1981. Concepts and problems in the evaluation of screening programs. *J Chron Dis* 34:159–71.

Psaty, B.M., T.D. Koepsell, T.A. Manolio, W.T. Longstreth, Jr., E.H. Wagner, P.W. Wahl, and R.A. Kronmal. 1990. Risk ratios and risk differences in estimating the effect of risk factors for cardiovascular disease in the elderly. *J Clin Epidemiol* 43:961–70.

Raiffa, H. 1968. *Decision analysis: Introductory lectures on choices under uncertainty.* Reading, MA: Addison-Wesley Publishing Company.

Revicki D.A., and B.R. Luce. 1995. Methods of pharmacoeconomic evaluation of medical treatments in psychiatry. *Psychopharmacology Bulletin* 31:57–65.

Riddiough , M.A., J.E. Sisk, And J.C. Bell. 1983. Influenza vaccination: Cost- effectiveness and public policy. *JAMA* 249:3189–95.

Russell, L.R., W.C. Taylor, R. Jagannathan, and E. Milan. 1995. What statistical model best describes heart disease risk? Evidence from the NHANES I epidemiologic follow-up study. In *The Risk and Risk factor Modeling Project: Final report.* Prepared for the Agency for Health Care Policy and Research, U.S. Public Health Service, grant HS 07002.

Sacks, H.S., J. Berrier, D. Teitman, V.A. Ancona-Berk, and T.C. Chalmers. 1987. Meta-analysis of randomized controlled trials. *N Engl J Med* 316:450–55.

Scandinavian Simvastatin Survival Study Group. 1994. Randomised trial of cholesterol lowering in 4444 patients with coronary heart disease: the Scandinavian Simvastatin Survial Study (4S). *Lancet* 344:1383–89.

Schulman, K.A., H.A. Glick, H. Rubin, and J.M. Eisenberg. 1991. Cost-effectiveness of HA-1A monoclonal antibody for gram-negative sepsis. *JAMA* 266:3466–71.

Schultz, K.F. 1995. Empirical evidence of bias: Dimensions of methodological quality associate with estimates of treatment effects in controlled trials. *JAMA* 273:408–18.

Selby, J.V. 1992. A case-control study of screening sigmoidoscopy and mortality from colorectal cancer. *N Engl J Med* 326:653–57.

Shapiro, S., W. Venet, P. Strax, L. Venet, and R. Roeser. 1982. Ten- to fourteen-year effect of screening on breast cancer mortality. *J Natl Cancer Inst* 69:349–55.

Shwartz, M. 1981. Validation and use of a mathematical model to estimate the benefits of screening younger women for breast cancer. *Cancer Detect Prevent* 4:595–601.

Shwartz, M. 1978. A mathematical model used to analyze breast cancer screening strategies. *Operation Research* 26:937–55.

Sonnenberg, F.A., and J.R. Beck. 1993. Markov models in medical decision making: A practical guide. *Med Decis Making* 13:322–38.

Sox, H., M.A. Blatt, M.C. Higgins, and K.I. Marton. 1988. *Medical Decision Making.* Boston: Butterworths.

Spitzer, W.O. 1991. Meta-meta-analysis: Unanswered questions about aggregating data. *J Clin Epidemiol* 44:103–7.

Steering Committee of the Physicians Health Study Research Group. 1989. Final report on the aspirin component of the on-going physicians' health study. *N Engl J Med* 321:129–35.

Steering Committee of the Physicians Health Study Research Group. 1988. Preliminary report: Findings from the aspirin component of the on- going physicians' health study. *N Engl J Med* 318:262–64.

Tabar, L., C.J. Fagerberg, A. Gad, L. Baldetorp, L.H. Holmberg, O. Gröntoff, U. Ljungquist, B. Lundström, J.C. Månson, G. Eklund, N.E. Day, and F. Petteron. 1985. Reduction in mortality from breast cancer after mass screening with mammography. *Lancet* 1:829–32.

Tosteson, A.N., D.I. Rosenthal, L.J. Melton, and M.C. Weinstein. 1990. Cost effectiveness of screening perimenopausal white women for osteoporosis: Bone denistometry and hormone replacement therapy. *Ann Intern Med* 113:594–603.

U.S. Preventive Services Task Force (USPSTF). *1995. Guide to clinical preventive services* 2d ed. Baltimore, MD: Williams and Wilkins.

van Oortmarssen, G.J., J.D. Habbema, P.J. van der Maas, H.J. de Koning, H.J. Collette, A.L. Verbeek, A.T. Geerts, and K.T. Lubbe. 1990. A model for breast cancer screening. *Cancer* 66:1601–12.

Weinstein, M.C., P.G. Coxson, L.W. Williams, T.M. Pass, W.B. Stason, and L. Goldman. 1987. Forecasting coronary heart disease incidence, mortality, and cost: The coronary heart disease policy model. *Am J Public Health* 77:1417–26.

Weinstein, M.C., H.V. Fineberg, A.S. Frazier, D. Neuhauser, R.R. Neutra, and B.J. McNeil. 1980. *Clinical decision analysis.* Philadelphia: W.B. Saunders.

Weinstein and Stason. 1982. Cost-effectiveness of coronary artery bypass surgery. *Circulation* 66 (suppl):III56–III66.

Weinstein, M.C., and W.B. Stason. 1976. *Hypertension: A policy perspective.* Cambridge, MA: Harvard University Press.

Weiss, N.S. 1983. Control definition in case-control studies of the efficacy of screening and diagnostic testing. *Am J Epidemiol* 116:457–60.

Wells, B.L., and J.W. Horm. 1992. Stage at diagnosis in breast cancer: Race and socioeconomic factors. *Am J Public Health* 82:1383–85.

Willems, J.S., C.R. Sanders, M.A. Riddiough, and J.C. Bell. 1980. Cost-effectiveness of vaccination against pneumococcal pneumonia. *N Engl J Med* 303:553–59.

6

Estimating Costs in Cost-Effectiveness Analysis

B.R. LUCE, W.G. MANNING, J.E. SIEGEL
and J. LIPSCOMB

This chapter examines the theory and process of identifying, estimating, and valuing the resource costs associated with the current use and future consequences of health care interventions. A primary objective of cost-effectiveness analysis is to incorporate a consideration of resource consumption into decisions about health care. An explicit examination of resources allows an assessment of costs relative to the health benefits of an intervention.

In this chapter, we first categorize the types of resources that are associated with health care interventions and describe generally how they are included in a cost-effectiveness analysis. We then describe the process of developing cost estimates by identifying, measuring, and then valuing the resources associated with an intervention. It is the cumulative result of this process, rather than any single element of it, that comprises cost. Although we focus much of this chapter on the construction of measures of costs from the components of resource units and their values, sometimes called *micro-costing*, we also comment on more aggregative *gross-costing* approaches that may be a useful alternative for some analyses.

We emphasize the estimation of costs for the Reference Case—that is, from a societal perspective. For this purpose, we rely primarily on the concepts of efficient production and social opportunity cost. In addition, we include a discussion of costing when other perspectives are taken.

A Graphic Illustration of Economic Consequences

The introduction and use of a health or medical intervention has potentially far-reaching economic implications, whether that technology is a behavioral or health educational intervention, a new drug, a screening test, or treatment device or procedure. Figure 6.1 illustrates these effects, beginning with the intervention (Box A)—for example, a screening procedure. The intervention itself requires health care resources such as a lab test and pathologist's time (Box E), and may require other types of resources such as transportation (Box F) or an informal (unpaid) caregiver's assistance (Box G). Usually, the intervention will require "time" inputs from the individual receiving the intervention (Box H).

The purpose of the intervention is to improve health or to delay declines in health. This improvement can be measured as reductions in an undesired health state, such as morbidity and mortality, or increases in a desired state, such as improved life expectancy and quality of life (Box B). Changes in health status have three potential economic aspects. First, there is the inherent value of health itself that may be measured in economic terms, such as the maximum dollar amount that a patient would be willing to pay for certain health states (Box C). Second, changes in health status can affect the amount or type of work done and the way an individual uses leisure time. This change

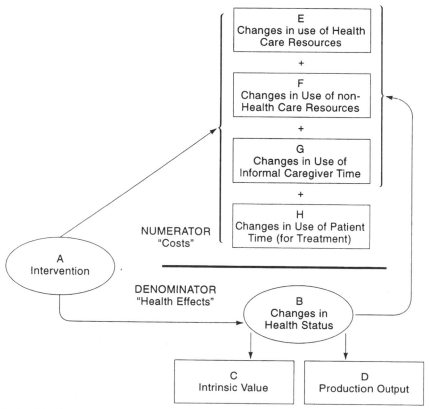

Figure 6.1. Economic consequences of health interventions: the cost effectiveness ratio.

is referred to as a change in productivity (Box D) and measured in dollar terms. Third, the changes in health status often result in a change in the subsequent use of resources. These include health care resources (Box E) and other resources (Box F). Sometimes informal caregivers, such as family members, will devote time to assisting ill patients (Box G).

Not all of these elements are used to calculate cost in a cost-effectiveness ratio—although they could be and, indeed, most are in cost-benefit analysis. In this chapter we will argue that the principal units of interest for calculating costs are those contained in the ''numerator'' in Figure 6.1: namely, in Box E, the change in health care resources from the intervention and from subsequent changes in health status; Box F, the similar change in use of non-health-related resources; Box G, the changes in use of informal caregivers' time; and Box H, the changes in the use of patient time related to the intervention. The reason for excluding a monetary value for Boxes C (inherent value) and D (productivity) in the ratio is that the denominator of the ratio, Box B (health status), if its measurement is sufficiently comprehensive, includes the concepts of the intrinsic value of health and ability to be productive. That is, in the Reference Case, Boxes C and D are captured completely by the measure of health effect or utility in the denominator, Box B, and to include their monetary value in the numerator as well would be to double-count them.

An ideal cost-effectiveness analysis begins by identifying all of the consequences of adopting one intervention or another, including use of resources (medical services use, public health program costs, informal caregiving, and patient time costs—Boxes E–H) and the effects of the intervention on health status (Box B). The amount or magnitude of each change is measured. Finally, these changes are valued: Changes in resource use are converted into a summary cost using dollar values for each input. The incremental difference in input and product costs forms the basis for the cost element in the CEA. The changes in health status and life expectancy are converted into QALYs or another summary health effect measure. The ratio of the increment in the cost summary to the increment in the effect measure is the cost-effectiveness ratio.

Types of Resource Costs

Before turning to the estimation of resource costs, we examine the kinds of costs that should be considered. Resource uses and their costs have been traditionally divided into ''direct'' and ''indirect'' in the literature. ''Direct'' generally refers to changes in resource use attributable to the intervention or treatment regimen. The term ''indirect'' is used in economics to refer to productivity gains or losses related to illness or death. In this book, we have chosen to avoid the term ''indirect,'' because it has many interpretations. For example, in accounting it is used to describe overhead or fixed costs of production. We describe ''direct'' costs, which include certain time costs, and ''productivity'' costs, which are associated with morbidity and mortality. We exclude the "intrinsic value" of health, sometimes considered an indirect cost. While the intrinsic value of health can be assigned an economic value, it is fully subsumed in the measure of health-related quality of life in the Reference Case, as noted earlier.

The categories of resource use and cost have been included in CEAs in an inconsistent manner. Most CEAs exclude productivity costs, but some have included them. All CEAs include direct costs, but often not comprehensively and not necessarily the same ones. For example, the costs of the patient's time spent in treatment and the costs of care provided by family members are sometimes included in CEAs, but often excluded.

Direct Costs

Direct costs include the value of all the goods, services, and other resources that are consumed in the provision of an intervention or in dealing with the side effects or other current and future consequences linked to it (Fig. 6.1, Boxes E and F). These costs are often thought of as involving—or potentially involving—a monetary transaction, although it is the use of the resource rather than a monetary exchange that defines the direct cost. Direct costs encompass all types of resource use, including the consumption of professional, family, volunteer, or patient time. Because the intervention (e.g., screening) can affect both current and future resource use and costs, these costs should be considered a stream of resource use that can span time, from a year or less for a simple procedure, to a lifetime for a preventive intervention or a chronic disease treatment regimen. By well-accepted convention, direct costs are contained in the numerator of the cost-effectiveness ratio.

Direct health care costs (Box E) include the costs of tests, drugs, supplies, health care personnel, and medical facilities. For example, the direct health care costs of mammography screening include the costs associated with the screening itself, such as those of the mammogram and physician time. In addition, they include the costs of further tests to follow up both false-positive and true-positive results and the downstream costs (or savings) associated with cases of breast cancer, such as hospitalization and treatment costs.

An accounting of health care costs would be an incomplete reflection of resource costs associated with an intervention if other, non–health care resources are consumed as a part of the intervention or its follow-up. *Direct non–health care costs* (Box F) include, for example, child care costs for a parent attending a smoking cessation program, the increase in total costs required by a dietary prescription, and the costs of transportation to and from the clinic. The time family members or volunteers spend to provide home care (Box G), such as chronic nursing care for a disabled individual or care for a sick child, may also be considered a direct non–health care cost. It is easily recognized as such when the services are purchased, such as when a private duty nurse is hired to provide home care. The same services offered unpaid by family members or volunteers ("home production," to use the economics term) also represent a consumption of resources. Omission of these costs would bias the CEA against treatments that relied on inputs or outputs that were purchased and in favor of ones that relied on family caregivers or volunteers.

Patient time costs

As discussed in Chapter 2, the time a patient spends seeking care or participating in or undergoing an intervention (Box H) constitutes a real change in the use of a resource by the patient and society. It is, in effect, a part of the intervention itself. For this reason, we recommend that patient time costs be included as a direct cost in the CEA. Time costs do not include the value to the consumer of the intervention itself but do include the value of the time consumed in that treatment. Relevant time costs include travel and waiting time as well as the time actually receiving treatment. Failure to include these costs would bias the CEA against interventions that relied on inputs or outputs that were purchased and in favor of ones that relied on the patient's time. While these costs have been frequently omitted from studies in the past, time is clearly a resource in limited supply, and its consumption should be reflected in CEA.

As described in Chapter 2, the cost of the patient's time associated with the intervention could be included in either the numerator or the denominator of a CEA. That is, it is technically correct either to convert the time into a monetary value and combine it with the other costs in the numerator or to delete time (suitably adjusted for lower quality of life during treatment) from the quality-adjusted life years in the denominator. These two approaches theoretically will yield the same ranking of treatments if the value of an incremental QALY is the opportunity cost of time and if thresholds for cost-effectiveness are allowed to vary across individuals with different opportunity costs of time (Garber and Phelps, 1995). However, if time costs for treatment appear in the numerator in some analyses and in the denominator in others, the resulting cost-effectiveness ratios will not be comparable. Switching the costs from the numerator to the denominator for a subset of CEAs will alter the estimated C/E ratios for the interventions considered, changing their ranking relative to interventions evaluated with the time costs in the numerator.

As long as the conditions are met for the equivalence between the two approaches, the only reasons to prefer one approach over another are concerns about reliability or bias in the measure of the quality adjustment for treatment time (if deducted from QALY) or in the dollar value of time (if added to other costs). We recommend that for the Reference Case, the analyst estimate the monetary value of time expended for the intervention and add that value to the other costs in the numerator of the C/E ratio. We have chosen this approach because adjustment for time in treatment is not common or accepted practice in the measurement of health-related quality of life. However, the placement of time costs in the numerator is not without problems, as discussed later in the section on valuation.

Sometimes the time spent receiving health care can have a negative or positive effect on health status, an effect distinct from the simple consumption of time. The time cost in the numerator is only the opportunity cost of time in treatment, and it does not include any adjustment for the unpleasantness of the intervention. To the extent that an intervention is unusually unpleasant or painful, an adjustment in the denominator QALY is necessary, while the time component remains in the numerator. For example, if prevention of heart disease involved a regimen of daily swimming, the value of the time spent would be included in the numerator, and any appreciable increase (or decrease) in health-related quality of life from enjoyment (or dislike) of the swimming would be assessed in the QALY.

Although the costs of time in treatment are real costs of an intervention, they may be omitted from an analysis if (and only if) they are small or the alternatives being analyzed involve very similar time costs. In this respect, costs of time receiving an intervention are like other costs: If they are trivially small or do not differ across regimens, their inclusion will have little effect on the final results of an analysis, and they may therefore be omitted at the analyst's discretion. (We refer to this criterion as the "rule of reason.") Analysts should take note, however, that if costs have been excluded in an analysis because they are similar across regimens, total program costs of the intervention would need to be reevaluated if the program is assessed in relation to a different comparator.

Productivity Costs

Two types of time costs comprise the category frequently labeled "indirect costs" but which we refer to as "productivity costs" (Fig. 6.1, Box D). These are (1) the costs associated with lost or impaired ability to work or to engage in leisure activities due to morbidity and (2) lost economic productivity due to death. Because the two categories are conceptually distinct and are handled differently in CEA, we distinguish "morbidity costs," the lost economic productivity due to sickness, from "mortality costs," the lost economic productivity due to death.

Morbidity costs

Morbidity costs are the costs associated with lost or impaired ability to work or to engage in leisure activities due to morbidity, such as time for recuperation and convalescence. As discussed in Chapter 2, the time cost associated with morbidity, like patient time invested in an intervention, could be monetized and incorporated into the numerator or it could be assessed in the QALY and placed in the denominator.

For the Reference Case, we recommend the latter convention—namely, that productivity costs associated with morbidity be included in the denominator. Thus, the full impact of morbidity is included in the calculation of the QALY. (See also Chapter 4.) The main reasons for this recommendation are, first, that it is difficult to separate the health-related quality-of-life impact of being ill from effects on role function and other experiences associated with the use of the time. Second, on balance, the inclusion of these effects in the denominator conforms more closely to the principle of cost-effectiveness analysis—namely, that "effects" are included in a nonmonetized form in the denominator. While monetization of these effects is theoretically equally acceptable, this can be accomplished using a cost-benefit framework.

We note that the division of time into treatment and nontreatment time involves a somewhat arbitrary approach to the valuation of time. Time spent in recuperation or convalescence is fully captured in the denominator, while time devoted to an intervention is captured in the numerator (and sometimes, if it is particularly pleasant or painful time, in the denominator as well). This approach also requires a distinction between treatment time and morbidity time that is not always clear. However, it is difficult to identify a preferable alternative for handling time expended for an intervention that maintains the distinction between opportunity costs in the numerator and health outcomes in the denominator. As a general rule, when time could be categorized equally well as treatment time or as morbidity time we suggest that analysts consider it to be morbidity time and incorporate it into the denominator in a Reference Case analysis.

Some analysts have developed QALY measures that expressly exclude the effects of morbidity on the use of time, asking individuals to assume they are fully compensated for any financial impact of the illness. When these measures are used, morbidity costs must be included in the numerator to avoid excluding them entirely. Technically, this approach is as correct as assessing and including financial and health impacts together in the denominator. However, cost-effectiveness ratios from analyses that treat these costs differently will not be directly comparable. Our Reference Case recommendation to include all effects of morbidity in the denominator is thus intended to improve consistency across analyses.

Productivity effects related to the reduction of morbidity time may be of particular importance in some analyses. For example, the effect of an alcohol abuse prevention program on improving the productivity of work time and the number of work hours may be one of the main benefits of the intervention. For an analyst wishing to highlight these effects in a Reference Case analysis, there are several recommended options. The first is to separately track and report the productivity effects, quantifying these effects in monetary terms if desired, but not including them in calculations of cost-effectiveness. The analyst can also conduct a secondary analysis incorporating the productivity cost in the numerator and excluding it from the denominator. (See Chapter 9.) Finally, the analyst might conduct a secondary analysis from the employer's perspective, highlighting the savings in productivity from the vantage point of the particular workplace setting. While these secondary analyses will not be comparable to Reference Case CEAs, they may provide useful information to the audience of the study.

It should be noted that when QALYs are not the measure of effect in a (non–Reference Case) CEA, the costs of morbidity that would have been factored into the health-related quality-of-life adjustment in the denominator are not captured in the analysis. The analyst might then obtain a monetary measure of health status and productivity effects to include in the numerator, without risk of double-counting. We do not encourage this approach in general for CEA, again because the inclusion of these costs in the numerator converts the analysis into a form of cost-benefit analysis. Instead, the analyst could follow the same approaches recommended above: Productivity costs could be estimated and presented separately, or the analyst could conduct secondary analyses. The financial impact of morbidity, as well as health-related quality of life effects, would be missing from the "baseline" analysis, and these omissions would need to be discussed in the CEA report. When the intervention's effects on morbidity and health-related quality of life are important, a Reference Case CEA using QALYs or a cost-benefit analysis would likely prove a more useful form of analysis.

Mortality costs

Changes in life expectancy resulting from an intervention are included in the denominator of a cost-effectiveness ratio. The natural unit of time incorporated in the QALY captures the full value of the time lost in death. As discussed further in the valuation section of this chapter, a person's time is frequently assigned a value based on what the individual can produce in that time, using the wage rate to indicate productivity. In CEA, because the denominator captures the full value of the time, it is not necessary—and would in fact be double-counting—to value that time in terms of its productivity.

Just as for productivity costs related to morbidity, the analyst may wish to demonstrate mortality effects in monetary terms. However, this calculation should be presented separately and *not* be included in the cost-effectiveness ratio because the denominator already includes mortality effects if QALYs (or life expectancy) are the measure of effectiveness. For example, an intervention to prevent neural tube defects would save lives, and the monetary value of these lives or years of life can be presented for illustrative purposes in a CEA. If the analyst wishes to incorporate the monetary value into the calculation of the ratio, we recommend that the analyst instead perform a cost-benefit analysis and present the net benefit of the intervention. As discussed in Chapter 3, a cost-benefit analysis may complement cost-effectiveness results, or, in some cases, it may be a preferred alternative.

Friction costs associated with productivity changes

Although the productivity gains and losses associated with illness or lost life are not included in the Reference Case cost-effectiveness analysis, *friction* costs associated with these events should be counted when relevant. Friction costs are direct, non–health care costs—transaction costs—associated with the replacement of a worker. For example, if substitute labor is never quite as productive as the labor it replaces and the difference in productivity is not fully captured by wage rates, then the discrepancy is a cost. Similarly, if there are training costs for new or temporary employees, friction costs accrue to the employer, and these are real societal costs.

A Clarification: Transfer Costs

Income transfers, involving the redistribution of money, are not real costs to society and should not be included in the cost-effectiveness ratio. The exchange of money per se does not necessarily indicate that resources have been consumed. Programs that provide welfare or disability payments transfer money from one group of people to another (e.g., from the working population to the disabled), but these income transfers do not change the aggregate value of resources available to society. No opportunity cost is incurred. We do encourage analysts to track and report transfers when they are significant, because redistributional effects of interventions are often of concern to the audience of a CEA. (See Chapter 9.) When describing transfer costs, it is important to emphasize that they should not be added to the real societal resource costs in the analysis.

When analyses are conducted from a viewpoint other than societal, transfer costs may represent lost or gained access to resources from the perspective of the analysis. In this case, the transfer costs should be included in the C/E ratio. For example, Javitt et al. (1988) incorporate avoided disability payments for blindness in an analysis on preventive ophthalmology conducted from a governmental perspective.

While transfers themselves are not costs to society, the process of transferring money may involve real resource costs that should ideally be included in the analysis. For example, determining eligibility for transfer programs and monitoring continuing eligibility requires administrative expenses, and the participant incurs application and compliance costs. Raising the money for transfer payments (i.e., with taxes) often requires real administrative costs. Another cost results when the payment of a tax or receipt of a subsidy changes the work choices of those involved.

Strictly speaking, these costs should be included, although the transfer payment itself is not. Often, however, the costs associated with transfer payments will not be important enough to merit inclusion. The author can assess whether, for example, deadweight losses from inappropriate financial incentives or the administrative cost of operating a tranfer program will affect the results of an analysis, and proceed with an analysis of these effects if they are significant. See Starrett (1988) for approximations to the welfare cost of using taxation as a source of funding in the context of cost-benefit analysis; similar qualitative conclusions also apply to cost-effectiveness analysis.

Identifying Resources

The identification, measurement, and valuation of resources are distinct steps. Although it is often easier to omit a step—for example, by collecting cost data without separately enumerating the changes in physical quantities of goods and services and then valuing the units—the full three-step approach will more likely lead to a comprehensive accounting and valuation of the costs and consequences of an intervention. In addition, this process demonstrates the actual resources consumed.

The first step in identifying the relevant resources for a CEA is to describe the *production function* involving the intervention: how the intervention will be used and how it will affect the disease of interest, its treatment, and the health status of the patients receiving it. The production function combines the epidemiology of the disease and the interactions of affected populations with the health care system, including the specific clinical management strategies that will be relevant to the intervention or the illness in question. Much of the event pathway relevant to the study will have been laid out in the initial steps of designing the study. (See Chapter 3.) Here, the analyst outlines in furthur detail the resources consumed in implementing the intervention (e.g., labor, equipment, and supplies), accounting for the manner in which these resources are combined. Similarly, resource consumption is examined for all of the sequelae potentially produced, including changes in health status and other outcomes.

The event pathway for the analysis typically will extend over the course of the episode of illness under study, and resource consumption may occur at every stage along this pathway. For example, in an analysis of the treatment of hypertension, the analyst would identify the drug and provider resources consumed, reductions in the future likelihood of a stroke, and the related reductions in the stream of treatment-associated health care resources and caregiving time associated with stroke. If radiation and chemotherapy increase susceptibility to other diseases (e.g., pneumonia) in a cancer patient, the resources expended to treat these sequalae are also included in the analysis. In prevention programs, epidemiologically based models are often used to depict the probability that clinical events (and thus resource use and costs) will occur over time. These effects may occur over as much as a lifetime (Oster and Epstein, 1987).

Deciding Which Resources To Include

All resource consumption that may be either individually or collectively large enough to have an impact on a decision should be included. Small amounts of resources consumed by large numbers of individuals, or a large number of small differences across resource elements can add up to sums that may be too large to ignore.

In the initial phase of the identification of resources, it is helpful to enumerate all resources consumed, even small ones and those difficult to value in monetary terms. It is important to identify less obvious resources, such as patient transportation to health facilities or time spent in counseling sessions, avoiding the temptation to give less quantifiable resources lower priority or to disregard them altogether. While some of the resources identified may prove nonessential to the analysis, ease of measurement should not be the initial criterion for identification. Listing the elements comprehensively will allow the analyst to make a considered decision of whether each resource should be included.

Study Perspective and Estimation of Resource Consumption

As described in Chapter 3, the perspective of the analysis is an important determinant of which resources to identify and measure. While we recommend the societal perspective for the Reference Case analysis, analysts may often report secondary analyses from the point of view of specific interests. Some societal resources, such as patients' travel time, may not be relevant from a different perspective, such as that of an insurer or a hospital. If differing perspectives are presented in the analysis, we encourage the analyst to identify, measure, and value the resources for each, and compare the results side by side. Table 6.1 summarizes the resources included for a number of perspectives.

Future Costs

Identifying the full range of resource use stemming from an intervention will include the cataloguing of resource use occurring as a future consequence. As discussed in Chapter 2, there is a longstanding controversy about whether future resource use includes costs for diseases unrelated to the intervention in question, which occur during added years of life. Theoretically, a case can be made for their inclusion in the Reference Case, because the intervention is in fact affecting the way in which resources are used in the future. If heart disease is reduced, morbidity for cancer and other major causes of death clearly will increase.

However, many question the appropriateness of considering resource use in added years of life in a CEA. Would decision makers really wish to oppose a smoking prevention program on the basis of a CEA that included the costs of future health care for individuals who were spared a premature death from lung cancer and other smoking-related illness? The users of the CEA could, of course, ignore its results, but then it would be hard to argue that the CEA had served its audience.

In addition to this difference of opinion, there are practical difficulties in including costs for unrelated illness in added years of life. Existing data may not be adequate to capture future resource use of all unrelated diseases; in addition, it may be unduly difficult to ascertain the effect of an intervention on the range of future causes of morbidity and death. Finally, if these costs are included, non–health care costs in added years of life should also be included. As discussed in Chapter 2, the exclusion of non–health care costs is acceptable if these costs add a constant cost to each year; however, no research has been done to determine whether this is the case.

Because of the practical concerns and unresolved theoretical issues surrounding the inclusion of health care costs for unrelated illness in added years of life, our recommendation for the Reference Case is that analysts use their discretion in including or excluding these costs. Like other costs and consequences, the rule of reason applies to these costs: If they are small compared to the magnitude of the C/E ratio, they can be omitted without affecting the analysis results in any case. If they are large, we recommend that the analyst conduct a sensitivity analysis to assess their effect.

When analysts do intend to include the costs of care associated with unrelated diseases in added years of life, age- and gender-specific medical spending rates from the general population can be used as a first step to predict what expenditures would be if

Table 6.1 Costs Under Alternative Perspectives

Cost Element	Societal	Patient and Patient Family	Self-Insured Employer[b]	Public or Private Insurer[a]	Managed-Care Plans
Medical care (aggregate)	All medical care costs	Out-of-pocket expenses	Covered expenses[b]	Covered payments	Covered services
"Units"	All units	Those paid out-of-pocket	Those covered	Those covered	Those covered
"Price"	Opportunity cost (including admin. cost)	Amount paid out-of-pocket	Amount paid + admin. cost	Amount paid + admin. cost	Marginal cost
Patient time cost for treatment or intervention	Cost of all time used	Opportunity cost to patient	Only if affects productivity, paid sick time, admin. costs	None	—[c]
Marketed caregiving	All costs	Out-of-pocket expenses	Covered payments	Covered payments	Covered payments
Unmarketed, informal care giving	All costs	Opportunity cost to caregiver	None	None	—[c]
Transportation and other nonmedical services	All costs	All costs	None	None	None
Sick leave, disability, other transfers, (taxes?)	Admin. costs only	Amount received	Amount paid by employer + own admin.	Amount paid by insurer + own admin.	If any paid

a. Third-party insurers.

b. Net of tax treatment.

c. If high, this could lead to a loss of enrollment and business.

the individual lived longer. The results of the National Medical Expenditure Survey (NMES), performed by the Agency for Health Care Policy Research, can be used as a data source for U.S. studies.

This approach is likely to be biased (and to require adjustments) in two cases. First, if the health care needs of a targeted population are different from the general population, then estimates based on age and gender from the general population could be seriously biased. For example, transplant recipients might be more frail or susceptible to infection during years of extended survival than members of the general population at the same ages. In this case, the costs associated with the additional frailty or susceptibility to illness should be assessed.

Second, if the illness under study represents an appreciable part of average health care spending, these data will not accurately estimate future unrelated costs. For example, if a treatment would alter the course of heart disease, using average medical spending to approximate costs in future years would lead to a double-counting of costs for heart disease. The analysis would explicitly model the change in the costs of heart disease treatment over time that followed the treatment, but the age- and gender-specific expenditures for all health care would also include a significant proportion of resources spent on heart disease. To avoid such double counting, we suggest that analysts subtract the costs of the disease being investigated from the estimate of the "unrelated" costs. In the example, one would use the non–heart disease costs of health care for the relevant age and gender as an estimate of the "unrelated" future cost.

Measuring Resource Consumption: General Considerations

As noted earlier, the numerator in a C/E ratio reflects the difference in resource use resulting from implementation of the intervention versus its comparator. This increment in resource use can be measured directly by determining specifically the amount of increased (or decreased) resource use. Alternatively, the analyst can sum resource use under each scenario and subtract the total cost associated with the comparator from the total cost associated with the intervention. In either case, it is the incremental use of resources that is of interest rather than the total cost of an intervention. Thus, if a blood pressure reading is added to a physician visit that would have occurred anyway, the time and equipment for the test, and not the entire visit, are attributed to the intervention.

The appropriate perspective in measuring changes in resources is the long term. If new resources must be added in the long term to conduct an intervention, or if resources must be maintained that would otherwise have been taken out of commission, the amount added or maintained is the relevant quantity.

The approaches to measurement of long-run, incremental resource use and to the assignment of cost to these resources vary along a spectrum of specificity. On one end of the spectrum, there are approaches that call for the direct enumeration and costing out of every input consumed in the treatment of a particular patient. On the other end of the spectrum are such gross approaches as estimating the cost of an event—for example, a hospitalization for a heart attack—by assigning a national average figure such as the Medicare-derived (diagnosis-related group [DRG]) reimbursement rate. We refer to the former approach as ''micro-costing'' and the more aggregative method as ''gross-costing.''

Micro-costing starts with the detailed inventory and measurement of resources consumed. The cost estimate for a myocardial infarction, for example, might be broken down into estimates of the resources used in the emergency room, hospital room and board, specific types of physician visits, drugs, and cardiac tests. Gorsky (1995) describes this process in the context of an HIV prevention program, detailing such resources as provider time for counseling sessions, materials costs per client, and follow-up telephone calls. Eisenberg et al. (1984) use a micro-costing approach to detect very small differences in the production costs of a commonly administered intravenous antibiotic. These investigators use the principles of industrial engineering and time-and-motion studies to compare the actual inputs into the ''production'' process of three different antibiotics. The production functions for acquiring, preparing, and administering the drugs are broken into discrete work-steps, which are analyzed to determine which steps varied across the drugs. Personnel time, supplies, and equipment are measured within each step.

An implicit assumption in micro-costing is that the mix of inputs and the quality of the product or service will generalize to the next application of the approach in a new setting. If this assumption is not valid, then some adjustment in the micro-cost estimate will be required.

''Gross''-cost estimation uses cost estimates for units of input and output that are large relative to the intervention being analyzed. For example, cost estimates might be obtained for hospital stays or doctor visits rather than for the procedures and professional time expended during these encounters. The advantages of gross-costing are its simplicity, practicality, and, if data are obtained broadly, robustness to geographic, institutional, and other sources of variation. Its disadvantage is that relatively little attention is given to examination of the interventions involved in treating illnesses, the site of health care delivery, or other details that contribute to cost.

The choice between gross-costing and micro-costing must balance the needs of the analysis—the sensitivity of the results to the bias and precision in the cost estimates—with the difficulty and expense of obtaining a cost estimate. In principle, micro-costing is preferred, because it allows others to see how well the analysis matches their situation, where patterns of care may differ. It is particularly important to use micro-costing when the cost of an input is integral to the analysis. For example, if examining different protocols for autologous bone marrow transplant, use of a previously collected cost-per-case measure would obscure cost differences related to the protocols under consideration. Or, if it is thought that differences in resources consumed per service or unit of output are small, but volume is large, then it would be appropriate to account painstakingly for the small differences. Micro-costing is also clearly indicated when the gross measure (such as a DRG or an average payment for a service) corresponds poorly with resource cost. For example, a more intensive cholesterol counseling program within a physician's office would require additional resources but might not affect a gross measure such as reimbursement rates for the office visit.

For many analyses, gross costs provide an adequate estimate, and, because they do not require the intensive research that may be needed to generate micro-cost estimates, they are generally much easier and less expensive to obtain. Gross costs are acceptable when using a more exact micro-cost estimate cost will not have an important effect on the analysis. Precision is generally less critical in estimating resources that will be consumed far in the future, as even fairly low discount rates (e.g., 3%) drastically diminish the importance of small differences over the course of time. Estimates of future consumption are necessarily inexact in any case; while we can be assured that technology and thus the cost of treating disease will change in the future, we seldom can validly speculate on exactly how it will differ from current practice.

Micro-costing and gross-costing can be and frequently are used within a single analysis. In general, micro-costing will be more important for aspects of the alternatives under consideration that are likely to diverge in cost, and for interventions and events occurring in the present. So, for example, in an analysis of a smoking cessation program, it would be important to micro-cost the intervention but impractical and unnecessary to micro-cost the costs associated with future cases of lung cancer, stroke, heart disease, emphysema, and other illnesses. Sensitivity analysis will always be necessary to illuminate the importance of imprecise estimates.

The processes of measurement and valuation of resources, which are reasonably distinct in micro-costing, are more blurred in gross-costing. Below, we first describe the processes separately, as they pertain to micro-costing. These sections are followed by a discussion of measurement and valuation strategies and data sources for gross cost estimates.

Measuring Resource Use For Micro-Cost Estimates

Perhaps the most highly specific micro-costing approach, which is frequently associated with primary data collection within randomized clinical trials or observational research studies, involves the prospective collection of data on the exact number and type of each resource consumed by the patient. These designs track resource consumption and intervention effects as they occur. Unit cost multipliers are applied to the quantity of each type of service consumed, and the results are summed to obtain total cost, either for the entire inpatient stay or for that subset of inpatient services germane to the analysis at hand.

Data on medical care utilization may be collected manually or electronically from encounter or billing systems. Increasingly, managed care settings have computerized, integrated patient-based data systems that permit efficient enumeration of these data.

When computerized data are not available or are incomplete, data must be collected manually, using medical chart review, diaries, or periodic interviews.

In fee-for-service settings, itemized and summary bills are excellent sources of encounter data. When bills are used, it is tempting to use charges as the primary source of data, although, as discussed below, charges are typically not good proxies for cost and may need to be adjusted. In addition, however, some categories of relevant resource use are not routinely captured by bills. Out-of-plan utilization generally requires separate data collection efforts, such as diaries or interviews, since neither nonmedical direct resource consumption nor time consumed in treatment are routinely tracked by any administrative systems.

While the level of precision obtainable in this kind of analysis is exemplary, the caveats noted in Chapter 5 for estimating effects from RCTs and observational studies apply equally to measuring costs for a CEA from these data sources. First, these studies generally do not continue long enough to capture the full economic (and health) consequences of the intervention. Models are therefore required to estimate the likelihood of utilization and health events occurring in the future. Second, such studies often include protocol-induced resource consumption, such as a level of monitoring in excess of what would be employed in practice. For example, if a study requires more frequent blood work or other tests, it would likely include resource consumption in addition to what would occur in regular practice that would be inappropriate to include in the analysis. Finally, the resource use and health outcomes observed in these research studies may differ from ''real-world'' practice because of varying community practice patterns and differences in patient compliance, limiting generalizability.

Although secondary data sets are more often useful for gross-costing, some forms are amenable to micro-costing approaches. Needing sound estimates of resource costs to survive in competitive markets, a number of the nation's larger hospitals have adopted sophisticated cost-accounting systems designed to provide detailed, service-specific estimates of average and marginal cost. These detailed management information systems (e.g., Transition Systems I) take a ''bottom-up'' perspective. The cost of each service in each product line is computed as the sum of the labor and nonlabor inputs estimated to be used in that service's production; overhead and other joint costs are typically allocated through state-of-the-art simultaneous-equation techniques.

Micro-costing systems have recently begun to be used in clinical policy analysis. (See, e.g., Wong et al., 1989.) These systems have the potential to yield relatively precise estimates of inpatient costs; see Ashby (1992) and the preliminary analyses of coronary artery bypass and angioplasty cost by Lipscomb et al. (1994). One limitation for CEA is that because such systems are costly to acquire, set up, and maintain, it is likely that they will continue to be found only in the larger, more complex institutions; this may prove problematic for multisite studies requiring a diverse provider mix.

There are several problems associated with the use of secondary data for measuring resources. The potential selection bias affecting who did and did not receive an intervention may limit the value and generalizability of any data collected, including data on resource use. Many resources, both medical and nonmedical, may not have been tracked in a given database and may be difficult to identify after the fact. For example, out-of-pocket costs, time expended for treatment, and informal caregiver time are rarely available retrospectively. Other services that are not itemized (frequently, those that are not separately charged to a payer) can be overlooked. For example, taking a blood pressure is covered by a standard office charge but may or may not have occurred during a specific visit. To solve these problems, analysts using secondary data sources may need to rely on other data sources to fill in additional information needed for a CEA.

The advantage of using secondary data such as from claims databases is that unlike primary data collected from an RCT, the data are drawn from actual "real-world" experience with the use of an intervention. Thus, they can provide externally valid estimates of medical resource utilization and costs. Another advantage of using secondary data sources is that they are available with little additional expense to the CEA analyst. Finally, these analyses can be particularly useful for the insurer's or provider's perspective.

Valuation of Resources in Micro-Costing

Having identified and measured the changes in resources used as a result of alternative interventions, the next task in the three-step process for estimating cost is to convert those changes into summary cost measures. In this section, we consider how to value or "cost-out" the inputs to health care interventions and the resources saved or consumed as a result of their implementation.

As discussed in Chapter 2, the real cost to society of a given resource is its opportunity cost, the value of the resource in its next best alternative use. For most purposes, market prices provide a reasonable estimate of opportunity cost. For example, the wages of a registered nurse or the charge for an office visit generally provide an adequate measure of the value of the resources consumed.

There are some cases, however, in which market imperfections are evident, suggesting that a price will not provide a valid estimate of opportunity cost. Sometimes, market prices may still serve as the initial ingredient for an estimate of opportunity cost, if an appropriate adjustment is made. In other cases, adequate adjustment is not feasible. In these cases, the analyst may need to investigate alternatives to using current market prices.

While an elaborate search for the true opportunity cost of all resources is generally beyond the reach of a CEA, the analyst should attend to important biases in market prices. In general, the effort the researcher devotes to adjusting or finding an alternative to a market price should reflect the importance of the estimate to the analysis. Below, we discuss common issues encountered in using market prices (handling geographical variation, the exclusion of fixed costs when assigning costs to an intervention, and the handling of first-copy costs), common adjustments required when using market prices (adjustments for profit and for time differences), and circumstances in which alternatives to market prices are desirable (critical market imperfections and cases when the real cost of resources has changed as a result of an implementation decision).

Using Market Prices to Estimate the Value of Resources

Selecting geographically appropriate prices

The prices used in a CEA should reflect the prevailing prices in the location where the intervention is or will be implemented. Many CEA studies have been based on prices prevailing in a specific community or at a specific hospital. If the regimen will be implemented locally, then this use of local prices is wholly appropriate: What matters is local gains (e.g., Boston QALYs) versus the local opportunity cost (e.g., Boston costs) of the change in resources consumed. However, if the analysis applies to a larger region or the nation, then the relevant prices and costs are those prevailing regionally or nationally. The use of local prices for a national problem could be misleading if they differ from regional or national prices, as they often do.

The analyst can consult the *Statistical Abstract of the United States* for an indication of the variation in the cost of living across areas and the *Area Wage Index* for the variation in labor costs across areas to determine the appropriateness of using local prices (U.S. Bureau of the Census, 1995; U.S. Bureau of Labor Statistics, 1995). Information on the costs or charges for specific procedures or services by region may require sampling providers, the use of third-party insurance claims data, or data provided by relevant trade organizations.

If the cost-effectiveness analysis is done from a perspective other than societal, the relevant price or value for a change in resource use will differ systematically from the full societal resource cost. Typically, the relevant ''price'' is the one paid by the decision maker or payer in that analysis. Table 6.1 lists several examples.

Variable and fixed costs

The cost to be included in a CEA is the value of all those goods, services, and inputs that may change because of the intervention being considered. These are defined as ''variable'' costs. ''Fixed'' costs—those that are held at a constant level, independent of the level of production and the time frame of the analysis—should be excluded. Thus, costs should not be included for inputs or outputs that are unaffected by changes in the intensity or frequency of an intervention or are unaffected by decisions to do or not to do the intervention at all. In any event, costs for these fixed resources will cancel out when incremental cost differences between regimens are calculated.

Overhead costs, such as utilities, custodial services, and adminstration, are frequently thought to be ''fixed'' because they are not itemized and directly allocated to a specific service. One implication of the above definition of fixed costs is that one should exclude administrative expense and overhead in a CEA if and only if such costs do not increase with the introduction of a new service or change in volume of an existing service. Because administrative and other "overhead" expenses usually do increase with additional output or new services, some allowance for overhead is usually appropriate. Like other costs in a perfectly competitive market that is in long-run equilibrium, overhead costs will be covered by the price for a good or service. In this case, a separate consideration of overhead is not necessary.

Most input costs that are fixed in the short run will in fact be variable in the long run. Examples are the cost of the equipment used for mammography screening or the start-up costs for a new health program. In these cases, the prices used in the CEA should be the costs that would prevail in the longer run, when these types of inputs would be related to the stage or level of implementation of the intervention. Unless the decision being considered is purely a short-run decision, the relevant time frame for a CEA is the long run when all inputs are variable.

Although the Reference Case analysis takes a long-run perspective (and, therefore, considers costs to be fixed only if they are fixed in the long run), in some instances, a secondary analysis taking a shorter-run perspective may provide important information for a decision. This may be the case, for example, when a factor is temporarily in excess supply. For example, if a surveillance program has established a laboratory at a certain site, the laboratory technician's labor for conducting tests not related to the original program might truly be "free" to the decision maker for the duration of the technician's contract. In considering short-term program options, the cost of the technician's time should reflect the excess capacity of this resource. The consumption of a resource that is in excess supply would not be counted as a cost for the short run, except to the extent that it is perishable or to the extent that wear and tear reduces its value in the longer run.

A short-run perspective has an important potential for misuse. For example, an analysis reflecting low short-run costs of magnetic resonance imaging (MRI) when the technology was in excess supply might be used to justify an unwarranted increase in interventions using that technology over the long term. For this reason, the determination of whether a cost is fixed should be based on a long-run perspective for the Reference Case, and use of a short run perspective for a secondary analysis should be carefully explained.

Research and development (R&D) costs and other first-copy costs

Research and development costs for a new drug or procedure provide very common examples of first-copy costs, a type of cost that CEA analysts have debated how to handle. First copy costs are defined as costs incurred in establishing a regimen—the costs of developing the first copy of an item, independent of the number of units provided once the first unit is produced. (These costs are sometimes considered to be a type of fixed cost, but technically, fixed costs are constant regardless of the level of production, and first-copy costs are not, because they depend on whether zero or one unit is produced.)

The appropriate handling of first-copy costs, such as for research and development, depends on the perspective of the analysis, the type of decision being made, and when the decision is made. Strictly speaking, R&D costs should be included if the decision addresses whether to provide the intervention at all. That is, if the intervention is not already in existence, the appropriate, long-run perspective includes the expected R&D, production, distribution, and provision costs.[1] If, however, the technology has already been developed and the decision addresses the use of the intervention, such as dosage of a drug or frequency of a screening test, then the price should exclude R&D costs. Instead, the relevant costs are the incremental production, distribution, and provision costs.

For perspectives other than societal, the price paid by the decision maker for the good or service is the relevant one, inclusive of whatever return on investment in R&D or rent to patent- or copyright-holder has been incorporated into the price. If a patient or insurance carrier pays a price for zidovudine (AZT) that reflects patent restrictions, for example, the relevant price for a CEA is the one paid, not the opportunity cost of the inputs that went into producing the actual units of AZT consumed. Similarly, if a health maintenance organization (HMO) obtains large bulk discounts or uses generics in its formulary, then those discounted transaction prices are the relevant ones.

We encourage analysts to conduct a formal sensitivity analysis to determine the impact of R&D costs on the price to be used in the analysis. In the case of pharmaceuticals, the marginal costs of production and distribution of a drug are often significantly less than the market price, especially during the period of patent protection, and the handling of these costs can affect the outcome of an analysis. However, for many cost-effectiveness analyses, this level of effort is beyond the resources available for analysis. Because the class of drugs must break even—have revenues large enough to cover R&D, production, and distribution costs—prevailing transaction prices will usually act as a serviceable way to value consumption of the drugs. The Average Wholesale Price (AWP), which approximates prices in discount pharmacies, is one source of such information (Drug Topics Red Book, 1994).

Capacity utilization and occupancy rate assumptions

Certain costs accrued in delivering a service depend on the capacity available at a given facility for delivering that service. Decisions about capacity are based on the demands the facility will need to meet, the repercussions of having inadequate capacity, and the costs of extra capacity. For example, emergency rooms are constructed to handle an expected number of visits, with an expected waiting time and some limit to their capacity. An emergency room where patients never had to wait would be overstaffed and idle much of the time; one designed to meet ''average'' utilization would be unable to handle peak demand.

There is no universal answer as to the correct capacity utilization rate. For example, one may be willing to have an "underused" screening device located in a small town in a rural setting because the alternative is the expenditure of even more resources on time and travel by people traveling to a more distant and more fully utilized piece of equipment. However, two facilities across the street from each other probably ought not have machines that are both used less than 50% of the time.

In general, services should be provided with as little excess capacity as possible in order to use resources efficiently. Capacity that is not routinely used is not necessarily "excess," however; the socially optimal amount of capacity depends on a consideration of the full costs of providing the service. As noted, emergency rooms are built and staffed in excess of the average load that they serve in order to meet peak demands— a multicar accident, or some other extreme case of injury and illness—where treatment cannot be deferred without substantial risks or losses to the patient. Whether peak demands are predictable or random, it may be socially rational to have the capacity to meet them if the willingness to pay for the service exceeds the cost of maintaining the additional capacity.

In using micro-costing to develop an estimate of the cost of an intervention or service, the analyst's assumptions about capacity and occupancy rate will influence the resources included in the analysis: the size of a structure, the number of units of a certain type of equipment, the level of staffing. If these costs are a large part of the total costs of an intervention, the assumptions about capacity could have a major impact on the estimated cost-effectiveness of that regimen.

The literature suggests that 80% utilization of capacity in hospitals and other health care facilities is a norm. When information on capacity utilization is not available, we recommend that analysts use this rate as a benchmark assumption. When better information is available, that information should be used. This assumption does not apply to cases such as the rural example above or to services for which demand is highly stochastic. When a significantly lower rate of utilization is assumed, we encourage the analyst to discuss and justify this assumption.

Analysts can refer to the literature for guidance in dealing with capacity utilization under specific circumstances. Boiteux (1956, 1960) and Dreze (1964) discuss issues related to peak-load pricing. For a generic summary of the issues, see Starrett (1988). Joskow (1980) provides an example involving hospitals. In the case of stochastic demand, the problem has been dealt with in the operations literature on multiserver queues.

Adjusting Market Prices

Profit
A common concern in using market prices is that these prices may not reflect the true opportunity cost to society of the resources used to produce the good or service because they include a component of profit in excess of a fair rate of return on investment and

allowance for risk. For example, if hospitals on average are earning revenues greater than the costs of all inputs (including a return on capital), then the hospital's charge for a service, such as a coronary artery bypass graft or a neonatal intensive care unit day, will exceed the opportunity cost to society of the resources used. Similar concerns about the relationship between price and resource cost arise if there is any form of market distortion or imperfection, whether it be that the price is above marginal cost due to market power, the divergence of administrative prices (e.g., under Medicare's Prospective Payment System [PPS]) from the incremental costs of treatment, or the underpricing of some resources because they are produced under conditions of the commons (Hardin, 1968).

One frequently used solution to this problem for inpatient care has been to deflate the prices by a cost-to-charge ratio that removes the excess. In the United States, the Medicare Cost Reports provide easily accessible data that can be used to calculate cost-to-charge ratios. The analyst must consider the specific needs of the analysis when applying this remedy. An average correction for the difference between costs and charges for the hospital as a whole may not provide the right correction for a particular service provided by that hospital. Cost-to-charge ratios for the specific service should be obtained when necessary.

The cost-to-charge ratio may be subject to the vagaries of historical costs and other accounting practices. For example, if a cost-to-charge ratio is based on the original, nominal prices for capital purchases rather than on replacement costs, it will understate current opportunity costs. In this case, it is necessary to calculate replacement costs and reconstruct the cost-to-charge ratio.

Technically, the cost-to-charge ratio or any other correction to a price should be based on the incremental or marginal cost of resource use. If the economies of scale in producing (or returns to scale in providing) an intervention are not known, then it will be necessary to estimate a cost function and derive the correct marginal cost. For many health care interventions, the technology will exhibit no important economies or diseconomies of scale or scope. In these cases, average costs and marginal costs will be equal, and the correction may be based on average costs; estimates of incremental or marginal costs thus need not be developed.

In the section on gross-costing below, we discuss a number of the practical issues involved in using cost-to-charge ratios. Because of the shortcomings of cost-to-charge ratios, they may not be readily usable to obtain unbiased estimates of the value of resources consumed in some applications. These concerns underlie our preference for micro-costing, rather than gross cost estimation, when the difference between the estimates from the two approaches are likely to differ appreciably.

Correcting for price inflation

When the data on prices used in a CEA come from different time periods, or when the study is projecting costs for different time periods, market prices can vary because of general inflation or because some particular resource is becoming more or less scarce.

The usual approach for handling price changes is to bring the past prices into current terms so that they reflect the opportunity cost of the resources in common dollar terms; one can directly add 1995 dollars, but it is not meaningful to add 1983 dollars and 1992 dollars because their real purchasing power was different.

Analysts should select an appropriate index for use in adjusting the prices of various resources. If the price being brought up to date is a wage or some other measure that rises at the rate of general price inflation, then the Consumer Price Index (CPI) provides a servicable way to correct for inflation. However, if the good or input has a different rate of price change than the economy as a whole, then a more specific measure should be used. For example, the Medical Component of the CPI could be used for medical costs, because these costs have been rising faster than general inflation.

Changes in the medical good itself can affect price, as can general changes in price level. Methodological problems in the construction of the Medical CPI have tended to combine the two factors. If nominal medical care prices have risen by 10% (as reflected in the Medical CPI), but the productivity of health care has risen by 8%, then the relevant price correction is 2%, which is obtained by subtracting the change in effectiveness from the Medical CPI. To know whether the price change is inflation or a change in effectiveness requires knowledge of the specific intervention. If a significant change in productivity or efficiency may have occurred, the analyst can conduct a sensitivity analysis to determine whether the potential effect on the C/E ratio is large enough to merit a more detailed subanalysis.

Changes in relative future prices may also be a concern in CEA. If all prices and incomes are expected to rise at exactly the same rate, then the real purchasing power for goods and services is exactly the same as if there had been no increase in prices.[2] The cost calculated in current dollars will adequately reflect the real costs of using goods and services when they are consumed. However, if the prices of some of the inputs, goods, or services being consumed or produced as a result of the intervention will rise at a different rate than others, then the increase or decrease in the real price for that item should be included in the calculation. The adjustments should reflect relative prices net of inflation and increases in productivity or effectiveness: Let r be the real rate of interest, p be the current price of x, and π be the true rate of inflation in x relative to general inflation, after any adjustments for increased productivity or effectiveness. Then the current *real* value of next year's expenditure on x will be $px(1+\pi)/(1+r)$, instead of $px/(1+r)$.[3]

CEAs for prevention provide examples in which differential rates of inflation may be important. During the last two decades, the rate of medical inflation has exceeded general inflation, with the result that medical care has become relatively more expensive than other goods. Evaluations of preventive care now versus curative care later may be appreciably biased if they do not account for this trend, after adjustment for productivity changes. Failure to include future real increases in the price of curative care will tend to bias the comparisons in favor of curative care; such a bias could be quite substantial.

When Market Prices Are Inadequate

Under some circumstances, market prices are likely to provide a significantly flawed estimate of opportunity cost. If the value used may have an important impact on the analysis, the researcher should consider other means of valuation. In general, the analyst will want to conduct a sensitivity analysis on the prices being used to assess their importance in the analysis. If the analysis conclusions are sensitive to relatively small changes in price, a more thorough consideration of the value of the resources in question will be required. If the results are not sensitive, existing prices will provide a reasonable proxy.

Changes in price resulting from implementation decisions

As noted earlier, market prices may not give an adequate representation of the marginal costs of a good or service for CEA when the decision to implement an intervention would result in real changes in costs. This problem can occur when the new quantity of the intervention provided affects the availability of a resource.

For example, the availability of a resource could be affected by the large-scale implementation of an intervention that depended on intensive nursing services. If the resulting increase in demand for nurses were large enough, it would cause a shortage of nurses and an increase in nurses' wages. If the supply of nurses increased in response, the wage rate would return to its former level, and the wage rate before implementation would serve as a reasonable proxy for marginal cost before and after implementation. However, if, in the long run, it required a higher wage to draw people into nursing or to work more hours, the opportunity cost of a nurse's services would be higher after implementation. The real marginal cost of nursing services for CEA would be reflected in the post-implementation price of nursing services, rather than in the former price.

A significant increase or decrease in the level of an intervention provided can also lead to economies of scale, economies based on learning-by-doing, or economies due to the scope of related activity. Economies of scale depend on the level of current production or delivery of a service. Economies based on learning-by-doing reflect cumulative experience. For example, the real costs associated with ophthalmic laser surgery have decreased as physicians have mastered the technology. Economies of scope occur when the marginal costs of two services are lower if they are done in the same large hospital. When economies of scale, scope, indivisibilities, or learning-by-doing are present, marginal costs for units of a good or service are not constant, and current prices may not provide an adequate proxy.

In general, unless these effects are likely to be large, analysts can assume that the marginal costs of interest are constant. When these issues are important, analysts should consult the literature for appropriate adjustments. In the case of substantial economies achieved by learning-by-doing, for example, the analyst should account for the effect of the current quantity of an intervention provided on *future*, as well as current, costs.

Unmarketed goods and inputs

One of the most prominent examples of unmarketed resources in CEA involves the cost of the patient's time in treatment and the cost of family time spent in caretaking. If an intervention requires patient travel, waiting, and time spent away from other activities (including leisure), then there has been a change in the way resources are used, even if there is no monetary transaction. In such cases, there are opportunities forgone, and a "cost" results in the form of the loss of the benefits that would come from the alternative use of time.

Time costs. The dollar valuation of a person's time spent pursuing or receiving an intervention involves assigning a monetary amount to each unit of time in the analysis. Ideally, the opportunity cost of the time consumed is measured by determining the dollar amount that one would have to compensate the individual for expending that time on the intervention. Economic theory suggests that if the individual whose time is consumed is a worker facing a constant wage rate, with no sick leave, and having the freedom to choose the number of hours of work, then the opportunity cost of each hour spent is his or her hourly wage. (See Deaton and Muellbauer, 1980, chapters 10 and 11 for a discussion of the theory for labor allocation and household production.) If some of these conditions do not apply, the wage needs to be adjusted. For example, if a worker receives overtime pay or compensation for sick time, the unadjusted wage rate would not reveal the tradeoff the worker is considering in choices concerning working hours.

Although the practice of using wage rates to estimate the value of time has some drawbacks, we recommend it as a tractable means for obtaining estimates for the Reference Case analysis. We recommend that analysts obtain the appropriate wage rates for the population targeted by the intervention under study. For example, if an analysis examines the cost-effectiveness of cervical cancer screening for women ages 40–65, then the average wage for women of the appropriate age groups could be used to estimate their time costs. This level of specificity provides a more accurate estimate of opportunity cost than using an overall average population wage. The appropriate wage rates may be obtained from survey data or by using data collected in the Current Population Surveys (CPS) (U.S. Bureau of the Census).

In general, age- and gender-specific wage estimates will provide adequately specific estimates of opportunity cost. If the analyst determines that these wages provide a biased estimate for a particular targeted population, a more specific wage estimate can be used. For example, if an intervention affects only nurse's aides, and their wages are different from the age- and gender-specific wages that would apply to the general population, the analyst should use an average wage for this subpopulation if available. Similarly, if the intervention largely affects working-aged women outside of the labor force, then some explicit correction must be made for the bias in estimates of time values derived from wage rates for working women, as discussed further below.

Using the observed market wage rate as the basis for estimates of the opportunity cost of time introduces existing patterns of income distribution into CEA. The implications of this effect may be undesirable on distributional grounds. For example, consider two CEAs, one on breast cancer screening and one on prostate cancer screening. If the two interventions require equal amounts of patient time, yet one uses younger women's wages to value this time while the other uses the higher wages of men, part of the difference in the cost-effectiveness ratios will be due to this difference in the valuation of time. If the effect is small (i.e., if patient's time costs are not a significant component of the analyses), it can reasonably be disregarded. If it is large, it may make the results of the analysis suspect, depending on the ethical framework of the study's audience.

However, altering estimates of the opportunity cost of a resource because of social concerns will influence the results of the analysis in ways that may be unacceptable. If the national average wage is used to value time, the C/E ratio for breast cancer screening will rise, and the C/E ratio for prostate cancer screening will fall relative to the case where market-based wages are used. The use of the average valuation of time would thus make treatment of breast cancer appear relatively less attractive, even though women in fact could earn less during their waiting time (if spent working) than men. Some would argue that a CEA incorporating an unrealistic, although "fair," estimate of time is not particularly more desirable than one reflecting objectionable but actual conditions in society. In general, if average wages are used, a given intervention will appear less cost-effective for people with lower wages relative to higher-paid individuals than it would if targeted wages were used.

There are convincing arguments on both sides of the question of whether to use targeted wages to value the patient's time expended in treatment or to use an average wage that places an equal (or more equal) value on the time of different persons. Because the numerator in the C/E ratio measures the opportunity cost of the resources consumed by the health care intervention and its consequences, some believe that the value of time in treatment should reflect the value of time in the marketplace. In this view, the equitable treatment of individuals in CEA is adequately addressed in the construction of QALYs, where each individual life year receives equal weight, and needs no further attention in the calculation of opportunity costs. However, others are concerned about the ethical implications of using different time values for different people and find using the average wage for the general population to be more appropriate. The debate illustrates the inability of CEA to deal with both efficiency and equity concerns simultaneously.

Our recommendation, as noted above, is to use the targeted wage, in order to approximate opportunity cost as accurately as possible. If time costs are a significant component of the analysis, we recommend that the analyst conduct a sensitivity analysis using an alternative, average wage. Analysts can describe the effect of the estimate used on the results and encourage users of the analysis to consider this effect in their interpretation of the study.

There are certain cases, frequently encountered in CEAs of health and medical care, when observed or market wages are not likely to be an appropriate measure of the value of time. These are: (1) individuals of working age who do not work for pay; (2) individuals engaged in tasks that they strongly like or dislike; and (3) groups for whom there is no direct, standard labor market experience—that is, the elderly, children, and those unable to work.

In the first instance, when a person is of working age but does not work for pay (e.g., housewives or househusbands), one option for valuing time is to use the hourly wage of individuals with similar characteristics (age, gender, education, labor experience) who do work for pay. This imputed wage provides a lower bound on the opportunity cost of time[4] and it may be close enough to the real opportunity cost of time to be used in a CEA. However, if time costs are a major component of the CEA, the analyst should investigate models with which to adjust the wage that accounts for more specific characteristics of the population under study, such as those discussed in Zick and Bryant (1990), Gronau (1973, 1977, 1986) and Heckman (1980).

The use of wages to value time assumes that the person obtains no direct satisfaction from the provision of the time. The time consumed is lost leisure or lost work, but it is of no other intrinsic value. However, if one enjoys helping others or caring for children, or differentially dislikes waiting in a doctor's office, then the wage used should be revised appropriately.

Finally, for three groups of people (children, the unable to work, and the elderly), we cannot use labor market behavior directly to impute an estimate of the value of their time. For those unable to work and in general for children, there are no wage data. For the elderly, there are some wage data, but the wage is not an adequate reflection of opportunity cost because of incentives and requirements built into retirement and Social Security systems. For example, if, by working extra hours, an individual forfeits Social Security income (or faces higher taxes), these factors influence choices about the number of hours worked.

Given the difficulties in valuing time for these three groups, some practical alternatives are needed for studies where time costs are substantial elements. We encourage research into how to better value the time for these three groups. In the meantime, we make the following suggestions. For the elderly, one could use the wage of workers matched for age and gender. This rate will likely be biased because of other financial incentives operating, and, until empirical research demonstrates the extent of this bias, the analyst should use this approach cautiously. Or, one can use projections based on life-cycle estimates of the wage rate in this age group. For teenagers, one could use the solution used for housewives and informal caregivers—namely, basing the wage rate on teens in the labor force and adjusting as necessary for the selection bias of using observed market wages for teens not in the labor force. For younger children and those unable to work, there is no easy alternative. Another alternative applicable to all three of these groups is to use questionnaires to elicit willingness to pay for the time costs, which could be done on standard populations in much the same way that weights can be derived for health states. Given the potential importance of the costs of time-in-treatment for these three groups, we encourage research into methods and estimates of the opportunity cost of time.

It should be noted that the lower time costs for people with relatively low wages make a given intervention more cost-effective for this group than for higher-paid individuals. This effect is the opposite of what occurs in cost-benefit analysis, where the benefits rather than the costs of the intervention are affected by the level of wages.

Home production. A problem related to the valuation of time consumed in treatment is the question of how to value home production of goods or services (e.g., informal caregiving or caretaking). The valuation of time costs addresses the value of time for a person receiving a health care intervention; home production deals with the value of services provided in the home, which substitute for services that could be purchased. In both cases, the time of a person who does not work for pay is often involved. For people receiving a health care intervention, the time consumed in traveling, waiting, or receiving the intervention generally amounts to an incremental change in the way their time is used. However, home production of services may involve a permanent or semipermanent change in the person's relation to the labor market. For example, a person who decides to care for a child or elderly parent at home may leave paid employment to undertake this task.

One approach to valuing the time spent in home production is to value the time at its market or reservation price, similar to the methods suggested for valuing the time of housewives or househusbands. Another method is to substitute the market price of a marketed equivalent service. This approach is often used in cost-of-illness studies. We prefer the former approach, because the latter is likely to be too high; a decision to "make" a service rather than to "buy" it indicates that home production is less costly to the individual. However, in many analyses, substituting the price of a marketed equivalent service will prove an acceptable approach.

Measurement and Valuation of Resources
in Gross-Costing

The distinguishing features of cost estimates on the "gross" end of the spectrum of specificity are their simplicity, tractability, and their (intended) insensitivity to site-specific details. Depending upon the method and data used, gross-costing may generalize over the site of care delivery (e.g., teaching versus nonteaching hospital), the particular input mix employed (e.g., whether the contrast medium used for the angiography was ionic or non-ionic), and patient-level characteristics (e.g., age, number of diseased vessels). What is sought in using gross costs is a satisfactory estimate of the "typical" cost of the service or its associated health outcome. Frequently such cost estimates are to be input into a larger decision model in which the service in question (1) is only one of many incorporated in the analysis, (2) occurs only with some probability, or (3) would occur sufficiently "downstream" such that its present value at conventional discount rates is relatively small.

Gross cost estimates are based on a sequence of "economically significant" events associated with the intervention. These events may include one or more of the following: (1) acute care hospitalizations; (2) other institutional services (e.g., nursing home care); (3) outpatient-based care (e.g., surgical centers); (4) physician (and other professional-charge) services; and (5) drugs, outpatient supplies, and durable medical equipment. Gross cost estimation of the cost of the intervention requires estimating these component event costs, then summing. In this section we focus on the measurement and valuation of the real resources associated with these component events, with particular emphasis on direct health care costs.

As will be seen, resource measurement and cost assignment frequently are not distinct steps but rather constitute an integrated process in a gross-costing approach. Often, these techniques draw on readily available administrative prices. In what follows, we consider major cost components in turn and discuss briefly the alternative approaches that have been, or might be, applied to measure and value resource consumption.

Acute Care Hospitalizations

A variety of approaches has been used to estimate the economic value of the resources consumed during acute admissions. To illustrate, we draw upon applications in the area of cardiovascular disease.

Oster and Epstein (1986) in their multiperiod cost-effectiveness study of a cholesterol-lowering medication estimated gross costs for emergency assistance, hospitalization, and follow-on care components for categories of cardiac disease, such as myocardial infarction and angina pectoris. For example, their hospitalization estimates were based on national average DRG payments for the disease categories, while their calculation of emergency costs was based on ambulance and emergency room charges. These costs were combined to estimate lifetime costs for each category of illness. Similarly, the research team working under contract to cost out clinical practice guidelines sponsored by the Agency for Health Care Policy and Research has applied a methodology in which the cost of specific hospitalizations is estimated by the national mean Medicare DRG payment (Health Economics Research, 1994). For example, in determining the cost of guidelines for unstable angina, the estimate used for coronary angiography with complications was simply $3,728—the 1993 average payment for DRG 124.

A less aggregative estimate can be obtained when the analyst uses hospital administrative data—basically patient billing information and summary estimates of departmental-level expenditures—to derive the costs of inpatient admissions. With such data, a range of approaches can be pursued. At one extreme, hospital charges can be used as a proxy for costs (e.g., Dudley et al., 1993). This may be reasonable in a comparative analysis of interventions, assuming that charges per admission are roughly proportional to economic costs per admission (see Hlatky et al., 1990); however, the consensus view is that charges poorly approximate the economic cost of care (Ashby, 1992; Health Economics Research, 1994; Finkler, 1982).

As a result, a frequent practice is to use cost-to-charge ratios to adjust charges. A number of recent studies have used hospital administrative data to implement variants of the cost-to-charge ratio approach for converting billing information into economic cost estimates. In its simplest form, use of cost-to-charge ratios involves applying one overall hospital-level ratio (computed as the particular hospital's total accounting costs divided by its total billings per period) to the total charges for the inpatient admission of interest. (See Ashby, 1992.) In their most commonly used present form, cost-to-charge ratios are employed in a more fine-tuned fashion: (1) The patient's detailed bill is reconfigured into a set of exhaustive charge, or billing, categories; (2) each charge category is assigned to a specific hospital cost center; (3) the cost-to-charge ratio for each center is used to convert these assigned charges to their corresponding cost estimates; and (4) the latter are summed to yield the cost of the admission. This is the basic approach to inpatient costing adopted by several of the AHCPR-sponsored Patient Outcomes Research Teams (PORTs) (see Lave et al., 1994 for details); it is also the approach long used by Medicare to estimate hospital costs for purposes of establishing cost-based reimbursement rates, and it has been used in individual studies (e.g., Smith et al., 1994).

Within the detailed cost-to-charge ratio approach, there are at least two important variations on the theme. In estimating the hospital cost of Medicare eligibles, charges as categorized in the Medicare Provider and Analysis Review (MEDPAR) file are mapped to cost centers, as categorized in the hospital's Medicare Cost Report (MCR); the cost-to-charge ratio for each such cost center is applied to the mapped charges to estimate cost for that admission. This strategy has been employed by both the Stroke Prevention and Ischemic Heart Disease PORTs, among others (Lave et al., 1994). In applying the detailed cost-to-charge-ratio approach to estimate stroke costs in a mixed elderly–nonelderly population, Holloway et al. (1995, in press) used charge categories as defined within the Uniform Billing (UB)-82 system instead of the MEDPAR categories. These analysts linked each UB-82 category to a corresponding MCR-defined cost center, applied the MCR ratios, and finally summed across cost center to get cost for each stroke admission.

While the MCR (available to users in the form of Hospital Cost Report Information System minimum data sets) remains the only national-level information source on the cost of providing hospital care, it has been criticized on several grounds. In an analysis conducted at the request of the Prospective Payment Assessment Commission (ProPAC), Ashby (1992) concluded that because the MCR defines both capital and operating costs according to Medicare reimbursement principles, "it does not necessarily provide an accurate measurement of the overall cost of providing patient care.'' In addition, because Medicare does not require either uniform accounting or uniform reporting of revenues, there may be difficult-to-detect inconsistencies across institutions. Moreover, hospital charges actually play an important role in the cost-finding process, since they are used to apportion costs among ancillary services and between inpatient and outpatient service. As noted, charges themselves may vary for reasons unrelated to underlying costs, such as local market conditions and institutional factors. Also, MCR-based estimates are best regarded as average-cost rather than marginal cost values, since it is not possible to separate out the nonvariable components of a hospital's cost from the Hospital Cost Report Information System (HCRIS) files.

One response to such concerns about the MCR is to use cost-to-charge ratios derived from each hospital's own internal cost accounting data; see, for example, the analysis of coronary artery bypass costs by Mauldin et al. (1994). The approach is clearly most feasible in studies involving a small number of facilities, since the administrative cost involved increases proportionally with sample size. In addition, virtually any effort to construct cost-to-charge ratios from traditional hospital data systems must confront several general problems: traditional step-down methods of accounting that arbitrarily apportion overhead, the use of historical cost-based purchase price rather than replacement value to estimate capital costs, and omission of the opportunity cost of working capital. Moreover, any given cost-to-charge ratio (regardless of accounting data quality) is necessarily an average value for the cost category in question. Thus, for example, a ratio of 0.65 for Laboratory Services for a hospital would be typically applied to *all* inpatient laboratory charges at the facility, whatever the actual variation in the resource cost of producing different lab services.

Because most non-U.S. hospital systems do not routinely generate patient bills, cost-to-charge ratio approaches can rarely be applied outside of the U.S. Rather, if detailed inpatient cost estimates are desired, some form of ''bottom-up'' micro-costing will generally be required; see Krueger et al. (1992) for such an analysis of the cost of coronary artery bypass surgery in Canada.

Other Institutional Services, Including the Facility (Nonphysician) Components of Outpatient Care

Given current reimbursement arrangements and data systems, there are fewer cost finding options for these types of services (e.g., nursing home care) than for acute inpatient admissions. There are no DRGs, nor is it generally feasible to apply cost-to-charge ratio methods. The practical available options for estimating the cost of such care include: (1) treating the amount billed as an acceptable proxy; (2) treating the amount contributed by all payers (third parties plus patients) as an acceptable proxy; or (3) obtaining patient-specific data on resource utilization (e.g., nursing home days for each admission) and then applying previously computed unit cost multipliers (e.g., average cost per nursing home day) to arrive at cost per event.

In studies where claims data are available and appropriate, e.g., cost analyses by AHCPR's Patient Outcomes Research Teams, the most common approach is to estimate the costs of such services from the amounts reimbursed (Lave et al., 1994). In prospective studies, including clinical trials, the most common approach is to collect detailed data on utilization and then apply cost multipliers. Such utilization data may be derived from provider records, patient self-reports (including diaries), or self-reports confirmed (typically on a sampling basis) by provider records. For example, the Health Care Financing Administration's MEDPAR file provides utilization information on the use of skilled nursing facilities based on reimbursement records. The U.S. National Long-Term Care Survey (U.S. Bureau of the Census, 1993) yields self-report information on nursing home stays, which can be substantiated for respondents age 65 and over by linking with their Medicare records.

Physician and Other Professional Services

The cost-finding options just discussed can be applied to professional services generally. Thus, the focus is either on the amount billed, or on the amount reimbursed, or on the quantity of resources consumed (e.g., physician visits) multiplied by the estimated cost per visit. For physician services in the United States, there is an important national-level source of information on cost per visit—the new Medicare Fee Schedule, which was developed directly from the Resource-Based Relative Value Scale (RBRVS) (Hsiao, 1988). For each physician encounter registered in utilization records, or reported by the patient-respondent and later confirmed in the records, there is a Current Procedural Terminology 4 (CPT-4) code. Associated with each code is Medicare's national rate of reimbursement (which is subsequently adjusted for geographic location and a few other factors). These national-level physician reimbursement rates, fully phased in by 1996 for the Medicare program, offer a potentially important means to move toward standardization in the cost finding process (notwithstanding the criticisms leveled at the RBRVS itself).

Outpatient Drugs and Supplies, and Durable Medical Equipment

In studies where insurance coverage for these items is extensive, the analyst may approximate cost by either the amount billed or reimbursed, as above. However, in a given study, coverage may prove to be light or nonexistent. For example, Medicare pays for durable medical equipment but not outpatient drugs. A private health plan may cover outpatient drugs, subject to patient cost-sharing, but not medical equipment. The more shallow the insurance coverage, and thus the poorer the formal documentation of utilization, the greater will be the reliance on patient self-reports, which may take the form of mail surveys, telephone interviews, or diaries.

Nonmedical Costs and Time in Treatment for the Patient and (Unpaid) Caregivers

Rarely are the direct costs incurred for nonmedical goods and services associated with an intervention covered by insurance. For example, neither the electric bed purchased by a stroke victim nor the babysitting expenses incurred when one parent has to transport the other one to the doctor is likely to be insured. Hence, information on the type, frequency, and magnitude of such expenditures must generally be obtained through self-report channels: mail surveys, telephone interviews, or diaries.

The same conclusion holds for the patient's time in treatment and the time contributions of unpaid caregivers. Because there are no institutional records tracking these events, the only sources of data are the self-reports of the participants.

Conclusion

Resource limitations are the implicit or explicit constraint underlying health care decisions. The value of a CEA thus depends on the analyst's ability to accurately incorporate the resource consumption and savings attributable to an intervention into a study.

From the societal perspective, all resource costs and savings are at issue. Resource use is counted in a Reference Case analysis regardless of which individuals or institutions in society experience a gain or a loss, regardless of the type of resource (medical or nonmedical), and regardless of whether a monetary transaction accompanied consumption of the resource. The principle guiding the valuation of resources is opportunity cost, reflecting competing societal demands for resources. In this chapter, we have outlined two general approaches to assessing costs. Micro-costing reflects the ideal of identification, measurement, and valuation of resources. Gross-costing, which is more feasible in some cases, bases cost estimates on more aggregated information on resource use.

Because of the numerous contributors to cost, it is not feasible for an analyst to incorporate every relevant cost in a study or to research the precise opportunity cost of all resources. In practice, analysts must balance the expense and effort required to include and value a category or element of resource use in the analysis with its importance in the study. In the future, research to establish standard cost estimates for CEA may reduce the burden on analysts of obtaining comprehensive and accurate estimates of cost, and further improve the comparability of analyses.

Recommendations

1. Resource use and costs should be identified and valued from the societal perspective for the Reference Case analysis.

2. All resource use that is both germane to the analysis and nontrivial in magnitude should be included in the Reference Case analysis. Resource use should be reflected, regardless of whether a monetary transaction takes place.

3. Direct costs for health care resources (e.g., clinician time, hospital services, and laboratory test) and non–health care resources (e.g., child-care, transportation, and criminal justice resources) consumed as part of, or as a result of, an intervention are included in the numerator of the cost-effectiveness ratio.

4. The costs of caretaking and other services related to the intervention or illness that are provided by family or volunteers (home produced) are included in the numerator of the C/E ratio.

5. Time spent seeking care or undergoing an intervention is a resource and should be incorporated in the numerator of a cost-effectiveness ratio. If the intervention has a significant positive or negative impact on health-related quality of life, this impact should be incorporated into the denominator, leaving the time component in the numerator.

6. Morbidity costs of an intervention (its impact on productive time and leisure time) should be excluded from the numerator of the cost-effectiveness ratio, because it is fully captured in the denominator in the Reference Case. In some instances (e.g., when recuperating from surgery), time could be categorized either as morbidity time (in the denominator) or as input to the intervention itself (in the numerator). As a general rule, in a Reference Case analysis, this time should be considered as morbidity time.

7. The monetary value of lost life years should not be included in the numerator, because the effects of a health intervention on length of life are captured in the denominator.

8. Effects of lost productivity that are borne by others (e.g., employers, co-workers), when significant, including ''friction'' costs, should be included in the numerator of a Reference Case CEA.

9. ''Transfer payments'' (e.g., cash transfers from tax payers to welfare recipients) associated with a health intervention redistribute resources from one individual to another. While administrative costs associated with such transfers are included in the numerator of a C/E ratio, the transfers themselves do not since, by definition, their impact on the transferer and the recipient cancel out.

10. At the analyst's descretion, the Reference Case may either include or exclude health care costs for unrelated illness in added years of life.

11. Whenever the inclusion or exclusion of health care costs of unrelated diseases makes a significant difference to the analysis, a sensitivity analysis should be performed to assess their effect on the C/E ratio and to permit comparisons with CEAs in which these costs have been included.

12. Costs in CEA should reflect the marginal or incremental resources consumed, rather than average costs, from a long-run perspective.

13. In principle, the full three-step micro-costing approach to determining costs, entailing the identification, measurement, and valuation of resource use, is preferred. The choice between micro- and gross-costing approaches should reflect the importance of precise cost estimates, feasibility, and cost.

14. Changes in the use of resources caused by a health intervention should be valued at their opportunity cost.

15. To the extent that prices reflect opportunity costs, they are an appropriate basis for valuing changes in resources. If prices do not adequately reflect opportunity costs because of market distortions, they should be adjusted; when substantial bias is present and adjustment is not feasible, another proxy for opportunity cost should be used.

16. The prices used in a CEA should reflect the prevailing prices in the location where the intervention is or will be implemented.

17. Variable costs, reflecting the value of those goods, services, and inputs that change because of the intervention being considered, should be included in the CEA, while fixed costs, which remain constant in the long run regardless of the level of production, should be excluded.

18. For the Reference Case, research and development and other "first-copy" costs should be included if the decision addresses whether to provide the intervention at all. For prescription drugs, long-run marginal cost can be adequately approximated in most cases by the Average Wholesale Price. Analysts are encouraged to conduct a formal sensitivity analysis to determine the impact of R&D costs on the price to be used in the analysis.

19. When information on capacity utilization in hospitals or other health care facilities is not available, we recommend that analysts use the benchmark assumption that capacity is utilized at the rate of 80%, under a long run perspective. When better information is available, that information should be used.

20. CEAs should be conducted in constant dollars that remove general price inflation. If the prices in question change at a rate different from general price levels, this variation should be reflected in the adjustments used.

21. For individuals in the labor force, wages are generally an acceptable measure of time costs.

22. Wages corresponding to the target population should be used to approximate time costs. In general, age- and gender-specific wage estimates will provide adequately specific estimates. If the analyst determines that these wages provide a biased estimate for a particular targeted population, a more specific wage estimate can be used.

23. Use of group-specific wages may influence the conclusions of the anlaysis in ways that are ethically problematic. In these instances, sensitivity analysis should be conducted to explicitly indicate the nature of this influence.

24. The wage rate generally does not adequately reflect the value of time for persons engaged primarily in leisure or in activities for which they are not compensated. For individuals not engaged in compensated employment, wages used as proxies must be adjusted to reflect the full opportunity cost of time.

25. In valuing unpaid services provided by volunteers or family members (home production), the preferred approach is to use the hourly wage of individuals with similar characteristics who do work for pay.

Research Recommendations

1. Research to establish standard cost estimates for CEA will facilitate individual analyses and improve comparability among analyses.

2. Research to obtain reasonable values for the opportunity costs of time for population groups for whom traditional labor market methods do not apply—that is, children, the retired elderly, and persons unable to work—is encouraged.

Notes

1. If one were doing a cost-benefit analysis on zidovudine (AZT) research, one would under-take any research strategy where the marginal willingness to pay for another dose of AZT equaled the marginal cost of producing and distributing one more dose and then sum the consumer surplus for AZT (at that price) over all of the users of AZT. If this sum were sufficient to cover the first-copy costs of research and development, then the R&D would be justified. Note that in this case, we do not prorate the cost of R&D over the units consumed, and then ask the question: Is the marginal willingness to pay at least that large? Such an approach will lead to two errors: (1) a decision to provide AZT to fewer people than optimal (or at a lower dosage than optimal) if it is produced and (2) a decision in some cases to not produce a good or service when it is desirable to do so.

2. If all prices and incomes move *exactly* together, then the physical quantities that the con-sumer can afford are unchanged. For example, regardless of whether prices and incomes are measured in dollars, quarters, or dimes, the consumer can still afford to buy the same physical amount. An amount of $100 spent on two goods with prices of $1 and $5 will buy the same quantities as $1,000 spent on goods priced at $10 and $50.

$$100 = 1 \cdot x + 5 \cdot y$$

$$1,000 = 10 \cdot x + 50 \cdot y$$

Both imply that the consumer can afford $x = 100 - 5y$.

3. This discussion applies to the handling of future costs. It should not be confused with the practice of bringing past prices into current dollars. If the analyst needs an estimate of a price or cost, but does not have a current dollar price, he may rely on estimates based on past prices or costs and then convert those past prices or costs into an estimate of current prices or costs. The analyst is not dealing with a stream of past and current expenditures. Instead, he is using an inflation-corrected past price as a proxy or missing value replacement. In such a case, the missing value replacement is not discounted.

4. In a perfectly competitive market, the individual will work at a given wage if the value of that individual's time is less than the value of the goods and services that the wage will buy. In the absence of structural unemployment, not working at the given wage implies that the value of leisure time exceeds the wage. Thus, for a nonworker, the wage that the person could but

chooses not to, earn is a lower bound on the value of time. The wage rate at which the person would be willing to work (the reservation wage) is the actual value of the time.

References

Ashby, J.L., Jr. 1992. The accuracy of cost measures derived from Medicare cost report data. *Hospital Cost Management and Accounting* 3:1–8.

Boiteux, M. 1960. La tarification des demands en pointe: Applications de la théorie de la vente au coût marginal. *Revue Générale de l'Électricité* 33:157–79.

Boiteux, M. 1956. Sur la gestion des monopoles publics astrients a l'Équilibre budgétaire. *Econometrica* 24:22–40.

Deaton, A., and J. Muellbauer. 1980. *Economics and consumer behavior*. New York: Cambridge University Press.

Drèze, J. 1964. Some postwar contributions of French economists. *American Economic Review* 54:1–64.

Drug Topics Red Book. 1994. Montvale NJ: Medical Economics Company, Inc.

Dudley, R.A., F.E. Harrell, Jr., L.R. Smith, D.B. Mark, R.M. Califf, D.B. Pryor, D. Glower, J. Lipscomb, and M. Hlatky. 1993. Comparison of analytic models for estimating the effect of clinical factors on the cost of coronary artery bypass graft surgery. *J Clin Epidemiol* 46:261–71.

Eisenberg, J.M., H. Koffer, and S.A. Finkler. 1984. Economic analysis of a new drug: Potential savings in hospital operating cost from the use of a once-daily regimen of parenteral cephalosporin. *Rev Infect Dis* 6 (suppl 4): S909–23.

Finkler, S.A. 1982. The distinction between costs and charges. *Ann Intern Med* 96:102–9.

Garber, A.M., and C.E. Phelps. 1995. Economic foundations of cost-effectiveness analysis. National Bureau of Economic Research.

Gorsky, R.D. 1996. A method to measure the costs of counseling for HIV prevention. *Public Health Rep* (in press).

Gronau, R. 1986. Home production—a survey. In *Handbook of labor economics*, Vol. 1, ed. O. Ashenfelter and P.R.G. Layard, 274–304. New York: Elsevier Science Publishers BV.

Gronau, R. 1977. Leisure, home production, and work—the theory of the allocation of time revisited. *J Political Economy* 85:1099–1123.

Gronau, R. 1973. The effects of children on the housewife's value of time. *J Political Economy* 81:S168–S199.

Hardin, G. 1968. The tragedy of the commons. *Science* 162:1243–48.

Health Economics Research. 1994. Volume I: Technical proposal costing AHCPR guidelines. Waltham, MA.

Heckman, J. 1980. Sample selection bias as specification error with an application to the estimation of labor supply functions. In *Studies in female labor supply*, ed. J. Smith, 206–57. Princeton, NJ: Princeton University Press.

Hlatky, M.A., J. Lipscomb, C. Nelson, R.M. Califf, D. Pryor, A.G. Wallace, and D.B. Mark. 1990. Resource use and cost of initial coronary revascularization: Coronary angioplasty versus coronary bypass surgery. *Circulation* 82(suppl 4):208–13.

Holloway, R.G., D.M. Witter, Jr., K.B. Lawton, J. Lipscomb, and G. Samsa. 1996. Inpatient costs of specific cerebrovascular events at five academic medical centers. *Neurol* 46:854–60.

Hsiao, W., P. Braun, P.L. Kelly, and E.C. Becker. 1988. Results, potential effects and implementation issues of the resource-based relative value system. *JAMA* 260:2429–38.

Javitt, J.C., J.K. Canner, and A. Sommer. 1988. Cost effectiveness of current approaches to the
control of diabetic retinopathy in type I diabetes. *Opthalmology* 96:255–64.

Joskow, P.L. 1980. The effects of competition and regulation on hospital bed supply and the
reservation quality of the hospital. *Bell J Economics* 11(2):421–48.

Krueger H., J.L. Goncalves, F.M. Caruth, and R.I. Hayden. 1992. Coronary artery bypass grafting:
How much does it cost? *Can Med Assoc J* 146:163–68.

Lave, J.R., C.L. Pashos, G.F. Anderson, D. Brailer, T. Bubolz, D. Conrad, D.A. Freund, S.H.
Fox, E. Keeler, J. Lipscomb, H.S. Luft, and G. Provenzano. 1994. Costing medical care:
Using Medicare administrative data. *Med Care* 32:JS77–JS89.

Lipscomb, J., D.B. Mark, P.A. Cowper, D. Sumner, and L. Davidson-Ray. 1994. Comparison of
hospital costs derived from cost-to-charge ratios and from a detailed cost accounting
system for patients undergoing cardiac procedures. Proceedings, annual meeting of the
Association for Health Services Research, June at San Diego, CA.

Mauldin, P.D., W.S. Weintraub, and E.R. Becker. 1994. Predicting hospital costs for first-time
coronary artery bypass grafting from preoperative and postoperative variables. *Am J Cardiol* 74:772–75.

Oster, G., and A.M. Epstein. 1987. Cost-effectiveness of antihyperlipemic therapy in the prevention of coronary heart disease: The case of cholestyramine. *JAMA* 258:2381–87.

Oster, G., and A.M. Epstein. 1986. Primary prevention and coronary heart disease: the economic
benefits of lowering serum choleterol. *Am J Public Health* 76:6:647–656.

Smith, L.R., C.A. Milano, B.S. Molter, J.R. Ebeery, D.C. Sabiston, Jr., and P.K. Smith. 1994.
Preoperative determinants of postoperative costs associated with coronary artery bypass
graft surgery. *Circulation* 90(part 2):124–28.

Starrett, D.A. 1988. *Foundation of public economics.* New York: Cambridge University Press.

U.S. Bureau of Labor Statistics, Office of Compensation and Working Conditions. 1995. *Area
Wage Index* Washington, DC: U.S. Department of Labor.

U.S. Bureau of the Census. *Current Population Reports.* Washington, DC: U.S. Department of
Commerce.

U.S. Bureau of the Census. 1993. *National Long Term Care Survey.* Washington, DC: U.S.
Department of Commerce.

U.S. Bureau of the Census. 1995. *Statistical Abstract of the United States* (115th ed.). Washington, DC: U.S. Department of Commerce.

Wong, J.B., F.A. Sonnenberg, D.N. Salem, and S.G. Pauker. 1990. Myocardial revascularization
for chronic stable angina: Analysis of the role of percutaneous transluminal coronary
angioplasty based on data available in 1989. *Ann Intern Med* 113:852–71.

Zick, C.D., and W.K. Bryant. 1990. Shadow wage assessments of the value of home production:
Patterns from the 1970s. *Lifestyles: Family and Economic Issues* 11(2):143–60.

7

Time Preference

J. LIPSCOMB, M.C. WEINSTEIN,
and G.W. TORRANCE

There is broad agreement that, in cost-effectiveness analyses, all future costs and health consequences should be stated in terms of their "present value" to the decision maker. Only then will the interventions' cost-effectiveness ratios be appropriately adjusted for the differential timing of costs and consequences so that the decision maker can compare each from the same temporal baseline. Virtually all checklists of the methodological "commandments" on how to conduct CEAs include such injunctions (e.g., Drummond et al., 1987; Eisenberg, 1989).

At the outset, it is instructive to examine the computational process, called *discounting*, for obtaining the present values of cost and health consequences in a given application. Central to this process—and, indeed, central to this chapter—is the selection of a discount rate for cost, and for health consequences, that reflects in each case the social decision-maker's *time preference* for present over future outcomes (Olson and Bailey, 1981). Thus, if the decision maker happens to be indifferent between incurring $1 of cost today versus $1.10 in cost a year from now, this implies an annual rate of time preference over cost outcomes of 10%; this is operationalized by employing an annual discount rate of 0.10.

To illustrate, suppose a 3-year program has been proposed with the following anticipated streams of costs and health consequences relative to the status quo: year 1, $10,000 and 2 life years gained; year 2, $12,000 and 3 life years gained; and year 3, $8,000 and 4 life years gained. Then, given the (arbitrarily chosen) discount rate above, the present value of cost and of health consequences may be expressed, respectively, as

$$\Delta C = 10{,}000 + 12{,}000/(1 + 0.10) + 8{,}000/(1 + 0.10)^2 = \$27{,}521$$

and

$$\Delta E = 2 + 3/(1 + 0.10) + 4/(1 + 0.10)^2 = 8.04 \text{ life years}$$

so the cost-effectiveness ratio is $\Delta C/\Delta E = \$3{,}423$/life year gained.

214

As indicated above, we adopt the convention of assuming that costs and effects occur at the beginning of each time interval (year). One could just as easily assume that these outcomes accrue at the end of each interval, or at the midpoint, and many CEAs do one or the other. We prefer the approach above, however, because it is consistent with the frequently employed practice of not discounting costs and health consequences that occur in the first year of the time stream.[1]

Virtually all cost-effectiveness analyses in health to date have used some variant of the following "discrete-time" model. Let $E_j(t)$ be the health consequence (QALYs, years of life saved, or other measure) in time period t for a well-defined group of individuals who receive intervention j, and let $E_0(t)$ be the health consequence expected for the group under the comparator (baseline) intervention. Let $C_j(t)$ and $C_0(t)$ be the corresponding costs associated with these interventions for period t. If the interventions were initiated at period 1 and continued through period T, then the present value of costs and health consequences (from the vantage point of the start of period 1) can be calculated, respectively, as

$$\Delta C = \Sigma_1^T[C_j(t) - C_0(t)]/(1 + i)^{t-1} \tag{1}$$

and

$$\Delta E = \Sigma_1^T[E_j(t) - E_0(t)]/(1 + r)^{t-1} \tag{2}$$

where i and r are the discount rates selected to convert future costs and health consequences, respectively, to present value. Dividing Equation (1) by Equation (2) yields the cost-effectiveness ratio for the intervention relative to the comparator.[2] We maintain the distinction between the discount rates for costs (i) and for health consequences (r) throughout the chapter, although our recommendation will be that, in general, they should be equal.

There is consensus in economics that Equation (1) represents the appropriate vehicle for converting costs (and monetary flows, in general) to present value, given the assumption of a constant discount rate over time. However, there has been much debate—mostly in the literature on cost-benefit analysis—about the specific value of the discount rate i appropriate for social program evaluation (e.g., Robinson, 1990; Lind, 1982; Sugden and Williams, pp. 1978, 211–228; Feldstein, 1964; Marglin, 1963). That debate has narrowed sharply in recent years, at least among economists, so now there is a dominant view, if not consensus, on the conceptually appropriate way to choose this rate. Moreover, there is a rough consensus on the range of rates from which to select a discount rate in a given application.

By contrast, there remains considerable controversy about precisely how to convert future health consequences—expressed in nonmonetary terms—to present value (Krahn and Gafni, 1993; Cairns, 1992; McNeil et al., 1978; Gafni and Torrance, 1984; Ganiats, 1994; Katz and Welch, 1993; Horowitz and Carson, 1990; Coyle and Tolley, 1992; Olsen, 1993; Hammitt, 1993). Thus, for example, should a life year gained 10 years from now be valued differently than a life year gained 1 year hence? If so, should it have a lower (and thus discounted) value? And if so, by how much?

The appropriate discount rate for health consequences in a cost-effectiveness analysis from the societal perspective—which we emphasize here because of its centrality for the Reference Case analysis—may well be different from that for other decision makers, such as private insurers, the individual patient, or even the government under some circumstances.[3] While we will not explore all of these perspectives, we will carefully examine time preference and discounting from the standpoint of the individual, because individual preferences are crucial in determining social welfare under the welfare-theoretic foundation of CEA and because there is evidence that individuals have widely varying time preferences for health outcomes.

In current CEAs, it is the mainstream practice to discount future health consequences to present value, just as one would discount future monetary flows. Moreover, the prevailing practice is to set r (the discount rate for health consequences) equal to i (the discount rate for cost).

The principal purpose of this chapter is to examine the role of time preference in cost-effectiveness analyses of health programs. While a number of issues will be examined, much attention will be devoted to the assumptions, rationales, and reasonableness of setting the discount rate for costs equal to that for health effects and to the problem of selecting a reasonable discount rate for application.

In the sections that follow, we first examine the conceptual basis for selecting a discount rate for costs. Then we turn to the more complex and vexing problems that arise in determining the present value of health consequences. In particular, we review the standard arguments that support setting $r = i$ (one of which was presented in Chapter 2), and we evaluate a set of counterarguments that challenge this approach. We give special attention to the theoretically unsettled issue of how to reconcile diverse individual rates of time preference within the societal perspective. Next we discuss the practical matter of how to choose a discount rate for societal CEAs. In that regard, we discuss the policies and recommendations of several government organizations and private analysts regarding the choice of discount rates for health costs and consequences. We also stress the importance of choosing a base-case rate for the Reference Case analysis and conducting sensitivity analysis around the base case. The concluding section contains our recommendations on how to proceed amidst the complexities and controversies that characterize this area of cost-effectiveness analysis.

Discounting Costs

Economic theory implies that in a perfectly competitive, risk-free, tax-free world in which all commodities (including something called ''health'') are ''perfectly divisible''—so that individual decision makers could precisely adapt their consumption of goods and services over time—there would be but *one* interest rate. It would represent, simultaneously, two fundamentally different expressions of time preference. First, such an interest rate would reflect the *consumption rate of interest* for the individual. The consumption rate of interest is an index of an individual's preferences regarding present and future *consumption* as reflected, for example, in after-tax returns on savings accounts. At the same time, this very same interest rate would reflect the *marginal rate of return on private investment*. The marginal rate of return on private investment is an index of the amount of future consumption that could be obtained by *investing* resources productively in the economy instead of consuming them at the present time and is reflected, for example, in corporate pretax returns on investment. This single interest rate would be the appropriate "social discount rate" for use in all cost-benefit and cost-effectiveness analyses.

In reality, markets are imperfect, investments are risky, and taxes abound. Indeed, individual and corporate taxes alone are sufficient to drive a wedge between an individual's consumption rate of interest (that is, the after-tax rate at which he or she is just willing to trade present for future consumption) and the marginal rate of return on private investment (reflecting the before-tax return from postponed consumption). Thus, many market interest rates coexist. Which, if any, should be used to discount costs in CEA?

At this point it is useful to examine briefly the debate about the appropriate discount rate for economic evaluations of social programs generally. Over the years, two broadly different strategies have been debated, and within each a number of alternative practical approaches for selecting a discount rate have been proposed (Arrow, 1966; Lind, 1982; Robinson, 1990; Krahn and Gafni, 1993). One strategy, consistent with modern welfare economics, requires that the societal discount rate be derived on the basis of revealed preferences in the marketplace. The myriad market interactions of consumers and producers yield information in the form of interest rates, returns on capital, and the like. The assumption is that current market rates—especially long-term rates, which theoretically reflect expectations regarding future time preferences and returns on investment—convey the relevant information needed to derive the social rate of discount (Harberger, 1973).

The other strategy rejects market-generated rates as inadequate and proposes, instead, that the social rate of discount be derived through the political process. Among the many arguments that have been advanced, the rationale has typically run along one of two lines. First, current market rates (and the private transactions that determine them) reflect an inadequate concern for future generations; hence, the social rate needs to be set lower than prevailing market rates. Second, individuals tend to have preferences for societal outcomes (e.g., the distribution of health or wealth across generations) that are distinct from the preferences that drive their private consumption and investment activity. Thus, current market rates of interest, reflecting only these private transactions cannot adequately convey the societal time preferences of market participants (Sen, 1982). As Krahn and Gafni (1993) note, a number of philosophers have challenged the normative foundations of any effort to derive the social discount rate on the basis of the private market transactions of individuals.

Whatever the merits of these arguments, an overarching practical difficulty with any extramarket process for determining the social discount rate is the absence of a well-defined political process or some other mechanism for determining the rate. Much more explicit guidance for choosing a rate has been generated over the years by the strategy that relies on current market transactions. Two distinct approaches have been debated.

First, under what has been termed the *social opportunity cost* (SOC) approach, the discount rate for cost (*i* in Equation [1]) is constructed as a weighted average of discount rates applicable to the various sectors of the economy contributing resources to the programs under evaluation. As Lind (1982) notes, there have been several variants of this proposal. Thus, Haveman (1969) has argued that the social rate should be a weighted average that reflects (1) the consumption rate of interest to the extent that the public program displaces consumption and (2) the marginal return on private investment to the extent that the public program displaces private investment; see also Baumol (1968). Others, such as Harberger, have contended that public investment basically "crowds out" private investment. That is, borrowing for public sector use raises interest rates, ultimately shifting resources away from uses in the private sector. Hence, the social discount rate should be a weighted average of the rates of return on private investment applicable to those sectors of the economy contributing resources to the social program.

In recent years, however, the social opportunity cost approach for identifying a discount rate has been eclipsed by an alternative termed the *shadow-price-of-capital* (SPC) approach, which economists now generally regard as conceptually superior. Under this approach, one first transforms the stream of program *costs* over time into the corresponding stream of *consumption losses* that would be induced by the forgone investment and consumption opportunities. Next, one transforms the stream of program *benefits* into the corresponding stream of *consumption gains*. Finally, one discounts these streams to present value using the *social rate of time preference* (SRTP)—that is, the rate at which the social decision maker is willing to trade off present for future *consumption*. (See Feldstein, 1972, or Bradford, 1975, for an early systematic exposition of this approach.) The basic premise is that the ultimate purpose of all private investment (and economic activity, in general) is consumption; thus, the proper measure of the opportunity cost of a public program, in terms of foregone private activities, is the present value of the consumption that would be given up. In general, the SPC approach will yield a different social discount rate from the SOC approach if there are more than two time periods involved (Feldstein, 1972).

A linchpin question under the SPC approach, of course, is how to determine the social rate of time preference. Cost-benefit analysts working in environmental policy have proposed practical ways to approximate this rate. Based on an analysis of U.S. Treasury bills, Lind (1982) determined that the real rate of time preference on "safe investments" was 1%; the real rate of time preference on a "safe long-term asset," such as a government bond (which is at some risk to shifts in the level of rates), was pegged at 2%. More recently, Lesser and Zerbe (1994) argue that under reasonable assumptions, the social rate of time preference can be well approximated by market interest rates reflecting the cost of capital. They recommend indexing the latter by the rate of return on government bonds whose length to maturity is roughly equal to the duration of the program being evaluated. In recent years, they conclude, this implies a real annual discount rate ranging from 2.5% to 5%. We return to the practical question of choosing a discount rate for health-related cost-effectiveness analyses later in this chapter.

We have assumed, and there is a broad (if implicit) consensus, that whatever discount rate is appropriate for a cost-benefit analysis will likewise be appropriate for discounting costs in a CEA framework. On the other hand, there has been much debate about how to bring health consequences to present value. We turn now to these issues.

Discounting Health Consequences

Aside from appeals to simplicity and tractability (which should not be discounted here), two major substantive rationales have been put forth in support of setting the discount rate for health consequences (r) equal to that for costs (i). These are the "consistency" argument of Weinstein and Stason (1977) and the Keeler-Cretin paradox (Keeler and Cretin, 1983).

The "consistency" argument holds that

> the reason for discounting future life years is precisely that they are being valued relative to dollars and, since a dollar in the future is discounted relative to a present dollar, so must a life year in the future be discounted relative to a present dollar. . . . It is the discounting of dollar costs, *and the assumed steady-state relation between dollars and health benefits* [emphasis added], that mandates the discounting of health benefits as well as dollars.
>
> (Weinstein and Stason, 1977, p. 720)

The detailed example used by the authors to illustrate this proposition has been reproduced in Figure 7.1.

Viewed from the perspective of society (not the individual), Williams (1981) finds such reasoning persuasive:

> because it is possible, at the margin, to transform health into wealth, and vice versa, at any point in time, and since "wealth" is (ideally) allocated through time with reference to the rate of social time preference, then it would be inconsistent to apply a different rate of discount to 'health' from that being applied to "wealth."
>
> (p. 277)

Closely related to the consistency argument is the paradox of Keeler and Cretin, described previously in Chapter 2. Keeler and Cretin (1983) attack the problem from a somewhat different angle by setting up a simple, multiperiod cost-effectiveness problem in which a perpetual sequence of statistically identical cohorts are vying for dollars from a budget that must be allocated (once and for all) at the present moment (i.e., at

Figure 7.1. Illustrating the consistency argument for discounting costs and health consequences at the same rate.

.. For programs involving screening for disease, where the life years saved are far in the future, it matters a great deal whether expected benefits are discounted. Without discounting, a program that saves one quality-adjusted life year 40 years hence at a present-value cost of $10,000 would have a cost-effectiveness ratio of $10,000 per QALY. With discounting at 5 per cent per year, the present value of that future QALY is reduced to $1/(1.05)^{40}$ or about 0.14, and the ratio becomes $70,000 per QALY, a remarkable difference in the implied priority of the program in the range of possible alternative uses of health resources. . . .

. . . Consider the following example that illustrates the chain of logic for discounting future health benefits (Table 1). Suppose that Program A saves one year of life expectancy 40 years hence at a present cost of $10,000, and that Program B saves one year of life expectancy now at a present cost of $10,000. Which program should have higher priority? To answer this question, consider first a hypothetical Program A_1, which can save one year of life 40 years hence at a cost of $70,000 borne in 40 years. This result is equivalent to Program A because $70,000 in 40 years has a present value (at 5 per cent) of $10,000 and because the benefits of both programs, A and A_1, are the same. Now, consider Program A_2, which simply translates both the benefits and the costs of Program A_1 from the future to the present. Provided life years are valued the same in relation to dollars in the present as in the future, Program A_2 should be considered to have the same long-run priority as Program A_1. Finally, consider Program A_3, under which both the benefits and the costs are reduced proportionately in relation to Program A_2 and which, therefore, has the same priority. Now, it is clear that Program B is preferable to Program A_3, since the costs are identical, but the benefits of Program B, which accrue at the same point in time as those of A_3, are much more. Moreover, we have seen that Program A_3, which has the same priority as Program A, could have been derived from Program A simply by discounting the future health benefits. The cost-effectiveness ratio for Program A is thus the present value of cost divided by the present value of benefit, or $10,000 \div (1/(1.05)^{40})$, or $70,000 per QALY, which compares unfavorably to the $10,000 per QALY ratio for Program B.

Table 1. Hypothetical Programs with Varying Timing of Costs and Health Benefits.

Program	Cost	Benefit
A	$10,000 now	1 yr of life expectancy in 40 yr
A_1	$70,000* in 40 yr	1 yr of life expectancy in 40 yr
A_2	$70,000 now	1 yr of life expectancy now
A_3	$10,000 now	$1/7 = 1/(1.05)^{40}$ yr of life expectancy now
B	$10,000 now	1 yr of life expectancy now

*$70,000 = $10,000 \times 1.05^{40}$.

Weinstein and Stason, 1977

the beginning of period 1 in the notation of Equations [1] and [2]). They show that, under certain conditions, if program effectiveness and costs are discounted at different rates, paradoxes arise in program implementation. In particular, if r is set below i, then the cost-effectiveness of any candidate program can always be improved by delaying its start successively in time. The longer one delays the program, the better its cost-effectiveness ratio, so a decision maker guided strictly by the logic of CEA would be led to postpone the program indefinitely. The following simple example, adapted from CDC (1994), summarizes the essence of the argument:

Assume that an investment of $100 today would result in saving 10 lives (or 1 life per $10 of investment). If the $100 were invested at a 10% rate of return, in 1 year it would be worth $110; and with this $110, it would be possible to save 11 lives. If the original $100 were invested for 2 years at 10%, it would be worth $121, and 12 lives could be saved. If the social decision maker is attempting to maximize the health output obtainable from the original $100, *and* if the value of future lives saved is not discounted, then the cost-effectiveness of the investment is improved for every year it is delayed. Without further restrictions, the investment would be delayed indefinitely (or, from another perspective, postponed ''until next year'' on a perpetual basis). It is easy to show that the paradox persists if lives saved are discounted at any rate below 10%, the rate by which cost would be discounted here in a CEA.

Adding force to the rationale for setting $r = i$ in cost-effectiveness analysis is that it leads to resource allocations in a ''time neutral'' fashion. Potential program beneficiaries who are identical in every respect except for their positions in time relative to the moment the decision maker must act will receive equal treatment. In contrast, if $r \neq i$, these identical beneficiaries will be assigned unequal cost-effectiveness ratios once the present value calculations are completed. Hence, setting $r = i$ creates what economists term *horizontal equity* among potential beneficiaries.

Moreover, one can make a veil-of-ignorance type of argument that such time neutrality is the most reasonable stance for the social decision maker to adopt. (See Chapter 2 for discussion of veil-of-ignorance reasoning.) Imagine a potential beneficiary ''behind the veil,'' totally ignorant of what future generation she will join and, in general, of what moment in time a health intervention will be needed. It is arguable that this individual would wish that each generation, each cohort, and indeed each future moment in time could be treated by the social decision maker in a time-neutral fashion. An implication of time neutrality is that for any two cohorts vying for resources, what matters is not whether one, or both, are ''alive'' at the moment of decision; rather, what matters is the health payoff per dollar spent for the candidate programs—regardless of when they are assumed to occur. This result of setting $r = i$ is illustrated in Appendix 7.2.

In light of these arguments, is there any reason *not* to adopt the strategy of discounting health consequences at the same rate as costs in CEA? In fact, this approach can be challenged potentially on several fronts. Some of these challenges are ad hoc and not firmly grounded, in our view; we review these first. The remainder of this section critically examines several of the more compelling claims.

Claim: Prevention Is Different

Some observers aver that when CEA is being applied to prevention programs, a lower discount rate (possibly even zero) should be applied to health consequences than to costs. Otherwise, it is argued, important downstream benefits will be unduly devalued relative to up-front costs, and prevention will too frequently appear to be not cost-effective. The remedy for this undervaluation—if indeed it occurs—is not found in ad hoc manipulations of the discount rate. As Fuchs and Zeckhauser (1987) assert: ''Self-respecting economists should not adjust discount rates for externalities stretching to the future or use different rates because it is health that is being valued'' (p. 265). Rather, if one wants to give extra emphasis to the output of such programs, one should ''adjust . . . valuations of future benefits upward . . . not [the] discount rate downward.'' In this way, the decision maker confronts the allocative implications of such a choice squarely and executes the differential weighting (if there is a compelling case for it) in a precise and transparent fashion.

Claim: Discount Rates in CEA Must Be Adjusted for Inflation

By way of introduction, there are two cases to consider: (1) The components of medical cost—for example, health care workers' wages, drugs—inflate at the same rate (or approximately so), or (2) they inflate at significantly different rates over time. That is, inflation may be assumed to be either balanced or unbalanced.

In cost-benefit analysis, it is well known that regardless of the pattern of inflation, one has the option of conducting the calculations in either real or nominal terms. In the former, all monetary outcome measures *and* the social rate of time preference are expressed as inflation-adjusted values. In the latter, each component of cost and benefit is allowed to inflate at its own (projected) rate and the discount rate is likewise expressed in nominal terms (generally, as the real rate plus the overall inflation rate). In principle, the choice of approach hinges on the degree of inflation imbalance. That is, if the components of medical cost inflate at very different rates, the latter method would be preferred. In practice, virtually all CBAs take the simplifying route of assuming balanced inflation and proceeding in real terms.

Similarly, all CEA applications known to the authors have been conducted in real terms. The distinction, however, is that in CEA only a ''real'' approach appears to make sense. To conduct a CEA in nominal terms would require that program effectiveness (e.g., QALYs) be converted from its natural unit of measure—which is inherently ''real''—into some other, inflation-multiplied unit of measure. While the arithmetic for carrying this out is straightforward, the exact interpretation of the resulting ''nominal'' units of effectiveness is not. If unbalanced inflation among the components of cost was deemed a problem, then the cost stream for each component could be deflated by the inflation factor applicable to that component; then the total program cost for each period would be expressed in real terms as the sum of its (estimated) real components. We are unaware of any attempts to deal with unbalanced inflation in CEA.

Claim: Discount Rates Must Be Adjusted for Uncertainty

When a cost-effectiveness analysis formally acknowledges that both costs and health consequences are uncertain, how should this affect the present value calculations? Over the years, some cost-benefit analysts have advocated adding a risk premium to the underlying (riskless) discount rate in order to give less weight to future uncertain consequences; see, for example, the review presented in Krahn and Gafni (1993). But the currently prevailing view regarding public investments is quite different: first convert all uncertain costs and effectiveness estimates to their ''certainty equivalents,'' expressed in real terms; then discount these at the selected real riskless rate. (See Lind, 1982, and Viscusi, 1995, for discussions.)

We explore this approach a bit further. For any uncertain outcome (whether cost or health benefit) its certainty equivalent is defined as follows. Imagine a decision maker with a hypothetical choice between (1) the outcome of interest viewed as a random variable (which in fact it is) and (2) some selected value of this outcome variable that could be guaranteed to occur (with certainty). That particular outcome value in (2) that makes the decision maker indifferent between choices (1) and (2) is called the *certainty equivalent of the uncertain outcome*. In point of fact, virtually all CEAs (and CBAs) conducted from the societal perspective assume, usually implicitly, that the decision maker is ''risk neutral''—implying that the certainty equivalent for each outcome is equivalent in preference to the mean (or average) value of the outcome.[4]

Now let us turn to the more interesting challenges to the practice of setting the discount rate for health consequences equal to that for costs. In the process, we will examine further the assumptions and conditions which underlie the setting of $r = i$.

Claim: The Keeler-Cretin Paradox Is Not Relevant to the Real World

While their brief is elegant and mathematically unassailable, the practical import of the Keeler-Cretin argument has been questioned (e.g., Parsonage and Neuburger, 1992). Some have observed that bureaucrats who use CEAs based on a discount rate for health benefits that is less than that for costs ($r < i$) will be politically motivated (or forced) to commit resources to current programs regardless of the dictates of the analysis (Redelmeier et al., 1994). Additionally, the Keeler-Cretin argument loses force if the time horizon for budget allocation is finite. To be concrete, imagine the very specific problem of allocating a designated budget across 5 years to seven finite population groups competing to receive a screening program. Regardless of the relationship assumed between the rates used to discount program costs and health consequences to present value, this CEA yields an unambiguous allocation of dollars across the seven groups and 5 years. It may well be that the social decision maker wants to set $r = i$ in this CEA, but setting $r < i$ in this context leads to no ambiguity or indefinite postponement in the allocation of resources. It should also be noted that the less-discussed case of $r > i$ poses no such paradox; see Keeler and Cretin (1983) and Lipscomb (1989).

In our view, the Keeler-Cretin paradox adds force to the argument for setting $r = i$. As noted, one can easily envision real decision contexts in which the paradox is essentially overridden by political, economic, or administrative constraints on the decision maker. Yet, many (perhaps most) of the cost-effectiveness analyses in health are conducted in the absence of such context-specific information; future constraints are unknown and frequently unknowable. In such cases, it is sensible to compute cost-effectiveness ratios in a way that avoids the paradox.

Claim: It Is More Reasonable to Discount Future Health Outcomes at a Nonconstant Rate

Harvey (1994) argues that the two standard approaches usually considered for computing present value of nonmonetary benefits—constant-rate discounting using the geometric functional form in Equation (2), and no discounting—are both too extreme. Traditional constant-rate discounting gives too little weight to the future relative to the present, he says, while failing to discount does just the opposite.

Harvey contends that a more defensible approach is to replace the discount factors in Equation (2) with discount rates that decrease as a function of time. Specifically, he proposes replacing the usual discount factors, $1/(1+r)^t$ by functions of the form $a(t) = [b/(b+t)]$, where $b > 0$. Such proportional, or "slow," discounting would strike a more reasonable balance between the weight accorded to the short term and the long term, he argues. Harvey concludes that both psychological evidence and common political observation imply that the time stationarity assumption built into constant-rate discounting (Koopmans et al., 1964; Green, 1978, chapter 12, especially pp. 186–196) is unrealistic.[5] Rather, the relative importance attached to the difference between any two outcomes tends to recede as the outcomes recede into the future. Such a tendency is consistent with proportional discounting—and inconsistent with constant-rate discounting.

Empirical evidence supporting nonconstant discounting by individuals has been presented in behavioral studies by psychologists (Ainslie and Haslam, 1992; Loewenstein and Prelec, 1992, 1993) and in a survey by Cropper et al., (1994). The latter survey suggests that individual discount rates are higher when the time interval for making tradeoffs is shorter and the respondent is older.

Notwithstanding the descriptive evidence, there are serious theoretical problems with this seemingly appealing construct. Abandoning constant-rate discounting leads to a disturbing consequence: The rate of tradeoff between health improvements at two different future times depends on the temporal vantage point from which one views those future times. Under "slow" discounting, as a future time period approaches, the rate of discount between that period and a more distant future time period increases. This means, in effect, that one's time preferences change—and predictably so—as time itself advances. Harvey dismisses this "dynamic inconsistency" objection (which dates from Strotz, 1956), pointing out that individuals may indeed experience evolving time preferences as a manifestation of the perplexing dilemma of "multiple selves" in behavioral decision theory.

But to base a normative theory of social choice on a foundation of dynamically shifting preferences is to abandon a fundamental tenet of welfare economics—namely, the stability of preferences. As a normative matter, it seems odd that one would allocate resources between two future years according to one's current preferences, knowing all the time that these preferences will change, thus eventually rendering the allocation suboptimal. More significantly, this course establishes an allocation regime in which cost-effectiveness rankings initially established in a base period are at risk to shifting as time progresses *and only because time progresses*. (This is the analogue of Strotz's "dynamically inconsistent" consumer who is constantly revising his multi-year consumption plan with every passing year.)

Consequently, it is more reasonable for the social decision maker to bring costs and health outcomes back to present value using the standard exponential discounting formulae and setting $r = i$ (with the latter choice assuming that the consistency argument, and its philosophical underpinnings, are sufficiently persuasive).

Claim: If the Real Value of a Health Consequence Changes Over Time in Response to Changes in Real Income, the Discount Rate (r) Should Be Adjusted Accordingly

In particular, the claim is that if the real income elasticity of demand for a health consequence—for example, a QALY—is positive (implying that willingness to pay for QALYs increases with real income) and if real income is increasing over time, then the social decision maker should discount QALYs at a rate lower than the real market rate. For example, Viscusi (1995) notes that if (1) the income elasticity of health is 1.0 (consistent with his recent empirical finding and implying that a 1% increase in income leads to a 1% increase in the quantity of "health" demanded), and if (2) if real income is growing at a rate of g, then the appropriate discount factor for year t is not $(1+r)^{-t}$, but rather $(1+r-g)^{-t}$. Parsonage and Neuburger (1992) make the same point less formally as part of a larger argument that health consequences should not be discounted at all in CEA.

If the social decision maker did want to assume that the real value of program effectiveness was rising over time (relative to real income), an alternative approach, which is both more precise and conceptually cleaner, is to augment the effectiveness score directly rather than alter the discount rate. This option was acknowledged both by Viscusi and by Parsonage and Neuburger.[6]

We are unaware of a CEA that has attempted to incorporate dynamic wealth effects. Indeed, the possibility that individuals in a given cross section with different income (or wealth) levels might value health consequences differently has not been acknowledged in work to date.

Claim: Allowance Must Be Made for Possible Changes Over Time in the Real Relative Cost of Producing Health Improvements

This claim is closely related to the preceding one, except that it operates on the numerator (cost) rather than the denominator (effectiveness) of the C/E ratio. As Weinstein and Stason (1977) first emphasized, it is quite possible (even likely) that the relative resource cost of achieving gains in health will change through time. For example, technological advances may reduce the real cost of health improvements in certain areas. In general, the technology for producing health may be altered or the relative real prices of inputs to health care may change over time. To the extent that these influences can be confidently anticipated, the social decision maker can allow for them by appropriate adjustment of the real discount rate r.

An alternative approach—which permits a more targeted, fine-tuned adjustment to be executed while not tampering with the real discount rate—builds these anticipated relative cost changes into the stream of cost estimates used in the numerator of the cost-effectiveness ratio. In this way, such changes in the real opportunity cost of resources can be incorporated directly into the CEA in a way that is tailored to the particular programs under investigation. We are, however, unaware of published cost-effectiveness analyses that have included any adjustment for changes in the relative cost of producing "effectiveness" over time.

Claim: Individual Time Preferences for Health Consequences May Not Be Consistent With a Discount Rate for Effectiveness (r) Equal to the Market Rate (i)

Direct information about individual time preferences for health consequences in no way enters the calculations of the cost-effectiveness ratio. While health states are preference-weighted relative to one another in constructing the number of quality-adjusted life years gained within a given time period, weighting across time periods is done by using a universal discount rate, i, without reference to individual tradeoffs over time. In this regard, Weinstein (1986) asks: "How should within-patient time preference be reconciled with societal time preference, where the latter depends on an economic argument and the former has origins independent of any market or price system?'' (p. 196). We consider both empirical and theoretical evidence to address this dilemma.

Empirical considerations

Within the past decade, there has emerged a growing literature focusing on how individuals make choices among options with a strong time dimension (Loewenstein, 1987, 1988, 1992; Loewenstein and Prelec, 1992, 1993; Ainslie and Haslam, 1992; Loewenstein and Thaler, 1989; Ben-Zion et al., 1989; Stevenson, 1993). There have also been several applications to the problem of valuing health and safety over time (Fuchs, 1982; Christensen-Szalanski, 1984; Cropper et al, 1992, 1994; Redelmeier and Heller, 1993; Cropper and Portney, 1990; MacKeigan et al., 1993; Chapman and Elstein, 1995; Lipscomb, 1989; Rose and Weeks, 1988; Olsen, 1993). Most of these studies derive inferences about individual time preference based on responses to hypothetical (though intended to be realistic) survey questions. At least one series of analyses has demonstrated how individual time preferences for survival can be inferred statistically from labor market choices (Moore and Viscusi, 1990; Viscusi and Moore, 1989).

While the studies above differ greatly in their particulars, certain general trends emerge, whether the objects of choice happen to be money, consumer commodities (e.g., fancy meals), or health outcomes:

- Individual discount rates frequently lie outside the conventional 0–10% range. In the experiment by Redelmeier and Heller, over 62% of the estimated rates were equal to 0, 10% were less than 0, and nearly 16% were greater than 10%. Some of the discount rates determined by Chapman and Elstein were in excess of 200%.
- Despite the variation between individuals, the mean rates in many experiments do fall within the conventional range. In the Redelmeier-Heller study, the grand mean was 3.3%. Moreover, the various rates estimated (econometrically) by Viscusi and Moore fell in the range of 1–14%.
- Discount rates tend to be lower when large-magnitude outcomes are being traded over time (and conversely).
- Discount rates tend to be lower the longer the time interval over which the trades are considered (Cropper et al., 1994). (The ''slow'' discounting model of Harvey is intended to capture this horizon-varying rate of time preference.)
- Discount rates for losses are typically lower than for gains.
- When a given outcome is embedded in a sequence of outcomes, the discount rate tends to be lower than when the outcome is evaluated singly (and thus not in the context of its outcome sequence).
- The sequencing of outcomes can affect time preference: Some people ''savor'' good outcomes and wish to postpone them; some ''dread'' bad outcomes and wish to get them over with; some attach special utility to having outcomes

improve over time, even if this means that the total payoff (e.g., money) is suboptimal.

In sum, there is much behavioral evidence that individual preferences are not consistent with the constant-rate exponential discounting model. And while Viscusi and Moore have derived an economically plausible range of rates, their parsimonious statistical models (and the utility functions undergirding them) *assumed* constant-rate exponential discounting across the life cycle.

However, as noted in Chapter 2, one must distinguish between the descriptive and prescriptive purposes of CEA. The purpose of CEA is not to describe actual decisions, let alone hypothetical responses to surveys, but rather to serve as a prescriptive tool. We will appeal, therefore, to a theoretical basis in arguing that it is reasonable for the social decision maker to act *as if* individuals tend, on average, to discount future health effects at the same (real) rate they use to discount money and other easily transferable commodities. Thus, while individual time preference rates for health might demonstrate wide variability, the decision maker would not expect these rates to be systematically higher or lower than the consumption rate of interest—and, therefore, not *systematically different* from the rate i employed in Equation (1). These issues are pursued more formally below and in Appendix 7.1.

In this vein, it is worth reiterating that the mean estimates of individual discount rates, whether from surveys or from labor market behavior, do fall generally in the range 1–10%. The fact that individual responses to surveys depart from this norm is not surprising, especially in light of the variation induced by difficulties respondents must have had in interpreting and responding to these hypothetical questions.

Theoretical considerations

Given the perplexing range of empirical findings about individual time preference rates, it is instructive to analyze more formally the theoretical conditions under which one would expect the individual's rate of time preference for health consequences—call it s—to be equal to the market rate of interest i. The issue is important. If, indeed, s closely approximates i, then to set the (societal) discount rate for health consequences (r) equal to i is to choose a value of r that closely approximates the *individual's* rate of time preference for health consequences: There would then be no individual-societal conflict in the discounting of effectiveness. But if s and i diverge, then setting $r = i$ will discount health consequences in a way that is not in accord with individual time preferences.

As Viscusi (1995) points out, "The fundamental source of all discounting stems from an economic model in which an individual maximizes the present value of a stream of utility over time, subject to an intertemporal budget constraint" (p. 129); see also Fishburn and Rubinstein (1982). In this spirit, we present a simple theoretical model of intertemporal choice in Appendix 7.1.

The model's fundamental implication is that the economically rational individual will attempt to adjust investments in the commodity called "health" so that, over time, the (marginal) rate of time preference s equals the (real) consumption rate of interest i. For example, suppose s were less than i for an individual (so that with her current health stock, her discount rate for future health is lower than the rate at which she can exchange present for future consumption, in general). The model predicts that this individual will seek opportunities to trade present consumption (whether health itself or other goods and services) for future health; she could accomplish this by saving money at the rate i and then using the proceeds to buy health. In reality, of course, such health stock adjustments may be neither swift nor sure. As several writers have emphasized, individuals cannot simply raise or lower their health levels across time in a fine-tuned fashion (see Cairns, 1992; Krahn and Gafni, 1993); not only is "health" not easily transferable between periods, but the individual typically operates under relatively severe information constraints about the "technology" for health production. In economic terms, the market for health is "incomplete" (at least from the individual's standpoint).

Nonetheless, individuals behaving according to this model will *attempt* to adjust health levels so that s (the time preference rate) equals i (the market rate). For some, s will be greater than i at a given point in time; for others at that moment, s will be less than i; and still others will be in intertemporal equilibrium (or nearly so). It is in this spirit that the social decision maker is well justified, in our view, in assuming *for prescriptive purposes* that individual time preference rates tend toward, and are roughly centered about, the market rate—and that, therefore, setting $r = i$ creates no compelling conflict between individual time preferences for health outcomes (as embodied in s) and the social rate of time preference for these outcomes (as embodied in r).

To put these matters in further perspective, note that, in reality, we typically would expect to find economically rational individuals "being out of equilibrium but moving toward it," rather than always fulfilling the exacting conditions set forth in models like that in Appendix 7.1. This is the case even for the choice between different commodities at the same point in time. Consider, for example, a hypothetical consumer whose marginal rate of substitution between apples and oranges is not equal to the price ratio for apples and oranges—the standard equilibrium condition from economic theory. Instead, suppose that with apples priced at $0.50 and oranges at $1.00, the individual would trade only one apple (instead of two) to get an additional orange. According to theory, this is patently irrational if the individual can freely buy and sell fruit at market prices. But suppose that there are transaction costs (the nearest store that sells oranges is a mile away), or that there is imperfect information (the individual is not sure what the price of apples is today), or that all reasonably accessible stores are sold out of one fruit or another (so that substitution possibilities are limited), or that any of a number of other deviations from the assumptions of consumer theory (including the underlying assumption of optimizing behavior) arise. Then, at the end of the day, this individual's marginal rate of substitution between apples and oranges might be 1:1 instead of 2:1. For another individual, the marginal rate of substitution might be 3:1, or 10:1. On average, we would expect these departures from economic optimization to balance out so that on average the marginal rate of substitution would be about 2:1. But there would be wide disparities across individuals. Does this fact mean that, in a cost-benefit or cost-effectiveness analysis, we would be reluctant to assign relative prices of 2:1 to oranges and apples? Certainly not. Then why treat individual variation around the optimal allocation between periods any differently from individual variation around the optimal allocation between goods? This line of argument lends important support to the rationale for setting $r = i$ in cost-effectiveness analysis.

Suppose, nonetheless, that we do wish to reflect the time preferences of individuals in cost-effectiveness analysis, even acknowledging that these preferences are not consistent with the preferences that would be induced by exemplary economic behavior. In Appendix 7.2, we investigate an alternative formulation of time preference in CEA that would satisfy the approach of setting $r = i$ and incorporate information about individual time preferences for health consequences. This formulation involves a two-stage procedure. In the first stage, the health consequences under each intervention are brought to an initial present value from the perspective of the individuals vying for resources, using an estimate of the individual rate of time preference. In the second stage, these individual-level present values, which in general will be spaced at different time intervals from the moment of decision, are brought to a final present value by discounting at a rate r equal to the market rate i. As noted in Appendix 7.2, the two-stage approach has drawbacks, not the least of which is that it depends on a basically arbitrary definition of the starting date of a program and that it assigns different weights to health consequences occurring in different cohorts at the same point in calendar time.

Therefore, we recommend setting $r = i$ as the best approach in CEA but recommend further theoretical and empirical work in order to understand better the relation between individual and social rates of time preference.

Choosing the Discount Rate for CEA

If the social decision maker adopts the strategy of discounting costs and health consequences at the same rate, the question of how to incorporate time preference into cost-effectiveness analysis comes down to the question how to select i, the market-based rate. The following evidence and policy recommendations from elsewhere bear review.

In the Discounting Costs section, it was noted that:

- Lind (1982) estimated rates of 1% for ''safe investments'' (e.g., a U.S. Treasury bill), and he recommended 2% for ''safe long-term assets'' (such a government bond in general).
- Lesser and Zerbe (1994) estimated that the appropriate real discount rate for public projects lies in the range from 2.5% to 5%, based on recent historical trends in government rates.

These estimates are all based on the shadow-price-of-capital (SPC) approach to determining the discount rate for public projects. The estimates below, while roughly similar in magnitude to those above, may or may not have this same conceptual base:

- While acknowledging that many cost-effectiveness studies have used a 5% real rate, Viscusi (1995) concludes: "Although this approach is not unreasonable, real rates of return of 3 percent, or even less, appear more in line with U.S. economic performance in the past decade" (p. 142). He recommends that sensitivity analysis be conducted over the range from 1% to 7%.
- A real rate of discount of 6% currently applies throughout the British National Health Service (Parsonage and Neuburger, 1992).
- In recent cost-effectiveness analyses, the World Bank (1993) decided to discount its outcome measure, disability-adjusted life years (DALYs), at a real 3%—a rate which "could be entirely attributed to pure time preference" (p. 214).
- The Centers for Disease Control and Prevention (CDC, 1994) has recommended that all benefits (both monetary and nonmonetary) and costs be discounted at a real rate of 5%, with sensitivity analysis conducted over the range from 0% to 8%.
- The U.S. Office of Management and Budget (OMB, 1994) has issued guidelines for discounting in cost-benefit and cost-effectiveness analyses of government programs, and these deserve careful scrutiny for the case at hand. For discounting *costs* within a "cost-effectiveness" analysis of a public program, where the analysis is conducted in real terms, OMB recommends using "the real Treasury borrowing rate on marketable securities of comparable maturity to the period of analysis." The most recently published rates by OMB for this purpose are as follows:

3-year	5-year	7-year	10-year	30-year
2.1%	2.3%	2.5%	2.7%	2.8%

To obtain discount rates for programs with terms different than above, linear interpolation should be used, OMB advises; for programs longer than 30 years, the 30-year rate should be used.

This being said, it turns out that OMB defines a somewhat circumscribed role for CEA relative to its standard application in the health policy literature. Specifically, the guidelines state that

cost-effectiveness analysis is appropriate whenever it is unnecessary or impractical to consider the dollar value of the benefits provided by alternatives under consideration. This is the case whenever (i) each alternative has the same annual benefits expressed in monetary terms; or (ii) each alternative has the same annual effects, but dollar values cannot be assigned to their benefits. Analysis of alternative defense systems often falls in this category.

(p. 4)

This interpretation of CEA sounds generally similar to what many health analysts call *cost-minimization analysis*. OMB evidently recommends discounting by the real Treasury borrowing rate because the focus of *its* CEA is simply on finding the lowest-cost way for government to achieve some predesignated objective. (In a discussion of discount rates for government programs, Lind [1990] also uses this restricted definition of "cost-effectiveness analysis.")

For cost-benefit analyses, however, OMB now recommends that all costs and benefits be discounted at a real rate of 7%—a rate which "approximates the marginal pretax rate of return on an average investment in the private sector in recent years" (p. 9). Indeed, the widely quoted OMB discount rate of 10% appears to have been rescinded with the publication, in October 1992, of the revised Circular No. A-94.

Consistent with Lind, Lesser and Zerbe, and other recent writers, OMB regards the SPC approach as the "analytically preferred means for capturing the effects of Government projects on resource allocation in the private sector." But the guidelines appear to regard the SPC approach as experimental, because, "To use this method accurately, the analyst must be able to compute how the benefits and costs of a program or project affect the allocation of private consumption and investment." In fact, OMB concurrence is required if the SPC approach is to be used instead of adopting a 7% rate. Hence, there is no internal contradiction between the new standard OMB rate for CBA and the range of real rates recommended by Lind and by Lesser and Zerbe; they simply have different conceptual underpinnings. Moreover, in our view, the *empirical basis* for the range of discount rates derived by the latter analysts, based on the SPC approach, is at least as compelling as the *empirical basis* for OMB's selection of a rate of 7%. That is, it is not obvious why a carefully derived "representative" discount rate based on the SPC approach is necessarily more inexact or arbitrary than a "representative" rate based on the concept of average pretax rates of return.

Thus, we conclude: The preferred conceptual underpinning for deriving a discount rate for cost in the CEA of health programs is the SPC approach. Between the two "standard contenders" for the discount rate in the current literature, 5% and 3%, empirical studies based on the SPC approach provide stronger support for the latter. Hence, a real annual (riskless) rate of 3% should be used in the Reference Case analysis.

Because scores of existing CEAs have adopted 5%, we urge that C/E ratios be calculated at a rate of 5% in addition to 3%, in both the Reference Case analysis and in key sensitivity analyses. This will enable "league tables" (which summarize a wide range of existing C/E ratios for comparative purposes) to incorporate both new and existing analyses.

The determination of a "standard" discount rate should be subject to reconsideration as new evidence arises over time—for example, revised estimates of real economic growth. Having said this, we do not recommend that the standard discount rate be changed frequently. To do so would work at cross purposes to achieving comparability across analyses performed at different times. Therefore, we recommend that the base rate of 3% and an alternative rate of 5% be retained for a period of at least 10 years.

A reasonable range of rates for conducting sensitivity analyses is from 0% to 7%. The lower bound provides the social decision maker with insights into the effects of discounting by showing what happens in its absence; the upper bound represents a reasonable (if not liberal) ceiling on the real consumption rate of interest in current markets.

Recommendations

1. In cost-effectiveness analyses from a societal perspective, the costs and health consequences of all programs should be expressed in terms of their present value to society, as a prerequisite for generating C/E ratios and resource allocation recommendations.

2.1. In the Reference Case analysis, costs and health effects should be discounted at the same rate.

2.2. Because the theory and empirical evidence regarding the relation between individual and market rates of time preference are unsettled, sensitivity analyses based on models that allow health and cost consequences to be discounted at different rates may be conducted. These models may include two-stage procedures which consider individual time preference within cohorts but which use societal time preference between cohorts.

3.1. Costs and health effects should be discounted to present value at a rate consistent with the shadow-price-of-capital (SPC) approach to evaluating public investments.

3.2. Given currently available data on real economic growth and corresponding estimates of the real consumption rate of interest, we recommend 3% as the most appropriate real (riskless) discount rate for CEA.

3.3. Because of the large number of published CEAs that have adhered to the traditional discount rate of 5%, we recommend that analyses performed in the near future conduct the base-case analysis and critical sensitivity analyses using 5% as well as 3%.

3.4. The discount rate should be subject to review, and possible revision, over time in light of significant changes in the underlying economic data. However, to retain comparability with existing analyses, we recommend that both 3% and 5% continue to be used in analyses for at least the next 10 years.

3.5. Sensitivity analyses should be conducted on the discount rate used in a CEA; a reasonable range of rates is from 0% to 7%, given current economic trends.

In bringing costs and health consequences to present value, several other important technical issues arise. In this regard, we recommend:

4.1. Cost-effectiveness analyses should be conducted in real (inflation-adjusted) terms, regardless of whether one assumes that the components of costs will increase at roughly the same rate (balanced inflation) or at different rates (unbalanced inflation).

4.2. If one wishes to reflect a belief that the real value of health for the typical individual is increasing over time, because real income in increasing and the individual's income elasticity of demand for health is significantly positive, then it is preferable to execute an upward adjustment to the effectiveness score rather than a downward adjustment to the real discount rate. However, the case for such global adjustments in CEA conducted from the societal perspective has yet to be fully made, in our judgment.

4.3. Suppose the real resource costs of producing health are expected to change over time in a given CEA, whether through changes in the technology for producing health or in the real relative prices of inputs to health care. In response, we recommend adjusting individual estimates of real costs on a program-by-program basis rather than making a global adjustment in the real discount rate. In practice, reliable information for making such cost adjustments is rarely available.

4.4. When uncertainty in the estimates of costs and health consequences is formally acknowledged in a CEA, one should, in principle, convert each uncertain quantity (random variable) to its "certainty equivalent" and then discount at the chosen real riskless rate. However, since virtually all CEAs assume risk neutrality (albeit implicitly) in the valuation of costs and health consequences, the standard practice of using expected values leads (albeit implicitly) to the conceptually appropriate specification of certainty equivalents.

Notes

1. If one were to carry out these calculations using a more general "continuous-time" version of the present value formulas, the issue of where in the interval to "lump" outcomes would become moot. (See note 2.)

2. A more general "continuous-time" version of these formulas can be expressed as

$$\Delta C = \int_0^T [C_j(t) - C_0(t)]e^{-it}dt \tag{1'}$$

$$\Delta E = \int_0^T [E_j(t) - E_0(t)]e^{-rt}dt \tag{2'}$$

where the integration in each case is over the interval bounded by the beginning of period 1 (labeled 0 above) and the end of period T (labeled by T). In this calculus-based formulation, the issue of where to "place" the outcomes in an interval disappears, since each is arbitrarily small.

3. For example, Lind (1990) concludes that the appropriate discount rate for some government decisions may be influenced by the presence of fixed budget constraints and other exigencies of the moment.

4. In CEAs conducted under uncertainty at the level of individual decision making, matters become more complicated. Johannesson et al. (1994) have shown that for constant-rate discounting of the usual sort to be appropriate within a theoretically correct specification of the QALY model under uncertainty, it is necessary that the individual be risk neutral with respect to *discounted life years* (or, equivalently, exhibit constant proportional risk posture with respect to discounted life years.) As the authors point out, the empirical reasonableness of such restrictions has yet to be investigated.

5. The assumption of time stationarity means that the decision-maker's preferences for outcomes occurring at different points in the future do not depend on the temporal vantage point from which the future is viewed. For example, the rate of time preference between outcomes in 2010 and 2011 should be the same whether viewed from 1995 or 2005.

6. Thus, if $E(t)$ is the effectiveness score for year t, and if one assumes that the real value of effectiveness to society is rising over time at the rate g, then effectiveness in year t could be expressed as $E(t)(1+g)^t$, whose present value is $[E(t)(1+g)^t]/(1+r)^t$. The alternative expression for this present value, $E(t)/(1+r-g)^t$, is a close numerical approximation to the exact representation $[E(t)(1+g)^t]/(1+r)^t$ and, in our view, has less direct intuitive appeal.

Appendix 7.1:
A Theoretical Model of Intertemporal Decision Making Regarding Health and Other Commodities

To examine the conditions under which economically rational individuals will act so as to equate their rate of time preference for health (label it s) with the prevailing market rate of interest (i), consider the following simple resource allocation problem. Assume that the individual's decision horizon is only two periods and that the objective is to choose both the level of health (H) and the level of a composite consumption bundle (X) in each period that yields maximum satisfaction, subject only to the constraint that the individual's expenditures not exceed the available budget over the two periods. More formally, the individual maximizes a two-period utility function of H and X, subject to a two-period budget constraint:

$$\max U = U(H_1, X_1, H_2, X_2) \tag{A1}$$

subject to

$$p(H_1)H_1 + p(X_1)X_1 + p(H_2)H_2/(1+i) + p(X_2)X_2/(1+i) = B \tag{A2}$$

where each $p(*)$ is the real price of the commodity in the period indicated, and B is the 2-year budget. The problem is to find the best feasible values of H_1, X_1, H_2, and X_2. (Application of the discount factor begins with the second period, not the first, in line with the convention adopted earlier for discrete-time models. The choice of two periods is merely to simplify the notation; completely analogous results hold for the general decision horizon of N periods.)

Note that the utility function (A1) is perfectly general and has its origins independent of any market or price system. Note also that there is no discount parameter built into this functional form. Rather, the individual is assumed simply to have smooth indifference curves relating consumption of health (or consumption bundle X) in period 1 to health (or X) in period 2. (Technically, we assume that U is at least twice differentiable and concave in each argument.)

By maximizing (A1) subject to condition (A2), we derive the following decision rule regarding the selection of health levels: For an optimum, it is a necessary that H_1 and H_2 satisfy the condition:

$$\left(\frac{\partial U}{\partial H_1} \middle/ \frac{\partial U}{\partial H_2} \right) = (1 + i)[p(H_1)/p(H_2)] \tag{A3}$$

where the term on the left-hand side of (A3) can be recognized as the marginal rate of substitution (MRS) between H_1 and H_2.

Equation (A3) states that, in equilibrium, the individual's marginal rate of substitution between health levels in consecutive periods—which standard theory says is equivalent to the ratio of marginal utilities in consecutive periods—is equal to $(1+i)$ multiplied by the ratio of the prices of health in the two periods. But the marginal rate of substitution between H_1 and H_2 can be expressed equivalently as $(1+s)$. Hence, if the price (i.e., marginal cost) of attaining any health level is constant across periods, as assumed in most analyses, then we have MRS $= (1+s) = (1+i)$, so that $s = i$. Thus, on the margin the individual will discount health at the market rate i. (In fact, "first-order conditions" analogous to [A3] hold for all other commodity pairs in the utility function; since these equations bear only indirectly on the points here, they are omitted.)

An important caveat to this line of reasoning lies in the assumption of continuous substitution possibilities between H_1 and H_2; otherwise, the equilibrium condition (A3) cannot be achieved, in general. That individuals are quite restricted in their ability to transfer health across periods is obvious and has been broadly acknowledged in the recent literature. (See, e.g., Olsen, 1993; Cairns, 1992; Redelmeier et al., 1994; Williams, 1981.) Opportunities to buy and sell marginal changes in health occur irregularly and in large boluses, as in episodes of illness. However, opportunities for prevention do occur more or less continuously and provide some basis for "smoothing out" the production possibility surface for health.

Finally, this analysis has assumed that all data relevant to decisions are known with certainty and that all outcomes are available with certainty. If the problem were recast under uncertainty, first-order conditions similar to (A3) would emerge, but all equilibrium commodity levels would be stated in terms of certainty equivalents; see the discussion on adjusting discounting rates for uncertainty in the Discounting Health Consequences section above.

Appendix 7.2:
A Two-Stage Procedure for Incorporating Individual and Societal Time Preferences

In what follows we develop a simple numerical example to cast the issues of time preference in concrete terms while further examining their implications for cost-effectiveness analysis. Undergirding these illustrations are several general propositions: (1) Individuals, as multiperiod utility maximizers, will manifest rates of time preference for health; (2) the social decision maker conducting the CEA wants to respect these individual-level time preferences, though subject to meeting certain societal-level allocative criteria; and (3) the most salient of the latter is the $r=i$ proviso.

The Data

Imagine a certain subpopulation of women at risk of a particular disease D. The natural history for each woman at risk is as follows: D occurs with certainty at age 56. Throughout that year and the next 2 years, the woman is in a painful, debilitating health state Y. At age 59 the woman dies. Until the onset of D, the woman is assumed to be in excellent health (EH). Suppose that the annual medical cost associated with maintaining EH is $100, that the annual medical cost of state Y is $2,000, and that no cost is associated directly with death from D. All costs are expressed in real terms.

Now suppose there is a prevention program which, if initiated when the at-risk woman becomes age 51, will delay the onset of D by 1 year. That is, D still occurs with certainty even with the program, but not until age 57. Again, the woman is assumed to spend 3 years in state Y (ages 57–59 now) and to then die at age 60.

The prevention program requires an initial battery of tests, at a cost of $500, and a daily regimen of "anti-D" medication, at an annual cost of $50. These medical costs are in addition to those incurred otherwise prior to the onset of D; once the disease begins, all prevention medication ceases. Because this medication has side effects, the woman will be in a state only of "good health" (GH), permitting her to engage in a full range of daily activities but with mild, though persistent, discomfort.

Based on representative population surveys, the preference weights (per time period of occupancy) for states EH, GH, Y, and Dead are 1.000, 0.9000, 0.4000, and 0.0000, respectively. In addition, these surveys included questions (in the spirit of those posed by Redelmeier and Heller [1993], for example) allowing estimation of each respondent's pure rate of time preference (denoted by s) for health outcomes. Suppose that subsequent analyses showed that the distribution of calculated s values is bimodal, with peaks at 0.03 and 0.10.

Assume that the real market rate of interest (i), as measured by the return on long-term government bonds, is 0.03.

The Resource Allocation Problem

Imagine a social decision maker at the present moment (t_0) with the task of determining the cost-effectiveness of allocating dollars to the prevention program for disease D. While this will surely require the decision maker to consider the merits of this program relative to all others competing for resources, it is sufficient for our purposes to focus only on the cost-effectiveness ratios involving the disease D program in relation to the natural history (status quo) option.

Consider first the cohort of all at-risk women who are 51 at the present moment, t_0. Virtually all of the raw ingredients for computing the cost-effectiveness ratio at t_0 are found in Tables 7.1 and 7.2. At each age, the discounted preference weight is calculated as the undiscounted preference weight for the health state (EH, GH, or Y) divided by $(1+s)^{t-1}$. The central issue of this illustration relates to the choice or r—the social decision maker's rate for discounting health effects—and the relationship between r and s.

Table 7.1 Natural History Profile of Health and Medical Cost Outcomes for a Woman in a Cohort at Risk to Disease D

Age (1)	Time Period (t)[a] (2)	Health State (3)	Discounted Preference Weight			Discounted Medical Cost	
			$s = 0$ (4)	$s = 0.03$ (5)	$s = 0.10$ (6)	$i = 0$ (7)	$i = 0.03$ (8)
51	1	EH	1.000	1.000	1.000	100	100
52	2	EH	1.000	0.971	0.909	100	97
53	3	EH	1.000	0.943	0.826	100	94
54	4	EH	1.000	0.915	0.751	100	92
55	5	EH	1.000	0.888	0.683	100	89
56	6	Y	0.400	0.345	0.248	2,000	1,725
57	7	Y	0.400	0.335	0.226	2,000	1,675
58	8	Y	0.400	0.325	0.205	2,000	1,626
59	9	Dead	0.000	0.000	0.000	0	0
60	10	Dead	0.000	0.000	0.000	0	0
Total			6.200	5.722	4.848	6,500	5,498

a. Cohort's own perspective.

Table 7.2 Profile of Health and Medical Cost Outcomes with Prevention Program for a Woman in a Cohort at Risk to Disease D

Age (1)	Time Period $(t)^a$ (2)	Health State (3)	Discounted Preference Weight			Discounted Medical Cost	
			$s = 0$ (4)	$s = 0.03$ (5)	$s = 0.10$ (6)	$i = 0$ (7)	$i = 0.03$ (8)
51	1	GH	0.900	0.900	0.900	$500 + 100 = 600$	600
52	2	GH	0.900	0.874	0.818	$50 + 100 = 150$	147
53	3	GH	0.900	0.848	0.744	150	141
54	4	GH	0.900	0.824	0.676	150	137
55	5	GH	0.900	0.800	0.615	150	133
56	6	GH	0.900	0.776	0.559	150	129
57	7	Y	0.400	0.335	0.226	2,000	1,675
58	8	Y	0.400	0.325	0.205	2,000	1,626
59	9	Y	0.400	0.316	0.187	2,000	1,579
60	10	Dead	0.000	0.000	0.000	0	0
Total			6.900	5.998	4.930	7,850	6,167

a. Cohort's own perspective.

We now introduce one more facet of the problem that is both realistic and critical to the exposition: In making choices at t_0, the social decision maker adopts a multiperiod perspective. Specifically, the decision maker considers not only the 10-year profiles (natural history versus with prevention program) of the cohort that becomes clinically eligible for the program at t_0, but also the analogous profiles for the cohort that reaches age 51 one year hence (at $t_1 = t_0+1$), the cohort that reaches age 51 two years hence (at $t_2 = t_0+2$), and so on. Label these cohort 0, cohort 1, cohort 2, and so on. Assume that the data in Tables 7.1 and 7.2 apply identically to all members of each cohort.

Alternative Discounting Strategies

The pivotal questions regarding the role of time preference in CEA from a societal perspective revolve around the assumed relationship between the market rate i, the individual's rate of time preference s, and the social decision maker's rate of time preference r. (In reality, just as preferences for health states Y or GH vary across individuals, so will s. Thus, the s employed below should be regarded as a "representative" rate of time preferences, just as the health-state preference weights below—and in CEA generally—are assumed to be representative.)

To proceed, we consider the following cases:

Case (A): $r = i; s = i$

With $i = 0.03$, the computed present values for the costs of the natural history and prevention scenarios are found at the bottom of column (8) in Tables 7.1 and 7.2, respectively. Similarly, the present values of health consequences are at the bottom of column (5) of each table. Thus the cost-effectiveness ratio for cohort 0 is

$$CE(t_0) = (\$6,167 - \$5,498)/(5.998 - 5.722) = \$669/0.276$$
$$= \$2,424/QALY$$

Because we assume that the time preference rate of the representative cohort member coincides with the market rate, when the social decision maker adopts the $r = i$ proviso, there is no conflict with individual time preferences. If the individual were to compute $CE(t_0)$ strictly for herself, she would have discounted QALYs at 3% and arrived at the same C/E ratio (assuming concurrence with all the other data in Tables 7.1 and 7.2).

Consider now cohorts 1 and 2, in turn. From the decision-maker's perspective at t_0, both the numerator and the denominator of the C/E ratio for cohort 1 are identical to those for cohort 0, except that all present value calculations are advanced 1 year in time. Hence,

$$CE(t_2) = CE(t_1) = CE(t_0) = \$2,424/QALY$$

In addition, with $s = i$ ($=r$), there is no conflict between the individual and societal formulations.

Case (B): $r = i$; $s \neq i$

With an assumed divergence between the individual's time preference rate and the market rate, three basic options arise for computing cost-effectiveness ratios:

1. Adopt the $r = i$ proviso and ignore individual time preferences. The C/E ratios for all three cohorts would be exactly those computed in case (A).
2. Use the individual time preference rate to calculate the present value of effectiveness and the market rate for the present value of cost.

    Assume now that $s = 0.10$ while $i = 0.03$. For cohort 0 we use the cost calculations in column (8) of Tables 7.1 and 7.2 and the effectiveness calculations in column (6) to obtain

$$CE_0(t_0) \quad (\$6,167 - \$5,498)/(4.930 - 4.848) = \$669/0.082$$

$$\$8,159/QALY$$

For cohort 1 we compute

$$CE_1(t_0) = (\$669/1.03)/(0.082/1.10) = \$8,713/QALY$$

and for cohort 2 we compute

$$CE_2(t_0) = (\$669/1.03^2)/(0.082/1.10^2) = \$9,305/QALY$$

Hence, with $s \neq i$, the cohorts no longer have "equal standing" (see Whittington and MacRae, 1986) in the competition for prevention resources to be appropriated at time t_0. If $s > i$ (as in this example), the more distant the entry of the cohort from t_0, the worse its cost-effectiveness ratio. In addition, all

C/E ratios are larger here than under the $r = i$ proviso. Note also that if $s <$ i, the rank ordering of cohorts 0–2 would reverse; now, the more distant the cohort's entry from t_0, the better its standing in the competition for resources. This illustrates the Keeler-Cretin paradox. If benefits are discounted at a lower rate than costs, then cost-effectiveness can always be improved by targeting successively more distant recipient populations. Without further constraints imposed, there is an infinite regress: No single cohort can be identified as "best."

3. There is a third option that allows the social decision maker to adopt the $r = i$ proviso while formally acknowledging that individual time preference may differ from that implied by the market rate. Specifically, the decision maker could adopt the following two-stage procedure (Lipscomb, 1989). For each cohort, first use the individual rate of time preference s to discount each 10-year profile of QALYs (both with and without the prevention program) to an *intracohort* present value. This is a present value from the perspective of a typical cohort member, computed from the moment when the prevention program could begin *for her*. Then, in the second stage, discount these intracohort present values of benefit to a "final" present value at t_0, using a social discount rate r equal to i. All the while, continue to discount all cost streams at the rate i.

Given the data in Tables 7.1 and 7.2, the two-stage procedure leads to the following results. For each cohort here, the intracohort present value of effectiveness, assuming $s = 0.10$, is $4.930 - 4.848 = 0.082$ QALYs (as derived from column [6] of the tables). Similarly, the intracohort present value of the cost difference between the prevention program and status quo option is $\$6,167 - 5,498 = \$669$ (as derived from column [8] of the tables). Then for each cohort the intracohort C/E ratio is $669/0.082 = \$8,159/$ QALY.

Now, we can derive the final present value of the cost-effectiveness ratio for each cohort, in turn. For cohort 0, this is simply $\$8,159/$QALY, since this cohort enters the analysis at t_0. For cohorts 1 and 2, the two-stage procedure leads to

$$CE_1(t_0) \quad (\$669/1.03)/(0.082/1.03) = \$8,159/QALY$$

$$CE_2(t_0) \quad (\$669/1.03^2)/(0.082/1.03^2) = \$8,159/QALY$$

Thus, the two-stage procedure preserves the *intercohort* balance, or time neutrality, inherent in the $r = i$ proviso while allowing the health profile of the individual to be evaluated according to the individual's assumed rate of time preference.

Note that for each cohort, the social decision maker regards the health benefit (effectiveness) as beginning when the prevention program is administered to the cohort, not at t_0 when the multiperiod decision is made (except for cohort 0, of course). This observation leads us to identify a troubling aspect of the two-stage procedure. Specifically, suppose that cohort 2 receives the benefits assumed above, beginning at t_2, but in addition receives 0.0001 QALY at t_0. This has the effect of moving the "beginning" time of the intervention from t_2 to t_0, thus effectively changing the C/E ratio from $8,159/QALY to a fraction less than $9,305, the value calculated using $r = 0.10$ instead of $r = i = 0.03$. Thus, the program becomes *less* cost-effective (higher C/E) when an additional benefit is added at an earlier point in time! The identification of the point in time at which a program "begins" is essentially arbitrary.

There is another troublesome property of the two-stage method. To see this, note first that, in the standard approach, if two women in different cohorts occupy the same health state, say Y, at the same distance in time from t_0, the social decision maker will assign the same discounted present value to each—notwithstanding that state Y arises at different points in the life-cycle health profile of each woman. For example, a woman in cohort 0 who receives the prevention program would be in state Y at time $t_0 + 9$ (corresponding to her age 59), while a woman in cohort 2 receiving the program would be in state Y at time $t_2 + 7 = t_0 + 9$ (corresponding to her age 57). In either case, the decision maker computes the present value of state Y with respect to t_0 as $0.400/(1 + 0.03)^8 = 0.316$. Thus, under the standard approach one might say that equal QALYs are treated equally in the discounting process. Many would regard this as a strength of the standard approach.

In contrast, under the two-stage procedure, two identical health states occurring the same distance in time from t_0, but in two different cohorts, will be assigned different present values with respect to t_0. With $s = 0.10$, the present value of state Y occurring at $t_0 + 9$, in the ninth year of the profile of cohort 0, is $0.400/(1.10)^8 = 0.187$. But the present value of Y when this state occurs in the seventh year of the profile of cohort 2 profile is $[0.400/(1.10)^6]/(1.03)^2 = 0.213$.

While this may be unsettling, it is well to note the following. The CEA illustrated here was cast entirely in a QALY framework. If, instead, the health-state profiles depicted in Tables 7.1 and 7.2 were evaluated by the individual via an alternative, holistic preference procedure—such as the healthy-years-equivalents (HYE) approach (Mehrez and Gafni, 1989)—something akin to the two-stage procedure would *have* to be employed if the $r = i$ proviso were to be maintained. With HYEs, for example, the health profiles shown in column (2) of the tables would receive an overall utility score; for illustration, suppose the HYE score for the natural history profile is 5.200 and the score given the prevention program is 6.300. With each cohort still assumed to be identical, the intracohort score for the prevention program is $6.300 - 5.200 = 1.100$ (per recipient). This is the effectiveness score that a cohort member would attach to the prevention program were she "standing in time" at the moment the program began (t_0 for cohort 0, t_1 for cohort 1, and t_2 for cohort 2). From the social decision maker's perspective at t_0, the final present value of effectiveness for cohorts 0, 1, and 2 can be stated, respectively, as 1.100, $1.100/1.03 = 1.068$, and $1.100/1.03^2 = 1.037$.

Similarly, suppose that this prevention program had been evaluated through a cost-benefit analysis in which effectiveness was measured (holistically) in terms of one's willingness to pay to have the health profile depicted in Table 7.2 rather than the profile in Table 7.1. Again, something like the two-stage procedure would be required if the social decision maker wanted to bring all intracohort valuations back to present value at t_0 while adhering to the $r = i$ proviso. Embedded in all of these analyses is the assumption, noted earlier, that the decision maker dates the benefits of a future program from its moment of actual implementation, not from the moment the resource allocation decision is made.

References

Ainslie, G., and N. Haslam. 1992. Hyperbolic discounting. In *Choice over time*, ed. G. Loewenstein and J. Elster, 57–92. New York: Russell Sage Foundation.

Arrow, K.J. 1966. Discounting and public investment criteria. In *Water research*, ed. A.V. Kneese and S.C. Smith, 13–32. Baltimore: Johns Hopkins University Press.

Baumol, W.J. 1968. On the social rate of discount. *American Economic Review* 58:205–15.

Ben-Zion, U., A. Rapoport, and J. Yagil. 1989. Discount rates inferred from decisions: An experimental study. *Management Science* 35:270–84.

Bradford, D.F. 1975. Constraints on government investment opportunities and the choice of discount rate. *American Economic Review* 65:887–95.

Cairns, J.A. 1992. Health, wealth and time preference. *Project Appraisal* (March): 31–40.

Centers for Disease Control and Prevention (CDC), U.S. Public Health Service. 1994. *A practical guide to prevention effectiveness: Decision and economic analyses*. Atlanta: U.S. Department of Health and Human Services.

Chapman, G.B., and A.S. Elstein. 1995. Valuing the future: Temporal discounting in health and money. *Med Decis Making* 15:373–386.

Christensen-Szalanski, J.J.J. 1984. Discount functions and the measurement of patients' values: Women's decisions during childbirth. *Med Decis Making* 4:47–58.

Coyle, D., and K. Tolley. 1992. Discounting of health benefits in the pharmacoeconomic analysis of drug therapies: An issue for debate? *PharmacoEconomics* 2:153–62.

Cropper, M.L., S.K. Aydede, and P.R. Portney. 1994. Preferences for life saving programs: How the public discounts time and age. *J Risk and Uncertainty* 8:243–65.

Cropper, M.L., S.K. Aydede, and P.R. Portney. 1992. Rates of time preference for saving lives. *American Economic Review* 82:469–72.

Cropper, M.L., and P.R. Portney. 1990. Discounting and the evaluation of lifesaving programs. *J Risk and Uncertainty* 3:369–79.

Drummond, M.F., G.L. Stoddart, and G.W. Torrance. 1987. *Methods for economic evaluation of health care programmes*. New York: Oxford University Press.

Eisenberg, J. 1989. Clinical economics: A guide to the economic analysis of clinical practices. *JAMA* 262:2879–86.

Feldstein, M.S. 1972. The inadequacy of weighted discount rates. In *Cost-benefit analysis*, ed. R. Layard, 140–55. London: Penguin.

Feldstein, M.S. 1964. The social time preference discount rate in cost-benefit analysis. *Economic J* 74:360–79.

Fishburn, P.C., and A. Rubinstein. 1982. Time preference. *International Economic Review* 23:677–94.

Fuchs, V.R. 1982. Time preference and health: An exploratory study. In *Economic aspects of health* (National Bureau of Economic Research conference report), 93–120. Chicago: University of Chicago Press.

Fuchs, V.R., and R. Zeckhauser. 1987. Valuing health—a "priceless" commodity. *American Economic Review* 77(3):263–68.

Gafni, A., and G.W. Torrance. 1984. Risk attitude and time preference in health. *Management Science* 30:440–51.

Ganiats, T.G. 1994. Discounting in cost-effectiveness research. *Med Decis Making* 14:298-300.

Green, H.A.J. 1978. *Consumer theory*. Rev. ed. New York: Academic Press.

Hammitt, J.K. 1993. Discounting health increments. *J Health Economics* 12:117–20.

Harberger, A.C. 1973. *Project evaluation: Collected essays*. Chicago: Markham Publishing.

Harvey, C.M. 1994. The reasonableness of non-constant discounting. *J Public Economics* 53:31–51.

Haveman, R.H. 1969. The opportunity cost of displaced private spending and the social discount rate. *Water Resources Research* 5:1–24.

Horowitz, J.K., and R.T. Carson. 1990. Discounting statistical lives. *J Risk and Uncertainty* 3:403–13.

Johannesson, M., J.S. Pliskin, and M.C. Weinstein. 1994. A note on QALYs, time tradeoff, and discounting. *Med Decis Making* 14:188–93.

Katz, D.A., and H.G. Welch. 1993. Discounting in cost-effectiveness analysis of healthcare programmes. *PharmacoEconomics* 3:276–85.

Keeler, E.B., and S. Cretin. 1983. Discounting of life-saving and other nonmonetary effects. *Management Science* 29:300–306.

Koopmans, T.C., P.A. Diamond, and R.E. Williamson. 1964. Stationary utility and time perspective. *Econometrica* 32:82–100.

Krahn, M., and A. Gafni. 1993. Discounting in the economic evaluation of health care interventions. *Med Care* 31:403–18.

Lesser, J.A., and R.O. Zerbe. 1994. Discounting procedures for environmental (and other) projects: A comment on Kolb and Scheraga. *J Policy Analysis and Management* 13:140–56.

Lind, R.C. 1990. Reassessing the government's discount rate policy in light of new theory and data in a world economy with a high degree of capital mobility. *J Environmental Economics and Management* 18:S8–S28.

Lind, R.C. 1982. A primer on the major issues relating to the discount rate for evaluating national energy options. In *Discounting for time and risk in energy policy*, 21–94. Baltimore: Johns Hopkins University Press.

Lipscomb, J. 1989. Time preference for health in cost-effectiveness analysis. *Med Care* 27:S233–S253.

Loewenstein, G. 1992. The fall and rise of psychological explanations in the economics of intertemporal choice. In *Choice over time*, ed. G. Loewenstein and J. Elster, 3–34. New York: Russell Sage Foundation.

Loewenstein, G.F. 1988. Frames of mind in intertemporal choice. *Management Science* 34:200–214.

Loewenstein, G. 1987. Anticipation and the value of delayed consumption. *Economic J* 97:666–84.

Loewenstein, G., and D. Prelec. 1993. Preferences for sequences of outcomes. *Psychol Rev* 100:91–108.

Loewenstein, G., and D. Prelec. 1992. Anomalies in intertemporal choice: Evidence and interpretation. *Quarterly J Economics* 107:573–97.

Loewenstein, G., and R.H. Thaler. 1989. Intertemporal choice. *J Economic Perspectives* 3:181–93.

MacKeigan, L.D., L.N. Larson, and J.R. Draugalis. 1993. Time preference for health gains versus health losses. *PharmacoEconomics* 3:374–86.

Marglin, S.A. 1963. The social rate of discount and the optimal rate of investment. *Quarterly J Economics* 77:95–111.

McNeil, B.J., R. Weichselbaum, and S.G. Pauker. 1978. Fallacy of the five-year survival in lung cancer. *N Engl J Med* 299:1397–1401.

Mehrez, A., and A. Gafni. 1989. Quality-adjusted life years, utility theory, and healthy-years equivalents. *Med Decis Making* 9:142–49.

Moore, M.J., and W.K. Viscusi. 1990. Models for estimating discount rates for long-term health risks using labor market data. *J Risk and Uncertainty* 3:381–401.

Olsen, J.A. 1993. On what basis should health be discounted? *J Health Economics* 12:39–53.

Olson, M., and M.J. Bailey. 1981. Positive time preference. *J Political Economy* 89:1–25.

Parsonage, M., and H. Neuburger. 1992. Discounting and health benefits. *Health Econ* 1:71–76.

Redelmeier, D.A., and D.N. Heller. 1993. Time preferences in medical decision making and cost-effectiveness analysis. *Med Decis Making* 13:212–17.

Redelmeier, D.A., D.N. Heller, and M.C. Weinstein. 1994. Time preference in medical economics: Science or religion? *Med Decis Making* 14:301–3.

Robinson, J.C. 1990. Philosophical origins of the social rate of discount in cost-benefit analysis. *The Milbank Quarterly* 68:245–65.

Rose, D.N., and M.G. Weeks. 1988. Individual's discounting of future monetary gains and health states. *Med Decis Making* 8:334 (abstract).

Sen, A.K. 1982. Approaches to the choice of discount rates for social benefit-cost analysis. In *Discounting for time and risk in energy policy*, ed. R.C. Lind, 325–53. Baltimore: Johns Hopkins University Press.

Stevenson, M.K. 1993. Decision making with long-term consequences: temporal discounting for single and multiple outcomes in the future. *J Exp Psychol Gen* 122:3–22.

Strotz, R.H. 1956. Myopia and inconsistency in dynamic utility maximization. *Review of Economic Studies* 23:165–80.

Sugden, R., and A. Williams. 1978. *Principles of practical cost-benefit analysis*. Oxford: Oxford University Press.

U.S. Office of Management and Budget (OMB). 1994. *Guidelines and discount rates for benefit-cost analysis of federal programs*. Circular No. A-94 (revised to include 1994 discount rates). Washington, DC.

Viscusi, W.K. 1995. Discounting health effects for medical decisions. In *Valuing health care: costs, benefits, and effectiveness of pharmaceuticals and medical technologies*, ed. F.A. Sloan, 123–45. New York: Cambridge University Press.

Viscusi, W.K., and M.J. Moore. 1989. Rates of time preference and valuations of the duration of life. *J Public Economics* 38:297–317.

Weinstein, M.C. 1986. Challenges for cost-effectiveness research. *Med Decis Making* 6:194–98.

Weinstein, M.C., and W.B. Stason. 1977. Foundations of cost-effectiveness analysis for health and medical practices. *N Engl J Med* 296:716–21.

Whittington, D., and D. MacRae, Jr. 1986. The issue of standing in cost-benefit analysis. *J Policy Analysis and Management* 5:665–82.

Williams, A. 1981. Welfare economics and health status measurement. In *Health, Economics, and Health Economics*, ed. J. van der Gaag and M. Perlman, 123–32. Amsterdam: North Holland Publishing.

World Bank. 1993. *World Health Development Report*. Washington, DC.

8

Reflecting Uncertainty
in Cost-Effectiveness Analysis

W.G. MANNING, D.G. FRYBACK,
and M.C. WEINSTEIN

In conducting a cost-effectiveness analysis (CEA) to evaluate the desirability of a treatment or prevention regimen, the analyst combines information on the course of disease and treatment, the clinical effectiveness of the regimens, preferences regarding health outcomes, the costs of the intervention and its sequelae, and other aspects of the clinical problem. For many of these pieces of information, the analyst may have a very good sense of what the true values and relationships are, based on clinical trials and observational studies in the literature, or experience. For some aspects of the study, the level of certainty concerning the correct value or the form of the relationship may be very limited. If the analyst knew the true values of all of the parameters needed to calculate incremental effectiveness and costs, the true form of the relationships, *and* the characteristics of the population, then it would be possible to summarize the cost-effectiveness ratio with a single set of numbers. However, given the lack of information about the true values of key aspects of the problem, there will always be some reliance on estimates, and hence some uncertainty[1] about the true cost-effectiveness of the alternatives. At best, the analyst can hope to have unbiased and relatively precise estimates of the costs and effectiveness from well designed randomized trials and observational studies.

One of the least-addressed areas of CEA concerns how to incorporate the inherent uncertainties regarding parameters, relationships, and model structure into the estimated C/E ratios, or other intermediate calculations, and then how to represent to the user of the CEA the impact of this uncertainty on the elements of the analysis critical to decision making. In this chapter, we catalogue sources of uncertainty in a CEA and briefly review the methods that have been suggested for dealing with this uncertainty. We will assume

that the computation of a cost-effectiveness ratio is the end point of a process of estimation, synthesis, and modeling. Rarely is the C/E ratio estimated exclusively from a
single experiment. Instead, the estimates of costs and effects of the intervention and the
alternative being analyzed are constructed by using an amalgam of relevant empirical
observations and expert opinion. The C/E ratio is a ratio of estimated net incremental
costs and net incremental effectiveness of an intervention compared to some alternative,
and these quantities are in turn functions of more elemental parameters combined in a
mathematical model. Uncertainty may apply to aspects of the costs or effects of either
the intervention or its alternative, or both.

Uncertainty about estimates of costs, effectiveness, and the C/E ratio can arise in a
number of ways. A taxonomy of sources of uncertainty and analytic remedies is presented in Table 8.1. We distinguish between two major sources of uncertainty—parameter uncertainty and model uncertainty. *Parameter Uncertainty* is uncertainty about the
true numerical values of the parameters used as inputs. *Model Uncertainty* includes
both uncertainty about the correct method for combining these parameters (*model structure uncertainty*) and uncertainty introduced by the combination of decisions made by
an individual analyst (*modeling process uncertainty*). The overall uncertainty in the
final estimated C/E reflects all three sources, parameter uncertainty, model structure
uncertainty, and modeling process uncertainty. We will discuss each of these in turn.

Parameter Uncertainty

These uncertainties can arise in a number of ways. First, in some cases, some key
parameter or quantifiable feature of the CEA problem cannot be known because we
have not observed it or could not observe it. For example, the future rate of medical
inflation relative to other goods and services cannot be known before it occurs. Second,
in some cases, there is a disagreement about what the appropriate value is, and it is not
likely that we will be able to resolve the issue in time for the completion of the current

Table 8.1 A Taxonomy of Uncertainty and Remedies

	Qualitative Analyses	*Statistical Analyses*
Parameter uncertainty	One-way sensitivity analysis	Delta method
	Two-way sensitivity analysis	Joint confidence/credible intervals
	n-way sensitivity analysis	Bootstrapped estimates
	Max–min analysis	Monte Carlo simulation
Modeling uncertainty		
Model structure	Sensitivity analysis varying structure	Weighted combination of alternative analyses
Model process	Examine analyses by multiple analysts	

CEA. For example, the appropriate rate of discount for social decisions is a continuing problem of this sort. Third, in some cases, there is still some uncertainty concerning key elements of the process, such as the epidemiology of the disease or patterns of physician behavior and patient compliance. These could in principle be estimated if data from a study with a suitable design could be collected.[2] Fourth, in some cases, the analyst has (asymptotically) unbiased estimates of key parameters, but these estimates will have sampling variability. Examples include estimates of the response to treatment or screening obtained from clinical trials and observational studies. Finally, in some cases, we may have a relatively precise estimate of the costs and the treatment effects for some ranges of the data or subpopulations, but we are less sure about these values for other ranges and subpopulations. Examples of this occur when one tries to inter-polate or extrapolate costs and effects to treatments that have not actually been tried, or where one tries to generalize from a sample of convenience or the often relatively compliant participants in some randomized trial, or if the participants exhibit a ''healthy volunteer'' effect.

As with any other estimate, the use of the estimated cost-effectiveness ratio requires that the analyst provide some indication of what confidence can be placed in it, or how uncertain the result is. For instance, what would happen if the true cost or effectiveness per case were somewhat higher or lower than the mean or ''best'' estimate? How much would the C/E ratio change if the discount rate were higher than the estimate used— 5% instead of 3%?

Analysts since Mishan (1976) have recommended that the analyst provide some assessment of the uncertainty in the results. Traditionally, such uncertainties have been examined using sensitivity analyses. But in recent years, there has been an increased interest in developing statistical measures of uncertainty in the estimated C/E ratio. In this section on parameter uncertainty, we will first examine the use of sensitivity anal-yses as a way of dealing with uncertainty. Second, we will discuss a statistical approach for cases where one can incorporate sampling variability in parameter estimates. Third, we will present some preliminary thoughts on how these might be combined.[3] Finally, we will conclude with some recommendations on reflecting these sources of uncertainty in cost-effectiveness analyses.

Sensitivity analyses

The standard way of dealing with all of these types of uncertainties in the CEA literature has been to conduct sensitivity analyses.[4] Weinstein and Stason (1977) argue that sen-sitivity analyses are fundamental to cost-effectiveness analysis. In a sensitivity analysis, some critical component(s) in the calculation is changed by a meaningful amount or varied from worst case to best case, and the cost-effectiveness ratio is recalculated. The resulting difference in the ratio provides some indication of how sensitive the results might be to a substantial but not implausible change in that parameter.[5] If the major results are insensitive to a reasonable variation in a parameter, then the analyst can be relatively sure that the conclusions are insensitive to the working assumptions about that parameter. If the major results are sensitive to which in a range of plausible values of a parameter is used, then the conclusions are not robust. If the results are sensitive to some variable over part of its plausible range (but not over other parts of the range) then the analysis may provide some evidence about when the analyst should be concerned about the value for that parameter. If more precise data are not readily available, then the study cannot be considered definitive. But often sensitivity analysis is useful to focus attention to critical variables and thus to pose the question of whether the issues are sufficiently critical such that better or more data are needed. Whether the investment in additional data is worthwhile is only answerable in the context of policy decisions that depend on the CEA result.

Univariate sensitivity analyses

The traditional approach to sensitivity analysis is to examine one variable at a time. Some analysts have examined the C/E ratio for both high and low values of each key variable in the analysis, as well as their "best" estimate of that parameter. In other studies, the values have been altered by plus or minus one standard deviation of sampling error from clinical data (Goldman et al., 1991). Yet others have employed the 95% confidence intervals for key parameters to determine a plausible range for variation. Some have advocated the use of a clinically meaningful range (Weinstein and Stason, 1977). In many cases, analysts have used extreme values of the plausible range. In such cases, lack of sensitivity from the extremes is fairly convincing. But if the results do change appreciably, the use of extremes may not be very informative unless the extremes form close upper and lower bounds on the likely range of the parameter's value. If the results are sensitive to a value well beyond the likely range of the variable, we cannot tell whether the results are sensitive in the relevant range, or beyond it.

In some cases, it may be difficult to decide what a plausible range will be or to develop reasonable worst case extremes. Instead, the analyst can rely on a threshold analysis if there is only one problematic parameter; see Pauker and Kassirer (1980). In a threshold analysis, the analyst varies the parameter over a range to determine at what values of the parameter major changes in conclusions are warranted. If procedure X looks cost-effective by some norm (e.g., $40,000 or $100,000 per QALY) for part of its range, but not for others, then the conclusion is conditional. If the critical parameter falls in the former range, then it is cost-effective. But if it falls outside of that range, then it may not be cost-effective. Further analysis will be required to determine which range applies.

Where the analysts have had to make some assumption about the functional relationships to carry out a calculation,[6] alternative modeling assumptions can be tried as a sensitivity analysis. For example, studies of infectious diseases frequently assume independent probabilities of disease transmission during each exposure. These probabilities may in fact depend on a variety of risk factors, and the analyst should explore the effect of various modeling assumptions. Markov models are often used because of their ease of implementation. However, semi-Markov models, with time-varying transition probabilities, may yield quite different results. Similarly, sensitivity analysis can also be used to address the valuation of nonmonetized outcomes (e.g., measures of health-related quality of life if there is some concern about the validity, reliability, or other attributes of the quality of life instrument being used).

One of the most important parameters that requires a sensitivity analysis is the discount rate, because of the lack of consensus on the true or relevant real rate of discount for policies and treatments that have consequences over a number of years. If the costs and/or effectiveness of any of the interventions occur over several years, but with different patterns over time, then the cost-effectiveness of a specific program may depend critically on the rate of discount. Cretin's (1977) study of the treatment and prevention of myocardial infarctions provides a classic example. The costs of the cholesterol screening program (with its benefits many years after the initial costs) were quite sensitive to the discount rate, but the results for the other alternatives were much less sensitive. For a discussion of the range of discount rates to use, and other specifics, see Chapter 7.

Sensitivity analysis suffers from three weaknesses that may limit the usefulness of the approach. First, the analyst must choose which variables to vary and which to treat as known or fixed. Second, the analyst must choose the amount of variation around the base value of the parameter that is considered clinically meaningful or policy-relevant. Third, the analyst must determine how much of a change in the base result is acceptable or constitutes a robust finding. Thus, the results of the sensitivity analysis depend on many subjective choices by the analyst.

An unsettling but consistent finding in the cognitive psychology literature is that humans substantially underestimate the uncertainty in their subjective estimates—the subjective 95% confidence interval for a parameter may be much too narrow. Thus, basing determination of a plausible range of variation for parameters on subjective judgment is problematic. Although not documented in the medical literature, sufficient evidence of this phenomenon, even for experts' assessments, appears in the cognitive psychology literature to warrant caution (Alpert and Raiffa, 1982).

Multivariate sensitivity analyses

Although insightful, univariate or one-at-a-time sensitivity analyses *by themselves* are inadequate. Looking at one source of uncertainty at a time in the model provides an incomplete estimate of how uncertain the estimated overall cost-effectiveness ratio actually is.[7] Typically, the results from a one-at-a-time sensitivity analysis will understate the overall uncertainty in the C/E ratio. There are three related problems to be considered here: (1) The incremental cost and effectiveness depend on multiple parameters, not just one; (2) the interaction of certain factors may imply that the total effect may be something quite different from the simple sum of individual contributions; and (3) the cost-effectiveness ratio is a ratio of two uncertain numbers, with the result that the uncertainty in the ratio may be substantially larger than that of either of its elements.

In most cases, multiple sources of uncertainty will usually generate a less "certain" result than a one-at-a-time, univariate sensitivity analysis would indicate. The typical CEA is based on many parameters, not just a single "cost" and a single "effect." For example, the cost measure in the numerator may depend on the discounted sum of office visits, hospitalizations, drugs, and supplies, each multiplied by their respective "price" or "cost." To complicate matters, the costs will involve the initial treatment and treatments for any adverse reactions, weighted by the likelihood of such adverse reactions or iatrogenic effects, as well as impacts of the intervention on subsequent patient morbidity and survival. The total variability in the cost thus depends on the uncertainty in each of the components *and* the relationships among these variables; the relationships, in turn, can include correlations among uncertain estimates of variables or the possible effects of any nonlinearities[8] or interactions in the model (e.g., $p \cdot v$, where p is the price per visit and v is the number of visits). Examining one source of uncertainty at a time may thus grossly understate the overall variability in the estimate of the cost-effectiveness ratio. Conversely, singly combining the extreme values of parameters to gain an "overall" best or worst estimate can overstate the uncertainty. Ignoring the correlation among terms or the presence of interactions could have the same effect.

To illustrate the effects of uncertainty in the components of the C/E ratio, we examine the effect of uncertainty around some variable(s) by using a graphical approach employed by O'Brien et al. (1994). In Figures 8.1 and 8.2, we plot the difference in effectiveness (ΔE) between two treatments on the horizontal or x-axis, and the difference in costs (ΔC) on the vertical or y-axis. The point ($\Delta E, \Delta C$) describes the comparison of the two treatments, and the slope of the straight line from the origin to

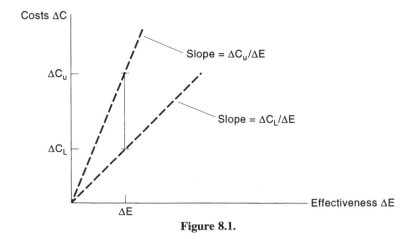

Figure 8.1.

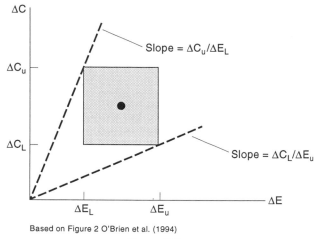

Based on Figure 2 O'Brien et al. (1994)

Figure 8.2.

$(\Delta E, \Delta C)$ is the cost-effectiveness ratio $(\Delta C / \Delta E)$. In Figure 8.1, the uncertainty is in some variable which affects only the incremental costs. ΔC_L and ΔC_U could be either plausible extreme values for incremental costs, or a 95% confidence interval for incremental costs, or some other measure of uncertainty. The two rays from the origin with slopes $\Delta C_L / \Delta E$ and $\Delta C_U / \Delta E$ indicate either the sensitivity of the cost-effectiveness ratio to a plausible change in the underlying variable, or a 95% confidence interval on the ratio if cost is the *only* uncertain aspect of the analysis.

A simple algebraic example will illustrate the problem. Consider a cost example where a treatment only affects the number of physician visits (v). The cost ($C = pv$) has two sources of uncertainty—the price (p) per visit and the number of visits (v). We can approximate the overall variability or uncertainty U in incremental costs by using a simple first order (linear) Taylor series approximation[9]

$$U(\overline{C}) \approx \overline{p} \cdot U(\overline{v}) + \overline{v} \cdot U(\overline{p})\qquad(1)$$

where we use U to indicate some measure of variability or uncertainty, and where the bar over C, p, and v indicates the average. If the concern is with the range of plausible estimates, for example, then $U(*)$ might be the absolute value of the difference between the high and low values. For example, if we want to use the range (max $-$ min, or 95% confidence interval), then the overall range of the cost is approximately:

$$\text{range in costs} \approx \overline{p} \cdot \text{range in \# visits}$$
$$+ \overline{v} \cdot \text{range in price per visit}$$

We will return to more-complex and more-complete solutions below.

Unless the uncertainty in the price p is trivially small (or negatively related to the uncertainty in v), a one-at-a-time or univariate sensitivity analysis provides an underestimate of the overall uncertainty in incremental costs. A univariate sensitivity analysis would indicate that the uncertainty in costs is either $\bar{p}U(v)$ or $\bar{v}U(p)$. But a multivariate sensitivity analysis would indicate that the overall uncertainty is *approximately* the sum of these two, which is larger than either component alone and illustrated schematically in Figure 8.2.[10]

The overall uncertainty need not be the simple sum of the uncertainty in each component, as was the case in the example above. For example, in our simple example, the price and quantity may be negatively correlated because providers will have an incentive to use less of a good or service when it is more expensive. If two parameters move together either negatively or positively, then it is possible for the overall uncertainty to be either larger or smaller thant he sum of the individual effects. In some cases, it may be possible for the overall effect to be less than the uncertainty due to any of the component parameters considered singly.[11] The relationship of the univariate sensitivities to the overall uncertainty will depend on the specific details of the treatments being compared.

Although univariate analyses are incomplete, they should still be done for two reasons. First, they are a logical, easy-to-grasp place to start understanding the structure of a particular CEA. Second, they provide the natural building blocks to do multivariate sensitivity analyses.

There are several ways to deal with multiple sources of uncertainty or variability. One alternative is to vary multiple parameters at a time; for such a bivariate sensitivity analysis, see Christianson and Bender (1982) and Vogel and Christianson (1986). A second alternative is to find the set of extreme circumstances across parameters—that is, the combination of parameter values that yield the worst (highest) and the best (lowest) cost-effectiveness ratios (OTA, 1981). Such an approach, however, is useful only if, as is rarely the case, it indicates that the results are insensitive to the combination of parameter values considered, as it did in the OTA study of influenza vaccination. If the results are sensitive to these extremes, then the results are not very useful bounds on the uncertainty in the cost-effectiveness ratio for two reasons. First, it is highly unlikely that all of the extreme values of key parameters will occur in any particular setting—that is, unlikely that we would reach the corners of the box in Figure 8.2. As a result, the conjoint extreme case does not provide a very good bound on the likely range of outcomes except in unusual cases. Second, under some circumstances, two or more sources of uncertainty may partially offset each other, due to the inherent structure of the problem. A special case of this is to select the combination of parameter values that would provide a worst-case analysis, rather than looking for all extreme values. If the intervention proves to be cost-effective under a worst-case scenario, then it will clearly be cost-effective if evaluated at the true values of the parameters. A third alternative is to use probabilistic (i.e., Monte Carlo) methods to simulate the model with assumptions about the variability in each of the parameters; see Critchfield and Willard (1986), Doubilet et al. (1985), and Dittus et al. (1989) for a discussion and citations. We will return to this suggestion later.

Statistical Approaches

Recently, there has been interest in applying statistical methods to examine the uncertainty in cost-effectiveness ratios if the source of the uncertainty is the sampling variation in estimates of the parameters used in the analysis. Like the multiple sensitivity analysis approach, the statistical approaches consider multiple sources of uncertainty simultaneously. Currently, there are three ways to provide an estimate of the uncertainty in the estimate of the cost-effectiveness ratio. The first relies on the delta method (Rothenberg, 1984) to calculate the variability of any composite measure. The second relies on simulating the variance of the estimated C/E ratio or the distribution of the estimated C/E ratio, based on estimates of the variance–covariance matrix of the parameter estimates. And the third is to derive a bootstrap estimate of the probability distribution of the ratio, its confidence interval, or the variance in the ratio.

To clarify the following discussion, we need a brief digression regarding nomenclature used in this chapter. We will generally use the term *confidence interval* to connote a numerical interval calculated to have a particular probability (typically 0.95) of containing the true value of a parameter of interest.[12] When we want to generalize the concept to two parameters at once we will refer to a *confidence ellipsoid*, meaning, generally, a smoothly convex region of a plane having one dimension determined by possible values for one of the parameters and the other dimension formed by possible values for the other parameter. These regions are referred to as *ellipsoids* (a family of shapes that includes circles) because this generally describes the shape of *contour lines* of likelihood in a graphical representation of a single-peaked joint probability density function of two parameters such as the bivariate normal density function. Ellipsoids such as these are depicted in figures in this chapter. This concept generalizes in a natural way to more than two parameters by using regions of higher dimension (e.g., three-dimensional solid ellipsoids, or even higher dimension constructs described mathematically instead of pictorially). *Confidence region* is the most general use of the construct as it allows arbitrary shapes of the set of values in which the true value of the parameter, or vector of parameters, is asserted to lie.

The adjective "confidence" in the term confidence interval comes from the frequentist (or "classical") statistics literature. There are well-known procedures for computing confidence intervals in most introductory statistics books; more advanced texts will give methods for computing confidence ellipsoids or higher dimensional confidence regions. The derivations of the formulae for confidence regions generally rely on the property that (regardless of their parent distribution) the sum of a set of independent and identically distributed random variables has approximately a normal distribution, with the approximation being better and better the more variables are added together and the mean of the normal distribution being equal to the sum of the means of the variables' parent distribution. (If each piece of data is an observation of the parameter in which we are interested, the mean of the distribution from which each observation is drawn is thought of as the "true" value for the parameter.) With some algebraic manipulation it is possible to use this relationship to derive a numeric interval whose end-points are functions of the mean and variance of a sample of data and which, with a particular confidence level, contains the true value of the mean of the parent distribution for the data. Although technically there are many possible, overlapping confidence intervals for a given parameter value, we speak of "the" confidence interval to refer to the particular confidence interval derived from the center, or highest-density region, of the distribution.

An alternative approach, using Bayesian statistics, to thinking about confidence regions will be described briefly later in this chapter. Although no less grounded in mathematical or statistical theory than the frequentist approach, the Bayesian approach is seen less often in the current medical literature. The Bayesian analogue to a frequentist's confidence region is called a *credible region* (or *credible interval*, or *credible ellipsiod*). The key difference between the two mathematically is that the confidence region is a function only of the observed data, while the credible region is a function of the data and a probability distribution summarizing everything known about the possible value of the parameter before the data were collected. This pre-data or "prior" distribution often reflects the subjective opinion of the analysts and/or decision makers. Although it can be reasonably argued that such subjectivity is overtly or implicitly a part of all empirical investigation (see Berger and Berry, 1988), explicit inclusion in statistical computations is controversial.

We believe that CEA computations will inherently involve many subjective choices by analysts and decision makers—for example, as discussed in Chapter 5. To convey this throughout this chapter we could have used the adjective "credible" wherever "confidence" modifies interval, ellipsoid, or region. Some members of the panel jointly authoring this book will argue strongly (to be opposed by other panelists) that the Bayesian approach is the only sensible one, thus continuing an intense debate that has roiled for nearly two centuries.

Luckily it is a fact that under many conditions confidence regions and credible regions for a parameter will be nearly the same. Generally the requisite conditions are that the prior opinion about the value of the parameter be not too strongly concentrated on a few possible values and that the data be numerous and fairly well concentrated on a narrow range of values. Under these circumstances the Bayesian and the frequentist will agree on the region's limits. (See De Groot, 1970, pp. 192–93, and Edwards et al., 1963, for extended mathematical discussions.)

In any event, our purpose in this chapter is to show that there are formal methods for dealing with uncertainty in complex computational analyses. Although our language in the chapter appears to favor classical frequentist statistics, the ideas here could be implemented using either the frequentist or the Bayesian method.

The confidence interval for the cost-effectiveness ratio can be calculated from the 95% confidence ellipsoid for incremental costs and effectiveness (ΔE, ΔC), as in Figure 8.3 (O'Brien et al., 1994); below we provide two approaches to constructing such an estimate. The analyst can construct a ray from the origin (OB) which is tangent to the

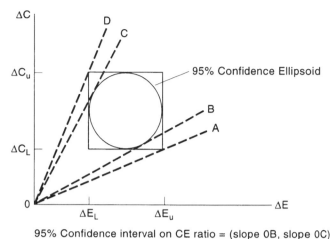

95% Confidence interval on CE ratio = (slope 0B, slope 0C)

Figure 8.3

southeast edge of the 95% confidence ellipsoid. The slope of this ray is the lower limit of the 95% confidence interval for the cost-effectiveness ratio. Similarly the analyst can construct a ray from the origin (OC) tangent to the northwest side of the confidence ellipsoid. The slope of this ray is the upper limit of the 95% confidence interval for the cost-effectiveness ratio. As Figure 8.3 indicates, the 95% confidence interval for the C/E ratio is smaller than what one would get by using a worst case analysis that relied on the southeast (ray OA) and northwest corners (ray OD) of the box given by the 95% confidence interval for cost and the 95% confidence interval for effectiveness. How different these are depends on the correlation between the two estimates. If the uncertainties in costs and effectiveness are negatively correlated, then there will be substantial uncertainty in the cost-effectiveness ratio, as in Figure 8.4. If the uncertainties in costs and effectiveness are positively correlated, then the two sources of uncertainty will tend to cancel each other out as far as the C/E ratio is concerned, as in Figure 8.5. In the extreme case of perfect positive correlation, there could be much less uncertainty in the cost-effectiveness ratio than there is in either incremental costs or effectiveness.

Given the critical role of the correlation between incremental costs and effectiveness, can we say anything about its sign? If the estimates come from different (independent) sources, then the two estimates should be independent of each other, and their partial correlation stemming from structure internal to the data collection itself should be zero. If the estimates of costs and effectiveness are based, in part, on the same data, then the estimates may not be independent. The direction of the correlation is not clear a priori. One might suspect that the two are negatively correlated, because cases with adverse effects are very likely to be more expensive than average. However, if a treatment increases life expectancy (and hence QALYs), the patients may incur higher costs over a longer period of time. This would tend to produce a positive correlation. Also higher quality, more effective care is likely to be more costly.

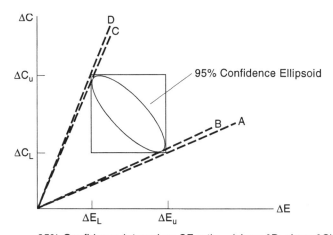

95% Confidence interval on CE ratio = (slope 0B, slope 0C).

Figure 8.4.

There are several ways to calculate a confidence interval or probability distribution for the cost-effectiveness ratio. O'Brien et al. (1994) suggest the use of the delta method, which is the second-order Taylor series approximation given in Equation (3) below. This is probably the easiest of the approaches to implement. Another alternative is the suggestion by Mullahy and Manning (1994) to use consistent estimates of the parameters and their variance–covariance matrix, or consistent estimates of the distribution of the parameters, to simulate a distribution of the cost-effectiveness ratio. The simulation approach is more difficult than the delta method approach, but its advantage is that it avoids an approximation bias that is inherent when the delta method is applied to ratios. The delta method may be excellent for linear combinations of variables, but

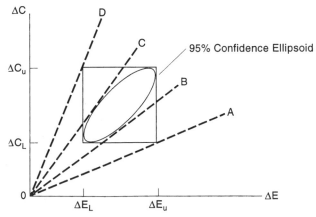

95% Confidence interval on CE ratio = (slope 0B, slope 0C).

Figure 8.5.

it has serious faults applied to nonlinear forms such as the C/E ratio central to CEA (Mullahy and Manning, 1994). A third alternative is to use the underlying primary data (if they are available) to obtain a bootstrap estimate of the cost-effectiveness ratio and its distribution. This is probably the most difficult of the three alternatives to implement.[13] However, recent changes in the cost of computing have now made the bootstrap approach accessible to most analysts, even those relying on personal computers in their efforts. Unfortunately, it is rare that analysts have access to sufficient primary data to employ the bootstrap.

The delta method

The delta method involves an application of a second-order Taylor series expansion to the estimation of the variance of some function, such as the cost-effectiveness ratio, or any of its components.[14] In the case of our $C = pv$ example earlier, the delta method yields

$$\mathrm{Var}(\overline{C}) = \overline{v}^2\,\mathrm{Var}(\overline{p}) + \overline{p}^2\,\mathrm{Var}(\overline{v}) + 2\overline{p}\overline{v}\,\mathrm{Cov}(\overline{v}, \overline{p}) \tag{2}$$

where $\mathrm{Var}(\overline{p})$ is the variance of the estimate of the mean of p, etc. In the case of the cost-effectiveness ratios with only two parameters—incremental cost C and incremental effectiveness E—then the delta method yields[15]

$$\mathrm{Var}\,(\overline{C/E}) = \overline{\left(\frac{1}{E}\right)}^2\,\mathrm{Var}\,(\overline{C}) + \overline{\left(\frac{C}{E^2}\right)}^2\,\mathrm{Var}\,(\overline{E}) - 2\overline{\left(\frac{C}{E^3}\right)}\,\mathrm{Cov}\,(\overline{C,E})$$

$$= \overline{\left(\frac{1}{E^2}\right)}\,[\mathrm{Var}\,(\overline{C}) + \overline{\left(\frac{C}{E}\right)}^2\,\mathrm{Var}\,(\overline{E}) - 2 \cdot \overline{\left(\frac{C}{E}\right)} \cdot \mathrm{Cov}(\overline{C,E})] \tag{3}$$

See O'Brien et al. (1994) for a derivation; Gardiner, et al. (1995) and Chaudhary and Stearns (forthcoming) provide examples. In general, there will be more than two parameters of interest. This requires the use of the general formula for the variance of a function $f(\theta)$, where θ is a vector of model parameters; the cost-effectiveness ratio $f = C/E$ is just such a function.[16]

One possible problem in using the delta method is that it is based on only a second-order Taylor series approximation. In the case of a ratio, especially one based on multiple parameters, the remainder term in the approximation may be substantial. The source of the problem is that the higher-order terms in a Taylor's expansion are still important.[17] In calculating a cost-effectiveness ratio ($= \Delta C/\Delta E$), the incremental effectiveness of a treatment (in QALYs or some other effect measure) enters as a reciprocal. Thus, the 95% confidence ellipsoid may include estimates of the change in effectiveness that may be close to zero, especially if the study was designed to have the usual levels of precision for the effect measure—for example, 80% power for a significance level of $\alpha = 0.05$. Under these circumstances, it is possible that the inverse of effectiveness will span a range from very small to quite large values if the increment in effectiveness is only moderately, though significantly, different from zero in its own right. As the estimate of the effectiveness approaches zero, the reciprocal ($1/E$) "blows up"—that is, produces an arbitrarily large cost-effectiveness ratio. Because of the reciprocal form of effectiveness, the second-order approximation in the delta method does not capture the behavior of the estimate of the reciprocal of effectiveness as effectiveness approaches zero. The result is that the delta method estimate may seriously understate the upper limit of the cost-effectiveness ratio, giving the analyst a misleading sense of confidence in a low estimate of the upper limit on the cost-effectiveness ratio. It could lead the analyst to believe that the 95% confidence interval is well within the acceptable range of cost per QALY when in fact there was a substantial probability that the true value was outside the acceptable range.

Mullahy and Manning (1994) provide a simulated hypothetical example to illustrate this problem with the delta method for the cost-effectiveness ratio. They examined a case where the estimated means for the incremental cost and effectiveness were distributed as bivariate normal with population means for both cost and effect normalized to 1.0, and the standard error of each mean equal to one-half. Thus, both the incremental cost and incremental effectiveness were significantly different from zero at slightly better than the 5% level. If the correlation between the estimated means were -0.5, then the delta method would generate a 95% confidence interval of $[-0.96, +2.96]$, while the true confidence interval is $[-0.26, +8.90]$. This example illustrates two points. First, the cost-effectiveness ratio is much less precisely measured than either incremental costs or incremental effectiveness.[18] Second, the delta method can provide a badly biased estimate of the true confidence interval, especially of the upper limit. Neither of these conclusions changes much if we alter the assumptions underlying the example until we get to situations where the denominator is very significantly different from zero (i.e., the numerical distance of the estimated net effectiveness from zero is large compared to the standard deviation of this estimated net effectiveness). However, the variability in the ratio can shrink as costs and effectiveness become positively correlated.

The quality of the performance of the delta method in the Mullahy and Manning (1994) example is the result of the fact that the numerator and denominator are significantly different from zero at only about $p=0.05$. As the two terms become more significant, the approximation problems shrink. When the p value falls to well below 0.01, the approximation in the delta method is substantially better.

Fieller (1954) suggested a refinement of the approach to be used for ratios. If the estimates of $\overline{C}$ and $\overline{E}$ follow a bivariate normal distribution, and if the C/E ratio is $R = C/E$, then the quantity $C - R{\cdot}E$ is normally distributed with variance:

$$\text{Var}(\overline{C}) + R^2 \, \text{Var}(\overline{E}) - 2R \, \text{Cov}(\overline{C},\overline{E})$$

As Chaudhary and Stearns (forthcoming) show, one can derive confidence intervals based on this relationship. This approach relies on the normality of the estimates but avoids some of the problems with the inverse of effectiveness.

A simulation approach

Mullahy and Manning (1994) suggest a simulation alternative to estimate the variance of the cost-effectiveness ratio or its distribution. Based on consistent estimates of the variance–covariance matrix of the parameter estimates or of the distribution of the estimates, one can simulate the cost-effectiveness ratio by repeatedly taking draws from the multivariate distribution of the estimates and then doing the cost-effectiveness analysis for each of those draws. The resulting distribution of the estimated cost-effectiveness ratios should provide a consistent estimate of the C/E ratio's distribution. This method is similar to the Monte Carlo method of probabilistic sensitivity analysis proposed by Doubilet et al. (1985) for decision analysis. Most commonly used medical decision analysis software (e.g., SMLTREE, distributed by Dr. James K. Hollenberg, New York, NY; Decision Maker, distributed through the Division of Clinical Decision Making, New England Medical Center, Boston, MA; and DATA, by TreeÅge Software, Inc., Boston, MA) supports this type of sensitivity analysis, as do some add-on's for spreadsheet software (e.g, @RISK, distributed by Palisade Corporation, Newfield, NY). Chaudhary and Stearns (forthcoming) provide an example of these techniques using data for Medicaid's Early and Periodic Screening, Diagnosis, and Treatment programs. In their example, the delta method generated a confidence interval that was smaller than that indicated by either Fieller's method or various bootstrap/simulation alternatives. Further, the confidence interval's lower and upper limits were less than for other estimates. This confirms the Mullahy and Manning (1994) result that the confidence interval is shifted to the left. Finally, the delta method confidence intervals are symmetric while those for other approaches are asymmetric and skewed right.

Assessing Overall Parameter Uncertainty

Nearly all cost-effectiveness analysis involves some combination of uncertain information, where some of the uncertainty is due to sampling variations and where other parameters have some range of plausible values but no formal statistical estimates of uncertainty. The univariate sensitivity approach can easily accommodate both kinds of uncertainty because variables are treated one at a time. The other two approaches, the delta method and simulation approaches, need to be modified to incorporate both types of uncertainty at the same time. What follows is a proposal for an approach that to the best of our knowledge has been only partially applied in the practice of CEA, although it has been used in decision analysis (Doubilet et al., 1985).

The heart of the modification is to treat the ranges used in univariate sensitivity analysis as if they provided some information on the underlying distribution of the parameter of interest, or as if one had some sense of the distribution of interest. The range used could be the worst and best cases, or some subjective or expert's sense of the 95% confidence or credible interval for that variable. The range could reflect a number of alternative distributions. If the values in the range seem equally plausible, one could assume that the resulting probability density function (pdf) of the parameter θ is given by a uniform distribution. If the distribution is more peaked in the middle of the range, then one might assume that the distribution is triangular or even normal. In the operations research literature on PERT/CPM (Program Evaluation and Review Technique/Critical Path Method), the beta distribution has been used frequently (Hillier and Lieberman, 1974). In the case of the beta distribution, if the minimum and maximum are a and b, respectively, then it is common to assume that the variance in θ is approximately:

$$\sigma_\theta^2 \approx [\frac{1}{6}(b - a)]^2 \tag{4}$$

under the rationale that the tails are about three standard deviations from the mean.[19]

Probabilistic sensitivity analysis

In the literature on medical decision making, a number of studies have used a similar approach under the rubric ''probabilistic sensitivity analysis.'' The uncertain parameters are assumed to follow some specific distribution, which is specified in terms of means, standard deviations, or other statistics. If the estimates of the parameters are independent of each other, then the outcome can be simulated by taking random draws from each distribution and calculating the outcome variable, such as the expected utility of following a particular strategy through a decision tree. Willard and Critchfield (1986) and Critchfield and Willard (1986) performed a probabilistic sensitivity analysis for deep vein thrombosis using both algebraic and simulation approaches with normal and beta distributions. Doubilet et al. (1985) used a logistic normal distribution[20] to examine three management options for patients with suspected herpes simplex encephalitis. Eddy et al. (1992) have described a Bayesian method for combining information from multiple sources, which can then be used as an input into the process described above.

Once the distributions have been specified for each of the parameters, one can proceed to assess the overall distribution of the cost-effectiveness ratio by either simulation or delta methods. If the distributions of parameters of interest are independent of each other, or approximately so, then one can set the covariance terms to zero. If subsets of variables are correlated, then the covariance terms within those subsets need to be specified. If the estimates follow a normal distribution, then the delta method can be employed to calculate the variance of the C/E ratio and then calculate the desired (e.g., 95%) confidence interval. If the estimates follow some other distribution, or if there is concern about the behavior of the delta method for ratios, then one should use Monte Carlo simulation methods to assess the overall distribution of the C/E ratio and then construct the desired confidence interval.

Bootstrap analysis

The delta method and simulation approaches require that the analyst know what the distributions of parameter values are or have consistent estimates from other analyses.

In one special case, there is a method that does not require the analyst to specify the distribution. If the data set for the analysis contains data on all the variables of interest—effectiveness and costs over the full span of time relevant to the analysis—then one can employ the bootstrap technique to estimate the distribution of the C/E ratio. If there are *n* observations in the database, then the bootstrap takes a sample of *n* observations at random with replacement to generate a pseudo data set. This pseudo data set is used to obtain an estimate of the parameter of interest, the C/E ratio. This process is repeated many times. The observed distribution of the resulting estimates across replicates provides an estimate of the distribution of the C/E ratio. Efron and Tibshirani (1993) describe how this can be done for simple ratio problems.

The bootstrap method can also be applied to the data for any subpart of the analysis. For example, there might be some concern about the distribution of estimates of mean health expenditures by treatment regimen, because the underlying distribution of the individual data is very skewed. In such a case, one could apply the bootstrap to the cost data to arrive at an appropriate empirical distribution for (some of) the incremental cost component. That distribution could then be used as an input into the Monte Carlo simulation described above.

Bayesian estimates of uncertainty

To this point we have drawn attention to the fact that besides the *point* estimate of the C/E ratio—that is, the best single estimated value for the C/E ratio—there is an associated *interval* estimate that is of interest to users of the CEA. The interval estimate is an estimated interval within which the true value is expected to lie with some specified probability.

Researchers typically report 95% confidence intervals for this purpose, and our exposition so far has been directed to this form of interval estimate. In the current literature these intervals are usually derived using classical statistical techniques. There is an alternative statistical methodology, Bayesian statistics, that also can be used to derive interval estimates to characterize the uncertainty in the C/E ratio; these intervals are termed *credible intervals* to emphasize their close relation to confidence intervals as well as their distinct pedigree.

The difference between the Bayesian and classical methods lies in what is considered to be relevant information with which to determine the estimated parameter values. For example, to estimate the sensitivity of a test (the relative frequency of a positive test result in patients who have the disease of interest), a classical statistician will observe the test results for a sample of patients who have the disease and then determine an estimate of the "true" relative frequency by computing the ratio of the number of patients with the disease with positive test results to the total number of patients with the disease with the disease who were tested. By contrast, in advance of collecting the data, the Bayesian statistician specifies a probability distribution over all possible values that the "true" sensitivity of the test could have; this *prior distribution* incorporates all the analyst (or relevant decision maker) knows about the likelihoods of the various values in advance of the experiment, collecting the data. The results of the experiment are then observed, and an estimate of the sensitivity is computed by formally combining the experimental data with the prior distribution. The result is the *posterior distribution*, a probability distribution that describes the likelihoods of all possible values for the sensitivity in light of both the prior distribution *and* the data. The mean of the posterior distribution is a Bayesian estimate of the parameter, and the central 95% interval of the posterior distribution forms the Bayesian 95% interval estimate for the parameter.

If the prior distribution is uniform across all possible values for the parameter, then the Bayesian and the classical point and interval estimates are generally the same (for all intents and purposes). If the prior distribution peaks somewhere, indicating a priori that some values of the parameter are more likely than others, the two methods will differ unless the data sample is large.

Excellent accessible references outside of medicine exist describing the differences between these methods (Edwards et al., 1963; Berger and Berry, 1988); in the medical context, interested readers are directed to a book on Bayesian methods by Eddy and colleagues (Eddy et al., 1992) and to a recent paper analyzing results of the Global Utilization of Streptokinase and Tissue Plasminogen Activator in Occluded Arteries (GUSTO) trial (Brophy and Joseph, 1995). Statistical treatment of the Bayesian approach is contained in texts on mathematical statistics (Degroot, 1970; Berger, 1980) and statistical decision theory (Pratt et al., 1995).

There has been nearly a century of debate about classical versus Bayesian approaches to statistical estimation and characterization of uncertainty. More recently a combination of the two—empirical Bayes technique—has also emerged (Louis, 1991; Maritz and Lwin, 1989). This is an intellectual area in flux and we cannot begin to cover the debate in this brief chapter. Nor do we endorse one method over another at the present level of knowledge and state of the art. However, we wish to underscore the fact that a great deal of parameter uncertainty exists in most analyses, and the analyst should use some credible method to characterize the resulting implications of the precision of the C/E ratio estimate for the end user. A major goal of methodologists in C/E analysis should be to further explore the methods mentioned here and to devise ways to make these methods more accessible to the community of CEA analysts and end users.

Uses of uncertainty analysis

These approaches to characterizing uncertainty should be useful for at least three reasons. First, one may wish to test hypotheses about the sign and magnitude of costs, effectiveness, and the C/E ratio. Second, decision makers may want to know how much confidence they should place on the results of an analysis. Third, uncertainty analysis can help guide decisions about further research. If the estimate of the cost-effectiveness ratio is as imprecise as the simulated example from Mullahy and Manning (1994) would suggest, then the proper conclusion of many of the studies in the literature should have been that the sample size was insufficient to provide *clinically and economically* meaningful power to choose among the treatments. Rather than rush to judgment, the decision maker may want to collect more information before reaching a decision. If the costs of waiting for additional data are low or the potential loss from a poor decision is high, waiting may be cost-effective. See Weinstein (1991) and Hay et al. (1991) for examples of the logic of deciding to do additional studies.

A Worked Example of Uncertainty in a C/E Ratio

To illustrate the effect of the joint parameter uncertainty underlying a C/E ratio, we use a simple illustrative analysis first presented by Mushlin and Fintor (1992). Neither the original authors (hereafter ''MF'') nor we intend this illustration to be a final and comprehensive CEA of mammographic screening for breast cancer. Instead, our pur-pose is to illustrate the issues and methods described above. With this caveat, we pro-ceed.

Problem setup

MF restricted their analysis to screening women 40–50 years old and based it on evi-dence available in a review of the literature through 1991. They analyzed the costs and consequences of 1 year of screening on the supposition that the purpose of screening is to find cancers incident in that year. Three parameters allow estimation of the positive and negative yields of the screening: the annual incidence rate of breast cancer in the target population ($i = 0.15\%$), the sensitivity of mammography to detect these ($s = 80\%$), and the false-positive rate ($1 -$ specificity) of mammography in this population ($f = 3\%$). In a population taken for convenience to be 10,000 women, this means that $10,000 \times i = 15$ will have an incident cancer. Of these 15, on average we will detect $15 \times s = 12$. Among the 9,985 women without incident cancer there will be 3%, or 300 false-positive screens.

The incremental analysis is built into one parameter: the ''efficacy of screening,'' which is taken to be the percent reduction in case mortality given detection by screening versus other manners of clinical surfacing ($e = 25\%$). This, with two additional param-eters, the case mortality rate without screening ($m = 65\%$) and the average incremental number of life years gained ($l = 23.8$ years), allows computation of an estimated number of life years gained by the screening program. Thus, the number of lives saved by screening is the number of cases found (12) times the mortality rate without screening (65%) times the reduction in mortality (25%), or $12 \times 0.65 \times 0.25 = 1.95$ lives saved on average. This represents $1.95 \times 23.8 = 46$ life years gained (incrementally) in the cohort by screening for breast cancer with mammography.

Putting this all together, the life years (LY) saved are

$$LY = (smile) \, 10,000 \qquad (5)$$

Costs were simplified by assuming that the additional costs of care averted for each life saved are $D = \$25,000$; the costs averted then are $1.95 \times \$25,000 = \$48,750$.

The costs of screening were assumed to be $M = $100 for each mammogram, totaling $1 million, and an additional $B = $900 per positive mammogram (both true positives and false positives) for follow-up biopsy, totaling $280,800. Net incremental costs are therefore $1,000,000 + $280,800 − $48,750 = $1,232,050. The formula for net incremental costs, $C, is

$$\$C = \{\$M(10,000) + \$B[is + (1-i)f](10,000) - \$D[isme(10,000)]\} \qquad (6)$$

The point estimate of the incremental C/E ratio for this simplified example is then:

$$R = \$C/LY \approx \$26,540 \qquad (7)$$

if we use the parameter estimates given in Table 8.2.

Uncertainty analysis: method

We take the MF analysis as our starting point and add uncertainty about the parameters. For this illustration, we subjectively estimated a hypothetical 95% confidence interval for each uncertain parameter. On the assumptions that the 95% interval covers a range of approximately four standard deviations and that the estimates are normally distributed we converted the original base-case parameter values and these ranges into a mean and standard deviation that described our uncertainty about each parameter suitable for entry into a simulation program.

The last two columns of Table 8.2 present the results of the univariate sensitivity analyses for each of the parameters in Equations (5) and (6). By and large the estimate of the C/E ratio is relatively insensitive to the uncertainty in individual parameters. The one exception is the effect of the estimate of the case incidence rate (i). For that variable, the C/E ratio varies from $19,700 to $40,220. In part, the sensitivity of the C/E to the

Table 8.2 Uncertainty Analysis for Mushlin and Fintor (MF)

Parameter	Symbol	Mean (from MF)	Estimated Range	Derived S.D.	S.D./ Mean	Univariate Sensitivity (S/LY) Lower	Upper
Number in the screened population	N	10,000	(fixed parameter)	0	0	—	—
Case incidence rate	i	0.15%	0.10–0.20%	0.025%	0.17	19,700	40,220
Test sensitivity	s	80%	75–85%	2.5%	0.03	24,930	28,360
Test false-positive rate	f	3%	2–4%	0.5%	0.17	24,600	28,470
Case mortality rate (no screening)	m	65%	60–70%	2.5%	0.04	24,570	28,840
Reduction in mortality rate due to screen (effectiveness)	e	25%	20–30%	2.5%	0.10	21,940	33,440
Incremental costs of care if not detected by screening	$D	$25,000	$20,000–$30,000	$2,500	0.10	26,330	26,750
Cost of mammogram	$M	$100	$80–$120	$10	0.10	22,230	30,850
Cost of biopsy	$B	$900	$800–$1,000	$50	0.05	25,870	27,210

estimate i is due to the fact that the range of estimates is plus or minus one-third the estimate of the parameter. However, part of the sensitivity is due to the impact of i on both the numerator and the denominator.

Using the range of parameter estimates from Table 8.2, we find that a worst-case analysis would indicate a range in the C/E ratio of from $12,940 to $59,830. This range corresponds to the slopes of the two rays in Figure 8.2, or OA and OD in Figure 8.3. This range is substantially greater than that indicated by the results of the univariate sensitivity analyses above.

If we assume that each parameter estimate in Table 8.2 is normally distributed and independent of every other parameter estimate, we can use the delta method for this example. Then the 95% confidence interval for the C/E ratio extends from $14,940 to $40,53(This range is larger than that of any of the univariate sensitivity ranges. Of the univariate results, only that for the case incidence rate i comes close to the delta method estimate of overall uncertainty.

We can also simulate a 95% confidence (or credibility) interval for the C/E ratio. The Monte Carlo simulation estimate of the range is $17,510–$43,570. That estimate is substantially larger than that indicated by even the worst of the univariate results. The simulation estimate of the confidence interval is slightly larger than that provided by the delta method. But more importantly, the simulation estimate is shifted to the right of the delta method, as predicted by Mullahy and Manning (1994). The simulation and delta method estimates have a smaller range than indicated by the worst case analysis. However, for all of the methods, the major contributor to the overall uncertainty in the C/E ratio is the individual uncertainty in the case incidence rate i.

Model Uncertainty

Model Structure Uncertainty

To this point, we have assumed no uncertainty about the functional form for the model by which the parameters are combined into estimates of costs and effectiveness. Under this assumption we have outlined a number of ways in which analysts have tried to incorporate and demonstrate uncertainty about parameter values. But what if the analyst, in addition to being uncertain about the values of particular parameters, is also uncertain about the mathematical forms by which they should be combined? For example, is the response to the treatment linear in dose levels, or does it exhibit decreasing effects as dosage increases? In Chapter 5 we mentioned that hazard functions may be estimated as either multiplicative or additive functions of risk factors and that choice of functional form can affect the resulting hazard estimate, which in turn can affect the computed C/E ratio. The choice of using multiplicative or additive functions is often made for mathematical convenience in the absence of clear evidence that one or the other of the functions is the appropriate one to use. (For example, see Kuntz and Weinstein, 1995.)

How should the analyst incorporate the uncertainty about which functional form is the correct one, or even which is the more accurate?

Unfortunately, it is difficult to incorporate formally this type of model structure uncertainty. Some alternatives can be combined into a single, more general model. For example, the specifications of the dose response in the last paragraph could be specified as

$$E = a_0 + a_1 D + a_2 D^2 \qquad (8)$$

where E is the effect and D is the dose level. Thus, uncertainty about a_2 captures the uncertainty in the functional form of the response. Unfortunately, the data or the design of the study may preclude a formal test of a_2 or the literature may not provide much insight about curvilinearity. For example, a study with only two dosage levels cannot distinguish between a linear and a curvilinear response. Thus, if the data or design were rich enough, we could convert a model of uncertain structure into one of uncertain parameter values. However, if the data or design is not rich enough, the issue remains one of uncertain structure.

Usually the analyst acknowledges where such structural choices were made in the report of the analysis. If there is sufficient worry about the magnitude of the error that might be introduced by structural assumptions, the qualitative remedy appears to be sensitivity analysis, computing the C/E ratio estimate under the alternative assumptions and reporting the magnitude of the effect. For quantitative analysis, a weighted average of the resulting estimates might be computed, with weights reflecting the degree of confidence in each structural form. Variances of the weighted average can be computed in a straightforward manner from variances of the two component estimates.

Beyond the suggestion to compute the estimates under each alternative structural assumption deemed reasonable, we can offer little more about this source of uncertainty in cost-effectiveness analysis.

Modeling Process Uncertainty

Our tour of sources of uncertainty would not be complete without a brief discussion of modeling process uncertainty. In the section on parameter uncertainty, we explored the variance in the cost and effectiveness estimates as a function of uncertainty in the parameters used in a specific C/E model. In the preceding section on model structure uncertainty, we noted that in addition to incorporating uncertainty about parameter values, it will be desirable to incorporate into the C/E estimates uncertainty about model structuring assumptions. Having shown the effect on the analytic results of these sources of uncertainty, the job of the individual analyst, or team of analysts, who produced the study is at an end.

But from the viewpoint of the user of the analytic results, there is one remaining source of potential error: the entire process by which the CEA was completed in this particular instance by this particular analyst or analytic team. It may be the case that if the analysis were to be conceived, structured, parameterized, and computed by another analyst, the results would be different. In this view, the particular analysis presented is but one sampled from a universe of possible analyst–analysis pairs.

We know of no simple method to test the reproducibility of the modeling process. Would the same analyst come to exactly the same computational result were there some way to start over without knowledge of the first result? We doubt the results would be the exactly the same, although they should be similar. Many, many choices are made in the course of developing a complex analysis. It is likely that some choices would be made differently, leading to different results—which we hope would not be *too* dissimilar from the first result.

Additionally, what would happen if a completely different analyst were to complete the CEA for the problem? Rarely in the literature do two completely independent analyses of the same problem appear. One instance, two analyses of costs and effectiveness of coronary bypass surgery, has been discussed by Weinstein, et al. (1980).

There have been ''dueling'' models—instances in which one team of analysts has produced what they believe to be their best estimate of costs and effects of an intervention, and another team of analysts has disagreed with or updated the assumptions and parameter values sufficiently to produce another model which they advocate as producing a substantially better estimate. For example, Fleming et al, (1993) produced an analysis of costs and benefits of alternative methods for treating localized prostate cancer and concluded that there is little benefit to aggressive treatment for most men. An alternative model, using other values for some critical parameters, was developed and published after the Fleming et al. model (Beck et al., 1994). Using this model, the authors concluded that radical prostatectomy has substantial benefit for many men.

Taking this further, we can imagine as a thought experiment a number of analysts completing analyses for the same problem and then comparing results. To our knowledge this has not been done in the CEA literature.

Brown and Fintor (1993) reviewed 16 studies purporting to compute a C/E ratio for routine mammographic screening to detect breast cancer. According to Brown and Fintor, ''Four of the sixteen studies . . . share a common assumption that is almost surely fallacious''; this assumption presumed a very large differential in the lifetime treatment costs for early versus late-detected stages of breast cancer. The remaining 12 studies exhibited a 25-fold difference in computed C/E ratios. Most of these differences could be ascribed to variations in the definitions of screening, to the confusion of average versus marginal C/E ratios, to the time horizon of the studies, and to the scope of costs and benefits that are counted. These might be characterized as variance introduced by either model structure variation or modeling process variation or both.

Interestingly, Brown and Fintor conclude that the range of variation in C/E outcome among ''truly comparable studies'' is much narrower, although still a fourfold difference. The authors use two studies with comparable model structure, but one using data from the United States and one from the Netherlands, and adjust for the differences in parameter estimates. The original apparent difference of \$34,600/life year gained versus \$7250/life year gained is almost entirely resolvable in terms of parameter differences due to known differences in the two settings.

In the Brown and Fintor examination of these studies of mammogram screening the best studies seem to have equivalent structures, implying that the model structure uncertainty may be relatively small (in the hands of competent analysts) compared to model parameter uncertainty. But values for model parameters are selected and distilled from a sometimes-voluminous and contradictory literature. The remaining variation not examined in Brown and Fintor's preliminary analysis may well be ascribed to model process uncertainty as described in this chapter, and this uncertainty may well be similar in magnitude to the contribution of model parameter uncertainty.

Several paragraphs above we posed a thought experiment to evaluate modeling process uncertainty in CEA. To our knowledge this experiment has not been attempted in this domain. But as more and more resources are committed in health care on the strength of CEA studies, we feel that the time may have come for such a study to be purposefully designed and funded. We need to know the relative contributions of the three sources of variance identified in the rows of Table 8.1. If the contribution of modeling uncertainty is as important as parameter uncertainty, a concerted effort is in order to understand the processes by which analysts develop models and to find and eliminate major sources of variation in this process.

Recommendations

1. At a minimum, the analyst should conduct one-at-a-time, or univariate, sensitivity analyses to determine where uncertainty or lack of agreement about some key parameter's value or the functional form of the model could have a substantial impact on the conclusions.

2. Analysts should conduct multiway sensitivity analyses for important parameters.

3. If possible, where parameter uncertainty is a major concern, a reasonable confidence interval or credible interval should be estimated based on other statistical methods or simulation. If both the numerator and denominator are substantially different from zero, then the delta method may be convenient; otherwise we encourage the use of the simulation approach.

4. When there is substantial uncertainty other than parameter uncertainty, analysts may need to use simulation in a substantially more sophisticated way (e.g., sampling model structures) to represent the uncertainty in the CEA results.

5. When relying on expert judgment to inform variance estimates for computing confidence or credible regions, analysts must be acutely aware that the literature in cognitive psychology indicates that experts substantially underestimate the variance in uncertain parameters.

6. If uncertainty in the C/E ratio is very large, analysts and decision makers should

weigh the risks of taking action based on limited information against the costs of more targeted data collection to reduce the key uncertainties in the CEA.

Research Recommendations

1. Agencies that fund CEAs should realize that the nature of usual distribution of costs is such that larger studies will be needed to supply adequate samples for cost analysis than are necessary for effectiveness and efficacy. Individual trials intended to provide data on both costs and health effects should be large enough to provide adequate power for both costs and effectiveness.

2. Very little is known about the contribution of variations in the modeling process itself to the overall uncertainty in CEA results. We recommend that this be a priority area for research in the near future.

Notes

1. Some authors draw a distinction between risk and uncertainty. For example, Drummond (1980) uses "risk" to refer to cases where there is some evidence, and "uncertainty" to refer to cases where there is little evidence or the element is unknown. For our purposes, we will use uncertainty to refer to any case where we do not know the true value of a parameter or the structure of a process.

2. Whether one would choose to collect such data is itself open to a cost-benefit analysis. If the value of the information is small relative to the cost of collecting it, then it may not be worth it for society to actually collect the data. For example, if the results are not sensitive to a plausible range of values of a parameter, or if the intervention is never cost-effective, or always cost-effective, then spending research funds to establish a more precise measure of some parameter may be an inefficient use of scarce research funds.

3. In what follows, we will not address the questions that deal with the validity, reliability, or consistency of the information used. Good discussions about these and related design and estimation issues can be found in Campbell and Stanley (1963), Cook and Campbell (1979), IOM (1985), and Mullahy and Manning (1994).

4. See Briggs et al. (1994) for a review of the role of sensitivity analyses in economic evaluations such as cost-effectiveness analysis.

5. In this case, a substantial range of values for the parameter refers to the range of our uncertainty about the value, not to the clinical or economic significance of the value.

6. See Chapter 5 for a discussion about modeling effectiveness and Chapter 6 for a discussion of costs.

7. To further complicate matters, one is comparing an uncertain measure of cost-effectiveness against thresholds for policy decisions, which are themselves not always well articulated or certain.

8. For example, there may be a diminishing yield or effectiveness as the quantity of intervention per patient increases. The declining yield for screening as the frequency increases provides a well-known example (Eddy, 1990).

9. This is a starting point for assessing overall uncertainty. Most situations will require higher-order aproximations, bootstrapping, or simulations.

10. This example can be generalized to any function $y = f(\theta)$ by noting that:

$$U(y) \approx \sum_{i}^{k} U(\theta_i) \cdot \frac{\partial f}{\partial \theta_i} \tag{1}$$

where $\partial f/\partial \theta$ is the partial derivative of f with respect to the ith parameter θ_i, and $U(\theta_i)$ is a range or some other measure of uncertainty in θ_i.

In the case of either Equation (1) or its generalization above, the analyst could use a second-order expansion of the specific CEA required consideration of a nonlinearity, such as may be necessary to allow for the interaction of two parameters.

11. When we consider statistical approaches below, we provide an example where the incremental cost-effectiveness ratio is less variable than its components if they are positively correlated.

12. Strictly speaking, the classical definition of a confidence interval is framed in terms of the probability that a particular sample estimate lies within a range, given a true parameter value, rather than the other way around. However, the term *confidence interval* is commonly used *as if* the probability that the true value lies in the interval were 95%. Statistical decision theory can be used to show that the definitions are equivalent if a uniform prior distribution on the parameter mean and the logarithm of its standard deviation is assumed (Phillips, 1973). When the range of the parameter is infinite (e.g., a positive real number), so that a uniform distribution is impossible, then an "informationless" or "improper" prior distribution must be invoked.

13. It is also possible to use combinations of these approaches. For example, one can bootstrap some components to be used in either a delta method or simulation approach for the C/E ratio.

14. Derivation of the delta method: Consider a function $f(x,y)$. If we take a first-order Taylor's approximation around x_0 and y_0, we get:

$$f(x,y) \approx f(x_0, y_0) + f_x(\Delta x) + f_y(\Delta y)$$

where

$$\Delta x = x - x_0, \ \Delta y = y - y_0$$

and f_x and f_y denote the partial derivatives of the f with respect to the x and y, respectively. Thus,

$$\text{Var } (f) = E \ [f - \bar{f})^2] \approx E \ (f_x \ [\Delta x) + f_y \ (\Delta y)]^2$$

where the bar indicates the average. The last equation can be written as:

$$\text{Var } (f) \approx f_x^2 \ \text{Var } (x) + f_y^2 \ \text{Var } (y) + 2 \ f_x f_y \ \text{Cov } (x,y)$$

15. We suppress the Δ notation, $\Delta C = C_2 - C_1$, and $\Delta E = E_2 - E_1$, for ease of exposition.
16. The general formula is

$$\text{Var } (\hat{f}) \approx \left(\frac{\overline{\partial f}}{\partial \hat{\theta}} \right)' \text{Var } (\hat{\theta}) \left(\frac{\overline{\partial f}}{\partial \hat{\theta}} \right) \tag{1}$$

where $\text{Var}(\hat{\theta})$ is the variance–covariance matrix for the estimates of the vector of the parameters θ in the C/E ratio model and the bar over the vector partial derivative of f with respect to θ indicates the average of the estimate of the derivative, not the derivative evaluated at the average. If all the parameter estimates came from a single study, then the estimate of the variance–covariance matrix will include the variances of the individual parameters and the covariances among the parameter estimates. If the parameter estimates come from different studies, then the variance–covariance matrix would include the variances (or variance–covariance matrix) from each source along the diagonal, or as block diagonal. The off-diagonal elements would be zero, because the estimates of the parameters from different studies are independent. Thus if the cost and effectiveness estimates were based on different samples, then

$$\text{Var}(\hat{\theta}) = \begin{pmatrix} \text{Var}(\overline{C}) & 0 \\ 0 & \text{Var}(\overline{E}) \end{pmatrix} \tag{2}$$

and the variance of the estimated cost-effectiveness ratio $\overline{(C/E)}$ would equal

$$\text{Var}\,(C/E) = \begin{pmatrix} \dfrac{1}{E} & \dfrac{-C}{E^2} \end{pmatrix} \begin{pmatrix} \text{Var}(C) & 0 \\ 0 & \text{Var}(E) \end{pmatrix} \begin{pmatrix} 1/E \\ -C/E^2 \end{pmatrix} = \dfrac{1}{E^2}\,\text{Var}(C) + \left(\dfrac{C}{E^2}\right)^2 \text{Var}(E) \tag{3}$$

suppressing the bar notation for averages.

If the estimate of any specific parameter is based on a number of studies, as in meta-analysis, then the variance estimate of the variance across the structure is the variance of the parameter pooling the information across studies. The variance terms are the standard estimates of the variance of the difference in the means between two populations in the two-sample problem; for example:

$$\text{Var}(\Delta\hat{\mu}) = \text{Var}(\hat{\mu}_1 - \hat{\mu}_2) = \dfrac{(\hat{\sigma}_1^2)}{n_1} + \dfrac{(\hat{\sigma}_2^2)}{n_2} \tag{4}$$

where the subscripts 1 and 2 indicate different health interventions, the $\hat{\mu}$'s are consistent estimates of the parameters of interest, and the $\hat{\sigma}^2$'s are the consistent estimates of the variance for each intervention.

17. A similar problem occurs with nonlinear Wald statistics. See Phillips and Park (1988) for a discussion of that case, and in particular, of the role of the higher-order terms in a Taylor expansion.

18. The 95% confidence interval for either costs or effectiveness in this example is [+0.02, 1.98].

19. If a and b give the 95% percent credible interval, then the 6 should be replaced by 4. In some applications of the beta distribution, operations researchers in the PERT applications assume that the mean time to completion is given by a weighted average of the mode m and the average of the extremes $[2m+0.5(a+b)]/3$.

20. If the variable log $[x/(1-x)]$ is normally distributed and $0 < x < 1$, then $y = 1/[1+\exp(-x)]$ follows a logistic normal distribution.

References

Alpert, M., and H. Raiffa. 1982. A progress report on the training of probability assessors. In, *Judgment under uncertainty: Heuristics and biases*, ed. D. Kahneman, P. Slovic, and A. Tversky, 294–305. Cambridge: Cambridge University Press.

Beck, J.R., M.W. Kattan, and B.J. Miles. 1994. A critique of the decision analysis for clinically localized prostate cancer. *J Urol* 152(5, part 2):1894–99.

Berger, J.O. 1980. *Statistical decision theory and Bayesian analysis*. New York: Springer-Verlag.

Berger, J.O, and D.A. Berry. 1988. Statistical analysis and the illusion of objectivity. *American Scientist* 76:159–65.

Briggs, A., M. Sculpher, and M. Buxton. 1994. Uncertainty in the economic evaluation of health care technologies: The role of sensitivity analysis. *Health Econ* 3:95–104.

Brophy, J.M., and L. Joseph. 1995. Placing trials in context using Bayesian analysis: Gusto revisited by Reverend Bayes. *JAMA* 23:871–75.

Brown, M.L., and L. Fintor. 1993. Cost-effectiveness of breast cancer screening: Preliminary results of a systematic review of the literature. *Breast Cancer Res Treat* 8:113–18.

Campbell, D.T., and J.C. Stanley. 1963. *Experimental and quasi-experimental designs for research*. Boston: Houghton Mifflin.

Chaudhary, M.A., and S.C. Stearns. Forthcoming. Estimating confidence intervals for cost-effectiveness ratios: An example from a randomized trial. *Stat Med*

Christianson, J.B., and S.G. Bender. 1982. Benefit-cost analysis and medical care delivery system change. *Evaluation Review* 6:481–504.

Cook, T.D., and D.T. Campbell. 1979. *Quasi-experimentation: Design and analysis issues for field settings*. Boston: Houghton Mifflin.

Cretin, S. 1977. Cost/benefit analysis of treatment and prevention of myocardial infarction. *Health Serv Res* 12:174–89.

Critchfield, G.C., and K.E. Willard. 1986. Probabilistic analysis of decision trees using Monte Carlo simulation. *Med Decis Making* 6:85–92.

De Groot, M.H. 1970. *Optimal statistical decisions*. New York: McGraw-Hill.

Dittus, R.S., S.D. Roberts, and J.R. Wilson. 1989. Quantifying uncertainty in medical decisions. *J Am Coll Cardiol* 14(Supplement A):23A–28A.

Doubilet, P., C.B. Begg, M.C. Weinstein, P. Braun, and B.J. McNeil. 1985. Probabilistic sensitivity analysis using monte carlo simulation: A practical approach. *Med Decis Making* 5:157–77.

Drummond, M.F. 1980. *Principles of economic appraisal in health care*. London: Oxford University Press.

Eddy, D.M. 1990. Screening for cervical cancer. *Ann Intern Med* 113:214-26.

Eddy, D.M., V. Hasselblad, and R.D. Schachter. 1992. *Meta-analysis by the confidence profile method: The statistical synthesis of evidence*. Boston: Academic Press.

Edwards, W., H. Lindman, and L.J. Savage. 1963. Bayesian statistical inference for psychological research. *Psychol Rev* 70:193–242.

Efron, B., and R.J. Tibshirani. 1993. *An introduction to the bootstrap*. New York: Chapman and Hall.

Fieller, E.C. 1954. Some problems in interval estimation. *J Royal Statistical Society* (Series B) 16:175–83.

Fleming, C., J.H. Wasson, P.C. Albertson, M.J. Barry, and J.E. Wennberg. 1993. A decision analysis of alternative treatment strategies for clinically localized prostate cancer. *JAMA* 269:2650–58.

Gardiner, G., A. Hogan, M. Holmes-Rovner, L. Griffith, and J. Kupersmith. 1995. Confidence intervals for cost-effectiveness ratios. *Med Decis Making* 15:254–63.

Goldman, L., M.C. Weinstein, P.A. Goldman, and L.W. Williams. 1991. Cost-effectiveness of HMA-CoA reductase inhibition for primary and secondary prevention of coronary heart disease. *JAMA* 26:1145–51.

Hay, J.W., E. H. Wittels, and A.M. Gotto, Jr. 1991. An economic evaluation of lovastatin for cholesterol lowering and coronary artery disease reduction. *Am J Cardiol* 67:789–96.

Hillier, F.S., and G.J. Lieberman. 1974. *Operations Research* 2d ed. San Francisco: Holden-Day.

Institute of Medicine (IOM). 1985. Methods of technology assessment. In *Assessing medical technologies*, Chapter 3. Washington, DC: National Academy Press.

Kuntz, K.M., and M.C. Weinstein. 1995. Life expectancy biases in clinical decision making. *Med Decis Making* 15:158–69.

Louis, T.A. 1991. Using empirical Bayes in bio-pharmaceutical research. *Stat Med* 10:811–29.

Maritz, J.S., and T. Lwin. 1989. *Empirical Bayes methods* 2d ed. London: Chapman and Hall. Mishan, E.J. 1976. *Cost-benefit analysis*. New York: Praeger.

Mullahy, J., and W.G. Manning. 1994. Statistical issues in cost-effectiveness analyses. in *Valuing health care: Costs, benefits and effectiveness of pharmaceuticals and other medical technologies*, ed. F. Sloan. New York: Cambridge University Press.

Mushlin, A., and L. Fintor. 1992. Is screening for breast cancer cost-effective? *Cancer* 69:1957–62.

O'Brien, B.J., M.F. Drummond, R.J. Labelle, and A. Willan. 1994. In search of power and significance: Issues in the design and analysis of stochastic cost-effectiveness studies in health care. *Med Care* 32:150–63.

Office of Technology Assessment (OTA), U.S. Congress. 1981. *Cost-effectiveness of influenza vaccination*. Washington, DC: GPO.

Pauker, S.G., and J.P. Kassirer. 1980. The threshold approach to clinical decision making. *N Engl J Med* 302:1109–17.

Phillips, L.D. 1973. *Bayesian statistics for the social sciences*. New York: Thomas Y. Crowell.

Phillips, P.C.B., and J.Y. Park. 1988. On the formulation of Wald tests of nonlinear restrictions. *Econometrica* 56:1065–83.

Pratt, J., H. Raiffa, and R. Schlaifer. 1995. *Statistical Decision Theory* Cambridge, MA: MIT Press.

Rothenberg, T.J. 1984. Approximating the distributions of econometric estimators and test statistics. In *Handbook of econometrics 2*, Vol. 2, ed. Z. Griliches and M.D. Intrilligator. Amsterdam: North Holland.

Vogel, R.J., and J.B. Christianson. 1986. The evaluation of economic development projects where military conflict is present: Investing in health care in El Salvador. *J Policy Analysis and Management* 5:292–310.

Weinstein, M.C. 1991. The cost-effectiveness of orphan drugs. *Am J Public Health* 81:414–15.

Weinstein, M.C., H.V. Fineberg, A.S. Elstein, H.S. Frazier, D. Neuhauser, R.R. Neutra, and B.J. McNeil. 1980. *Clinical decision analysis*. Philadelphia: W.B. Saunders Company.

Weinstein, M.C., and W.B. Stason. 1977. Foundations of cost-effectiveness analysis for health and medical practices. *N Engl J Med* 296:716–21.

Willard, K.E., and G.C. Critchfield. 1986. Probabilistic analysis of decision trees using symbolic algebra. *Med Decis Making* 6:93–100.

9

Reporting Cost-Effectiveness Studies and Results

J.E. SIEGEL, M.C. WEINSTEIN,
and G.W. TORRANCE

The way a cost-effectiveness analysis is reported is a critical determinant of the impact and utility of an analysis. The comprehensiveness of a report affects the degree to which research can be reviewed or extended by other analysts. Its organization and clarity govern its accessibility to an audience, its credibility, and, ultimately, the likelihood that study results will play a part in policy discussions.

The contribution of CEA to decision making hinges on the ability of a CEA report to facilitate comparisons of the relative value of interventions. Cost-effectiveness analysis provides information on health care interventions, practices, and technologies that serves as an input to a process of relative ranking, as discussed in Chapter 1. The previous chapters in this book have outlined the Reference Case, a series of methodological recommendations that, if included dependably in cost-effectiveness analyses, will permit consumers of CEA to identify studies of consistent quality and comparable results. This chapter focuses on the reporting of cost-effectiveness analyses that incorporate the Reference Case.

Because cost-effectiveness studies address a wide range of topics and serve multiple purposes, it would be constraining and often unprofitable for analysts to adhere to a strict template for reporting all CEAs. However, it is important that the information needed to understand and evaluate studies be readily available to consumers and reviewers of cost-effectiveness analyses. The purpose of the recommendations in this chapter is to improve the transparency of analyses reported in the literature, aid the analyst in assuring the completeness of the cost-effectiveness report, and encourage the presentation of comparable C/E results.

We describe two types of reports, the *journal report* and the *technical report*. These reports serve complementary purposes. The journal article has been the primary means of communicating cost-effectiveness results to the study's audience, whether the CEA is intended to contribute to a policy discussion or to inform the clinical decisions in the practice setting. Of course, not all cost-effectiveness manuscripts are submitted for journal publication; they may be included in books or government reports, or be distributed through other mechanisms. Here, we will refer to any summary manuscript similar to a journal article (intended to communicate the context of the problem and the analysis, the main features of the analysis, its results, and the quality of the work) as a journal report.

Because of the space restrictions in most journals, journal articles generally contain limited detail concerning many aspects of cost-effectiveness analyses. Authors often find it difficult to outline data and assumptions adequately and justify methods in the space allotted. This problem affects reviewers, who may be unable to determine what has been done in an analysis. It also affects authors, who may receive unclear comments or unwarranted rejection of their studies.

To provide another avenue for the communication of the results of cost-effectiveness analysis, we recommend that authors prepare a *technical report*, described later in this chapter, containing additional information to be made available upon request to researchers and others interested in further details about the study. Readers of the technical report may be scrutinizing the analysis in order to evaluate the study, improve their understanding of specific data or methods, reproduce the work, or adapt it to local circumstances. The technical report is intended to provide adequate detail for any of these purposes. Ideally, the technical report should enable readers to replicate the analysis, if not exactly, at least in its essential features.

While the technical report will provide information essential to some consumers of the analysis, it does not entirely address the problem of space limitations in journal articles. The recent report of the Task Force for Economic Analysis of Health Care Technology (1995) encourages journal editors to allow adequate space for authors to present a full discussion of key assumptions and methods. In addition, to supplement the article specifically for purposes of review, we recommend that authors attach (and journals request) a concise *technical addendum* to the journal article when submitting the manuscript. The technical addendum, several manuscript pages in length, would explain and clarify assumptions, models, methods, or calculations for the reviewers of the study. Journals could have the option of publishing this technical material as an appendix to the article.

The Journal Report

We outline information recommended for the journal report in sections addressing (1) the framework of the analysis, (2) methods and data (including effectiveness, outcome values, and costs), (3) results, and (4) discussion. Most cost-effectiveness reports in the literature follow a format similar to this one. We offer this general structure as a guide for authors, since consumers and reviewers of analyses will find it easier to locate needed information when information is placed in predictable parts of journal reports.

Framework

An introductory section at the beginning of a CEA journal report commonly provides background for the subject under study and describes the framing and design of the analysis in general terms. The problem addressed by the analysis is described, as is the program or intervention being evaluated. Frequently, the author will be assessing the cost-effectiveness of a general type of program (e.g., mammography screening programs initiated in physician offices) rather than an identifiable project (a cervical cancer screening outreach effort located in a New York City urban hospital clinic). In either case the program description should be detailed enough to allow readers to determine the appropriateness of generalizing the results of the analysis.

The description of the intervention includes the characteristics of the target population. The target population may be identified by age, gender, race, socioeconomic status, physiologic risk factors, risk-related behaviors, clinical history, geographic location, or other descriptors, depending on the analysis. In some cases, the analyst will have undertaken subgroup analyses, and the groups studied can be indicated in this discussion. When relevant, the care setting (location, type of institutions involved—such as hospitals, ambulatory clinics, or primary care practices), the mode of service delivery (equipment, personnel, and other aspects of the strategy used), and the timing of the intervention will also serve to define the intervention under study.

The incremental cost-effectiveness ratio obtained will depend as much on the comparison program as on the intervention itself, and similar care should be devoted to outlining the comparator, or "baseline" program, in the analysis. In Chapter 3, we recommend that, as a minimum, the intervention be compared with existing practice. Depending upon whether the status quo is a single intervention or a mix of practices, the analyst will face different requirements in describing this comparator. For example, the analyst may specify a mix of practice patterns by describing the component practices and the proportion of each assumed in the comparator. Other comparators in the analysis should also be described and the reason should be given for including each in the study. Among the possible comparators are the best available alternative (e.g., as defined by clinical guidelines), a low-cost alternative, or a "do-nothing" alternative. A summary of how these alternatives relate to current practice will help orient the reader. If a "do-nothing" option is not formally evaluated, its exclusion will often be because it is not a feasible option; the author may wish to note the reasons—ethical, political, or otherwise—that it is not.

The journal report should clarify the boundaries (scope) of the analysis. For example, if an analysis of a sexually transmitted disease stops at the third generation of a patient's sexual contacts, this analytical boundary should be explicit. As described in Chapter 3, the analysis boundaries are defined by the groups of people included and the types of effects assessed. The author may also wish to note the time horizon of the study in conjunction with the definition of boundaries. The time horizon will clarify how far into the future resource use and effects are measured.

As previously discussed, the perspective of the analysis is an important feature of the study, defining the costs and effects relevant to the analysis. The study perspective should be stated explicitly, early in the journal report. This stipulation appears widely in the literature on cost-effectiveness methodology (Drummond et al., 1987; Udvarhelyi et al., 1992; Weinstein, 1990); nonetheless, a significant proportion of studies neglect to follow this guideline (Udvarhelyi et al., 1992). When the Reference Case analysis is used, by definition the perspective stated will be societal. If the study includes analysis from one or more additional perspectives, the analyst should also identify these.

It is often helpful to devote an early paragraph to a description of the general approach used in the cost-effectiveness analysis, a discussion that can relate the goals of the study to the strategy used in the analysis. Is this a ''what if'' analysis intended to demonstrate the impact of the intervention if a certain level of effectiveness is established, or is this a subject for which effectiveness and outcomes are well documented? The discussion can also indicate the extent to which modeling is used in the analysis and the types of inputs to the model. For example, are the estimates of costs, effectiveness probabilities, and outcome values obtained from primary data, from secondary data in the literature, from results of modeling, or from expert opinion?

Methods and Data

The methods section describes the analytic methods used in the CEA in greater depth than the paragraph in the introductory portion of the report, fully outlining the analysis strategy, structure, and important assumptions. The author will often begin by describing the event pathway in the study. The analyst can then trace the pathway, describing the links between the intervention, its immediate effects, and more ''distal'' health events with the ultimate outcomes. For example, in a study of an antihypertensive medication, the analyst may relate the direct effect of the drug in lowering blood pressure to a decreased probability of cardiovascular events, and then to reduced cardiovascular mortality and increased life expectancy. Events affecting health-related quality of life or giving rise to costs may occur along the pathway as well as at its end, and the researcher may wish to note states where health-related quality of life or resource consumption is measured. It is important to indicate explicitly the outcome(s) of interest—for example, an improvement in health-related quality of life. A diagram incorporating all important features of the analysis will often prove indispensable for illustrating the event pathway.

If the study employs a mathematical or simulation model, the author should describe the approach used. For example, does the analysis employ a simple decision tree, a state-transition model, or a probabilistic simulation? The discussion of the modeling strategy should relate the basic conceptualization of the model; for example, does it portray a cohort, a sequence of individuals, or several heterogeneous risk groups? The model states and mechanisms for movement between states in mathematical or simulation models are generally described in conjunction with the description of the event pathway.

Special features of the analysis that the author has had to address in the study should be communicated in the methods section. For example, were the probabilities modeled as additive or multiplicative with respect to risk factors, and what was the specific mathematical form of the risk equation? As another example, if probabilities of a patient's recovery change over time, how do the mechanics of the model capture this feature? For screening programs, handling of lead time and length bias should be delineated. It is useful to indicate the type of software used to conduct the analysis or program the model.

Some analyses—generally those using program-specific primary data—will involve little explicit modeling. In this case, the author should relate the general strategy used in the analysis and carefully articulate important assumptions implicit in the data. For example, data on annual costs for a hospital's cardiac patients will reflect specific medical practice patterns and the case mix of that institution. Or a particular method of survival analysis may have been used to extrapolate survival beyond the end of the empirical data. These assumptions should be laid out in reporting an empirically based analysis, just as they would be in reporting an analysis based on a simulation model.

Effectiveness

An understanding of the evidence of effectiveness underlying a CEA is fundamental to assessing the quality of an analysis and the appropriate use of its results. An analysis undertaken before studies of effectiveness are completed (a ''what if'' analysis) may be highly useful for guiding policy decisions, but consumers will need to interpret its results in light of the assumptions contained in the analysis. Similarly, consumers of an analysis may use the analysis differently if the evidence of an intervention's effectiveness is contradictory or inconclusive. For this reason, a thorough discussion of effectiveness, including a review of relevant studies, is an essential component of the journal report.

A discussion of effectiveness should ordinarily include a summary of the body of evidence on the effectiveness of the intervention, describing the nature of relevant controversies as well as the direction of the evidence. (See Chapter 5.) The major studies in the area may require more detailed description, including an assessment of the quality of the research as well as its results. For example, the analyst may discuss randomization, sample sizes, representativeness of the samples, and other aspects of study design and execution, and report effect sizes and confidence intervals for specific parameters from the study. This level of detail is particularly necessary when studies are used as a source of secondary data, as opposed to forming part of a more general summary of the literature.

If a specific study of effectiveness has been undertaken for the CEA, the characteristics of that study will naturally comprise a significant part of the discussion. In this case, as for cases when secondary data are used, the author should provide adequate information for assessing the strength of the study and for the interpretation of the study results in the journal report.

The author should describe the rationale and assumptions necessary to generalize from studies to provide estimates of effectiveness for cost-effectiveness analysis, whether in the case of primary research or of studies from the supporting literature. For example, the author might discuss the extent to which data from a clinical trial reflect efficacy rather than effectiveness, including unrealistic assumptions about patient compliance to a regimen. Or, if a study had inclusion or exclusion criteria, it would be important to discuss the relation of the study population to the target population of the CEA. If a survey was used, reporting its response rate would provide information about the degree to which the data obtained could be generalized to the type of population from which the sample was drawn.

The discussion of effectiveness also includes the assumptions required and the mechanisms employed to incorporate data into an analysis. For example, if the author is incorporating life tables that extend to age 75, what assumptions are used for probabilities of death after that age? Were life tables adapted to the demographic or socioeconomic composition of the target population? If data on disease progression are available for 5-year periods, how does the author model progression within that time period on a yearly or monthly basis? In an analysis based on a primary study of effectiveness, how is the analysis extended beyond the length of the trial—if, in fact, it is? It is useful to summarize estimates of effectiveness employed in the analysis in a table for easy reference by the reader.

Outcome values

For a Reference Case analysis, the author may have obtained information on health states by using data that have been collected previously, by measuring health states directly within the CEA study, or by asking clinician experts to describe the health states within the terms of the particular measurement instrument they are using. In all of these cases, the preference weights for those health states should then be taken from an existing measure that has gathered community weights. (See Chapter 4.) The measurement system that has been used (e.g., the Health Utilities Index or the EuroQoL) should be cited, and information describing the measure, including the method it uses to value outcomes (e.g., time tradeoff, rating scale), should be presented as part of the CEA report.

The author should discuss the adequacy of the measure for capturing health-related quality-of-life effects relevant to the intervention under study. For example, angina has symptoms that affect different domains, including pain, emotional functioning, and role functioning. How well does the measurement instrument encompass the range of health states experienced by persons with angina? It is useful to enumerate the different health states used in the study, presenting the preference weight associated with each. A tabular format is recommended.

In some instances, analysts will collect preference weights directly as part of a CEA. The analyst may wish to justify the choice of method and describe the process used to obtain the preference weights, explaining, for example, the sampling strategy and the rationale for selecting the valuation technique or the measurement instrument. In addition, the author can provide more details on preference assessment steps, including the mean and range of the preference weights and how they may vary by subpopulations (e.g., by preference structure or by sociodemographic characteristics). Because they are patient rather than community preferences, these preferences generally will not be suited for Reference Case analyses.

Costs

The journal report should include an explicit statement of the year in which costs are presented in the study and, if not obvious, the type of currency (e.g., 1995 U.S. dollars). The year is often omitted in cost-effectiveness articles, and as a result, it is difficult to interpret the cost-effectiveness ratio or compare it with the results of other studies. The author should also specify adjustments for inflation, such as use of the Medical Component of the Consumer Price Index. (See Chapter 6.)

As described in Chapter 6, we recommend that costs in the numerator of the Reference Case analysis include direct medical costs, direct nonmedical costs, and time costs associated with the intervention; the monetized values of lost work time associated with illness, disability, and mortality are not included in the numerator, as they are already reflected in the denominator. All of the costs included reflect resource use not only for the intervention itself (e.g., mammography) but also for the cascade of events that follows (e.g., breast biopsies, treatments for detected disease). Reasonably detailed information on these costs should be provided in the journal report, preferably in tables. For example, rather than providing a single estimate of the medical costs saved by preventing a neural tube defect, the author should identify major components of this cost, such as neonatal hospitalization, subsequent medical treatment, rehabilitative costs, and special education.

If the analyst has separately measured and valued resources, it is desirable to present both the cost per unit of each resource and the number of units consumed. The source of data for each estimate should be described, including the type of study, survey, or database from which it is derived and the characteristics of the source population, such as insurance status (e.g., if data are from a claims database) and geographic location. It is important to indicate whether data represent costs or charges, to describe adjustments that have been made (e.g., use of ratios of cost to charge at a particular institution), and to detail any other methods or models used to estimate unit costs. As with effectiveness, it is appropriate and necessary for the author to comment on the quality of the data.

Use of expert judgment

If experts are used to provide inputs to the analysis (estimate probabilities, costs, preference weights, etc.), we suggest that the author describe the basis for selecting the experts (the source of their expertise), the number of experts contributing, and the process used to elicit their input. For example, was a delphi or similar technique used to obtain estimates? Were averages, modified averages, or median estimates used? The author may also wish to discuss the reason for using expert judgment. Were the experts used to reconcile conflicting data, or were they used to estimate parameters in an area where no research has been done?

Discounting

As discussed in Chapter 7, we recommend the discount rate of 3% for both costs and health effects in the Reference Case analysis. Because many analyses in the literature either do not discount or discount costs and not health effects, we recommend an explicit statement in the journal report that both costs and health effects were discounted, as well as a statement of the rate.

Results

Model validation

If a model is used, the author should briefly describe tests performed to demonstrate the accuracy of programming and to establish the face validity of the model calculations. Appropriate tests will vary depending upon the model. Generally, they will include presentation of intermediate modeling results. For example, in an analysis using QALYs as a final outcome measure, the author might describe the model's predictions of the number of myocardial infarctions occurring with and without an intervention in an analysis. Tests of the model's performance using extreme assumptions will also demonstrate to the reader that the model obtains predictable results. When a previously validated model is used in an analysis, the author may choose to cite previous papers that provide evidence of validity.

Reference case cost-effectiveness results

The Reference Case results reported in the CEA should generally include tables of the costs and effects for each program or intervention, such as shown in Table 9.1. The suggested accounting of costs and consequences lists totals as well as incremental calculations. Users of the analysis may be interested in the totals—usually per capita costs and effects—per se. Of equal importance, totals allow the reader to follow and reproduce the computations in the analysis. We suggest that the tables include both dis-

Table 9.1 Reference Case Results

Intervention	Total Cost[a]	Total Effectiveness (QALYs)[a]	Incr. Cost	Incr. Effectiveness (QALYs)	C/E (Incr. Cost/Incr. QALY)
Discounted Results **(3%)**					
No screening	$ 4,600	16.4	—	—	—
Program A: Screen every 2 years	$10,000	17.9	$5,400	1.5	$ 3,600
Program B: Screen every year	$18,300	18.3	$8,300	0.4	$20,750
Undiscounted Results					
No screening	$ 5,000	23.0	—	—	—
Program A: Screen every 2 years	$11,000	25.9	$6,000	2.9	$ 2,069
Program B: Screen every year	$20,000	26.4	$9,000	0.5	$18,000

a. Costs and effects are per person in the target population.

counted and undiscounted total costs and total effectiveness. These main results should be presented using the Reference Case discount rate.

In most CEAs, we suggest that two measures of outcome—years of life saved and QALYs—be reported. QALYs reflect a more comprehensive range of health outcomes and allow for a broader range of comparisons across health care interventions; for this reason, it is the Reference Case outcome measure. Years-of-life-saved, however, is currently a more standard and reliably measured outcome. Consumers of CEA differ in their views about the relative merits of these two types of information and may prefer one of these, either in general or in a specific CEA. The reporting of both types of outcome measure provides readers with an indication of the relative importance of the life-lengthening versus the quality-enhancing benefits of the intervention. (Of course, if the main effect of an intervention is to improve quality of life, then reporting of life years alone is not useful.) In addition, this information may be particularly relevant to researchers or others interested in applying alternative preference weights to the analysis in question.

Cost-effectiveness ratios should be reported as a dollar (or other currency) cost per unit of effectiveness, stating the year of the cost—for example, $23,000 per QALY saved (1994 dollars). In tables like Table 9.1, costs and C/E ratios can be rounded to whole dollars, and measures of effect should also be rounded reasonably. Researchers frequently present results in CEA tables using more significant figures than warranted by the precision of the data in order to allow readers to understand and verify the calculations. However, when reporting C/E ratios in the text, an appropriate number of significant figures should be used to avoid giving a misleading sense of the exactness of a C/E ratio. In most CEAs, no more than two significant figures will be justified. The discounted incremental cost-effectiveness ratio for "screening every 2 years" compared to "no screening" in Table 9.1 would thus be described as "$2,100 per QALY (1994 dollars)" in the CEA report, in cost-effectiveness tables, and in works referencing the study results.

The main cost-effectiveness results to be presented are the discounted incremental cost-effectiveness ratios for the interventions evaluated. These ratios should be presented in the text of the report. Information on incremental costs and incremental effectiveness as well as the ratios are generally presented in an accompanying table (e.g., Table 9.1).

As described in Chapter 3, the cost-effectiveness ratios should compare each intervention to the next most effective option, after eliminating options that are *dominated* (i.e., have higher cost and lower effectiveness than some other option) to obtain incremental C/E ratios. Instead of attempting to calculate ratios for dominated options, it should be recorded in the table that the option is dominated. Similarly, options ruled out by extended dominance—that is, those with higher incremental C/E ratios than a more effective option—should be identified as such without reporting any incremental C/E ratio. An example of these calculations is given in Table 9.2. Using the algebraic method to identify dominated points is well documented (Cantor, 1994; Torrance et al., 1972; Weinstein, 1990) and is incorporated into cost-effectiveness software. The formats in SMLTREE and Decision Maker, for example, follow the recommended convention for reporting C/E results with dominance or extended dominance.

We caution against reporting average cost-effectiveness ratios—ratios calculated with respect to a hypothetical zero-cost, zero-life-expectancy scenario—in the journal report. For the hypothetical interventions in Table 9.1, for example, it is potentially confusing to readers to report the average cost per QALY saved by "no screening" as $4,600/16.4 QALYs = $280; instead, the top row of the C/E column should be left blank. All other interventions should be compared to the next most effective undominated option. In analyses that examine more than one intervention or program variation, therefore, only one will be compared directly with the least effective option—generally, the "status quo" comparator option. In Table 9.1, if there were a reason to compare program B to the "no screening" option (e.g., if program A were not an option in a particular decision-making context), then the author might elect to include this incremental comparison separately in the text or in a separate table, or readers could make this comparison themselves. As long as program A is an option, however, the ratio of ($18,300 − $4,600)/(18.3 − 16.4) = $7,210 overstates the true (incremental) cost-effectiveness of program B, and it would be misleading to present this calculation.

Conveying uncertainty

As described in Chapter 8, two sources of uncertainty in an analysis warrant consideration: parameter uncertainty, which arises from uncertainty about the true numerical

Table 9.2 Dominated Alternatives—Discounted Results (3%)

Imagine that the Reference Case shown in Table 9.1 contains two additional alternatives, program C and program D. Program C has a total cost of $8,600 and produces total QALYs of 17.1 years. Program D has a total cost of $12,600 and total QALYs of 17.7 years. In this case, program D is dominated by program A, which is both less costly and more effective. Therefore, program D should be ruled out of contention and not be included in the incremental cost-effectiveness calculations.

Program C is also ruled out, but by extended dominance rather than simple dominance. Under extended dominance, a program is not surpassed by any one alternative but by a mixed strategy of two other programs. For example, program C is dominated by a strategy of providing A to half of the target population and providing no screening to the rest. This particular mixed strategy would have a total cost of 0.5($4,600 + $10,000) = $7,300 and total QALYs of 0.5(16.4 + 17.9) = 17.15. It would be both less costly and more effective than program C, thus dominating it. This is not the only combination of programs that would dominate program C—and indeed it probably would not be an acceptable option. As an algebraic test, however, this example is sufficient to rule out program C as a cost-effective option.

Intervention	Total Cost	Total Effectiveness (QALYs)	Incr. Cost	Incr. Effectiveness (QALYs)	C/E (Incr. Cost/Incr. QALY)
No screening	$ 4,600	16.4	—	—	—
Program C	$ 8,600	17.1			dominated (extended dominance)
Program A	$10,000	17.9	$5,400	1.5	$3,600
Program D	$12,600	17.7			DOMINATED
Program B	$18,300	18.3	$8,300	0.4	$21,000

values of the parameters used as inputs, and model structure uncertainty, which concerns the manner in which elements in the analysis are combined.

The journal report should describe the tests done to assess the effects of uncertainty in the analysis and present the important results. At a minimum, as described in Chapter 8, these results will include one-way sensitivity analyses, and they will include multiway sensitivity analyses on important variables. They may also include a confidence interval or credible interval for the C/E ratio if the analyst has used statistical approaches such as the delta method or a simulation model that provides probability distributions on the results.

In considering sources of uncertainty, the analyst should not overlook methodological choices that, in the analyst's view, may have important ethical implications. For example, the Reference Case analysis specifies that a gender-specific wage would be used as a proxy for women's opportunity costs in analysis of an intervention affecting only women. Because of the disparity between men's and women's wages, the analyst may be concerned about the effect of this assumption, and would conduct a sensitivity analysis using the average wage or another estimate of women's opportunity cost. This analysis would demonstrate the influence of the difference in wages, holding constant all other aspects of the study.

Given the variety of cost-effectiveness analyses, it would be impossible to develop a comprehensive list of the variables or factors to evaluate in sensitivity analyses supporting a Reference Case analysis. However, some commonly encountered sources of uncertainty have been noted throughout this book.

Graphical representation of Reference Case results

If space permits, we suggest that incremental cost-effectiveness results be presented graphically as a plot of net cost and net effectiveness. Each intervention is represented by a point on this plot. If cost is displayed on the vertical axis and QALYs on the horizontal axis, then the inverse of the slope of the line segment connecting two consecutive interventions represents the incremental C/E ratio. The graphical method is to select the alternative with the lowest cost to be plotted at the origin and then plot all other alternatives relative to this one.

Dominated alternatives of both types are easily identified when the results are plotted on a cost-effectiveness graph (Figure 9.1). Dominated options fall inside the concave envelope of the plotted points. One can imagine draping a cloth over the points such that it rests on the upper points, as shown by the line segments in Figure 9.1. All points below the line are dominated, either by simple or extended dominance. The incremental cost-effectiveness ranking should use only the nondominated points.

The example in Figure 9.1 includes different intensities of the same program. De-

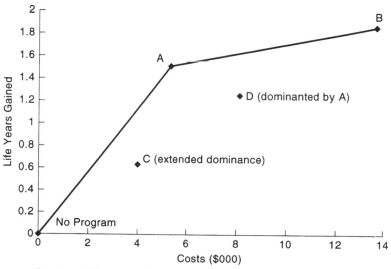

Costs and life years gained calculated relative to no program

Figure 9.1. Cost-effectiveness graph for Reference case results.

veloping a valid cost-effectiveness ranking becomes more complicated when more than one program, each having different levels of intensity, is considered. A simple numerical example of this case is provided in Drummond et al. (1993).

Aggregate cost and effectiveness in a defined population

Aggregate cost may constrain adoption of a program independent of the program's cost-effectiveness. Similarly, the total magnitude of benefit (whether to society or to an individual) can be a consideration additional to an intervention's cost-effectiveness. Estimates of aggregate incremental cost and effects at the national level or in various subpopulations thus may be useful to consumers of CEA.

Relevant aggregate costs are often different from the "total costs" presented for the Reference Case. The total cost category reflects a total calculated in the analysis; it depends on the analytic strategy. Usually, the total cost category represents the sum of costs for a single person. The aggregate cost, in contrast, is the present value of the expected program costs for an intervention if it were to be implemented for the population for whom it is contemplated. It is obtained by applying per capita costs to a target population.

If a cholesterol screening program is contemplated nationally, national aggregate cost information is likely to be relevant. Similarly, aggregate cost information can be calculated for smaller populations, such as a state, city, or institution. Annual program costs, annual drug expenditures, or total medical expenditures averted by the program are other examples of aggregate information. For effectiveness, total numbers of life years or QALYs saved in the relevant population may be of interest.

Disaggregated results

While the results of the cost-effectiveness analysis are summarized in cost-effectiveness ratios, the disaggregated cost-effectiveness results provide a great deal of information about what has occurred in the analysis. The journal report will not have adequate space for detailed presentation of these results, and most disaggregated information will be better placed in the technical report. However, the analyst may want to include selected results in the journal report.

For example, while total cost and effectiveness per person are part of the Reference Case CEA results (Table 9.1), the author may wish to provide a further breakdown of costs and effects per member of the target population, such as a differentiation of medical versus nonmedical costs or inpatient versus outpatient costs. Disaggregated information on health-related quality of life, such as preference weights for various states or subpopulations in the model or total QALYs associated with each state by year, may be of interest. Or, the author might present disaggregated information on costs, such as program expenditures per year or total hospital costs per year.

Secondary analyses

Depending on the analysis and its purpose, additional cost-effectiveness information will be relevant to include in the journal report. Some secondary analyses will differ from the Reference Case only in varying one particularly important parameter, while others will require changes in many aspects of the Reference Case analysis.

By definition, the results of secondary analyses will not be comparable to Reference Case analyses. In any context where users wish to compare the results of studies done according to the standard, Reference Case guidelines, it would be misleading to include the results of secondary analyses. Of course, this caution does not apply to a specific journal report, where secondary analyses will be compared to the Reference Case results to illustrate specific points relevant to the analysis.

The secondary analyses included in a journal report might include the following:

Perspectives other than societal. CEA studies are often motivated by policy choices relevant to specific institutions or individuals and in fact may be conducted by them. In these cases, the perspective of primary interest may be that of a managed care organization, hospital, employer, state health department, federal insurance program (Medicare or Medicaid), or other party—rather than the societal perspective.

One option for the analyst is, of course, to undertake a non–Reference Case analysis using the perspective of interest. However, it is our recommendation that the analyst conduct the study of interest as a secondary analysis, accompanying a Reference Case CEA. There are several reasons for recommending that results be presented from the societal viewpoint even in cases when the primary audience for the study is interested in a different perspective. Most importantly, use of the Reference Case in these analyses will contribute to standardization within the CEA literature. Readers will be able to identify readily Reference Case results, which are comparable to results from other Reference Case analyses, and secondary analyses, which are not. This convention should alleviate the current temptation to draw from an analysis that is not appropriate to use in making comparisons when no other results are available. At the same time, the Reference Case analysis will add to the pool of analyses supporting broad comparisons from the societal viewpoint.

The juxtaposition of a secondary analysis using a different perspective with the Reference Case analysis adds to the value of a particular study by highlighting the factors determining the differential cost-effectiveness. For example, if subscribers to an employer-based insurance plan leave the plan once they become eligible for Medicare, a breast cancer screening intervention would likely be less cost-effective from the point of view of the insurance plan than from the societal perspective. The importance of these incentives for the company's decisions would be quantified by comparing the cost-effectiveness from the two different perspectives.

It may not be advantageous to some stakeholders to have an analysis done from a societal perspective. For example, if a drug or device is cost-effective from a hospital's perspective as a result of costs transferred to other parts of the medical system, its manufacturer might want to use a cost-effectiveness analysis from the hospital perspective for marketing purposes but avoid an analysis from the societal perspective. Private groups can and will conduct cost-effectiveness analyses reflecting their own interests, and may well publish them in journals targeting their specific audience. However, because this information can be misleading, it is our belief that publication of an analysis done *only* from a viewpoint other than societal should be well justified, and the journal report should include the observation that the results are not comparable with those of Reference Case (societal perspective) CEAs.

Intermediate outcome measures. In many cases, the analyst will determine that it is important to present results using an intermediate outcome measure. These measures reflect relatively near-term effects of the intervention such as cases of rubella prevented, premature births averted, or smoker quit rates. Intermediate outcome measures allow decision makers to make direct comparisons among programs having the same objective. For example, a program planner could decide among HIV prevention strategies on the basis of their costs per transmission prevented.

The advantages of an intermediate outcome measure are that it provides information focusing on a decision criterion and that it avoids the need to analyze or project the pathway between the intermediate and final outcomes. Using the measure of HIV cases prevented, for example, avoids the need to incorporate into the CEA a model of the progression from HIV infection to development of AIDS and death. Using an intermediate outcome can therefore provide a result containing much less uncertainty than a Reference Case CEA, in which the cascade of effects is incorporated into the estimation of QALYs gained. (See Chapter 5 for discussion of the steps involved in extrapolating from intermediate to final outcomes.)

The primary disadvantages of intermediate outcome measures are that they may not capture all important aspects of the outcome of interventions and that they limit the types of interventions that can be compared across CEAs. A C/E ratio giving the "cost per case prevented" of measles or stroke will not reflect factors such as the length of cases of the illness prevented, the age of those affected by the intervention, or quality-of-life effects or medical expenditures associated with cases of differing severity. A C/E ratio of cost per premature birth avoided will not capture the course of events following birth or the associated costs; it will not convey the full impact of the intervention to a user of the analysis. A C/E ratio of cost per millimeter of blood pressure reduction will not incorporate differences in side effects of different antihypertensive treatment regimens and their associated effects on health-related quality of life.

The use of intermediate outcome measures is not a limitation if the purpose of the analysis is only to guide resource allocations among interventions having the same proximal outcome, and provided that the cascade of events following the intermediate outcome is the same across interventions. However, a screening program that detects cancers at an early stage may well save more quality-adjusted years of life than a screening program that detects the same number of cancers at a later stage. As a result, analyses using an intermediate outcome measure such as "cost per case of cancer detected" can provide practical information but not full information on the cost-effectiveness of an intervention.

Analyses using intermediate outcomes are not comparable to Reference Case analyses, a caveat that should be clearly stated when results of the analysis are presented. Caution must be exercised in comparing C/E ratios based on intermediate outcome measures to assure that these results are compared only with the results of studies using very similar outcome measures.

Additional final outcome measures. Final outcome measures in addition to those used in the Reference Case may be useful in some analyses. Cost per life saved, for example, provides a perspective different from cost per year of life saved. QALYs can also be calculated using alternative preference weighting systems as a type of sensitivity analysis.

Subgroup analyses. Subject to the availability of data, analyses may be performed with respect to important population subgroups, defined by demographic (e.g., age, gender, race, geographic location) and clinical (e.g., risk factors, stage of illness, clinical history) variables.

Productivity costs. As discussed in Chapters 2 and 6, productivity costs, the monetized value of work time lost due to morbidity or mortality, are not included in the numerator in the Reference Case analysis, because these effects are included in the denominator of the C/E ratio. There are reasons, however, to prefer monetary valuation of some or all of these effects. The analyst might therefore elect to do a secondary analysis that includes them in the numerator and excludes them in the measure of effectiveness in the denominator. Alternatively, the analyst might report productivity costs separately (apart from the calculations of cost-effectiveness) or conduct a cost-benefit analysis to capture these costs in monetary terms.

Secondary analyses can accommodate the monetization of the productivity effects of morbidity when the analyst is not satisfied that the QALYs in the denominator of the CEA are the best mechanism for capturing these effects. For example, a disability may decrease the number of hours worked annually, and the decrement in productivity may be more credibly captured by a monetary valuation than by eliciting a preference weight for the disabled state that includes the loss of financial compensation for lost work hours. In this case, a secondary analysis might use a measure of life years saved in the denominator and include the monetized value of productivity costs in the numerator.

Secondary analyses incorporating productivity costs can also be indicated when these costs are important from a perspective other than the societal perspective. For example, prevention of alcohol abuse or treatment of lower back pain can expand the work options open to an individual and reduce time missed from work. From the perspective of an employer, the value of what a worker produces is a specific gain against which the value of benefits offered to the worker may be assessed. This contrasts with the societal perspective, where the value of a worker's time is only partially reflected in the ability to produce goods.

Discount rates. In addition to presenting the Reference Case results using a 3% discount rate and no discounting, we recommend that authors also report detailed results using a 5% discount rate. (See Chapter 7.) This practice will help to assure comparability with a large body of existing analyses using this rate. Results of sensitivity analyses using other discount rates, such as rates higher than 5%, should be reported if the author has reason to believe that the higher rates are relevant and if the qualitative conclusions differ markedly from the Reference Case; otherwise, a statement that results were not sensitive to the discount rate is sufficient.

Discussion and Interpretation of Results

The discussion section provides the author an opportunity to communicate the study findings clearly to the reader. In this section, quantitative results are translated into a qualitative description of cost-effectiveness. Below, we discuss a range of subjects germane to the interpretation and summarization of a study, including limitations of the study, policy implications, and comparison of the CEA with other relevant studies. The discussion section should highlight the assumptions underlying the results and the robustness of results. As a general rule, authors should take care to identify and consider alternative points of view in interpreting the findings of their and others' studies.

Description of results
An important part of the discussion section is a description and interpretation of the meaning of the cost-effectiveness result. The results of the Reference Case analysis should be summarized, describing the overall effect of important assumptions and the sensitivity of results to key assumptions and estimates. If estimates known or suspected to contain bias have been used in the analysis, the author should explicitly discuss the effects of these data and the results of the reported sensitivity analyses on the parameters involved. For example, the analyst may have used a price as a proxy for the resource cost of a drug or device, even though the market for that item is not competitive. Or, the analyst may have assumed optimal treatment in response to a positive diagnostic test. The reader will want to know the effect of these assumptions, whether or not the results of the analysis are sensitive to them.

In addition, the analyst may wish to highlight the results of sensitivity analyses on assumptions having ethical implications that the analyst or readers might find objectionable. For example, as described earlier, the analyst may have conducted a sensitivity analysis to determine whether the use of population-specific life tables has an effect on estimates of the life-saving potential and cost-effectiveness of an intervention. This information may critically affect the way readers interpret the results.

Limitations
Discussion of the limitations of a cost-effectiveness study is intended to guide the reader in interpreting and generalizing from its results. For example, if the data underlying an

analysis are obtained from particular population subgroups, the analyst may recommend caution in applying the results to other groups, even if no significant differences are expected. The author may direct the reader's attention to assumptions based on expert opinion, theoretical models, or incomplete data as limitations affecting the analysis. Another frequently encountered limitation is that the analysis may not have been able to address all options relevant for a policy decision. While it is important that relevant comparators be included in the CEA, few studies will be able to examine the relative cost-effectiveness of all options for addressing a health problem. Omission of competing choices from the CEA should be discussed, and the possible effect of this omission on the C/E results should be explored. The discussion of limitations should highlight the analyst's efforts to compensate for the study's shortcomings.

Relevance of results

The discussion section allows the researcher to place the cost-effectiveness results in the decision context(s) identified when the analysis was initially framed. If the study addresses a particular decision, the analyst can describe the relevance of the results for that decision and for debates surrounding it. For example, if there is controversy over a decision to extend a breast cancer screening program to additional age groups, the report would highlight the C/E results bearing on this controversy.

Because a given cost-effectiveness study can ordinarily examine only a subset of interventions and comparators, it is useful to remind the reader of the more global set of options in order to place the C/E results in a broader context. For example, a CEA addressing alternative drug treatment programs might consider a variety of methadone maintenance and drug-free treatment programs. In the discussion section, the author would describe other methods of addressing drug abuse, such as school-based drug education and other prevention programs.

Reporting the results of other CEAs

The discussion section should include a brief review of cost-effectiveness results from CEAs of similar or related interventions. For example, the discussion of an analysis of breast cancer screening would describe the results of other studies on breast cancer screening, even if the frequency of the intervention, its setting, or other aspects of the intervention or target population were different. It is helpful in interpreting the various studies if the author explains important differences in the analyses and in the cost-effectiveness findings.

Cost-effectiveness results from other analyses should be converted to the currency year used in the author's study using the Consumer Price Index or appropriate component of it so that the results can be compared. If the year is not given in the cited analysis, we recommend that the author assume the year to be 3 years prior to the date of publication, reflecting a typical lag between the collection of data for a study, conduct of the CEA, review of the manuscript, and publication. While the year of the cited study will be available in the reference section of the report, the author may wish to call attention to changes in the intervention or the health condition it addresses, differences in the analysis itself, or other factors that bear on the interpretation of the cited cost-effectiveness ratio.

As described in Chapter 3, cost-effectiveness tables are sometimes used to summarize and rank cost-effectiveness ratios across interventions. If the analysis addresses resource allocations within a particular disease (e.g., heart disease prevention and treatment) or intervention type (e.g., screening for colon cancer, breast cancer, or cervical cancer), then the comparisons may be limited to those areas. These tables may be the focal point of review articles, or they may be included in journal reports as a means of placing the C/E ratio in the context of other competing uses of resources. If a cost-effectiveness table is used in a journal report, the Reference Case results should be presented, assuring consistency in the analytic perspective (societal), discount rate, and other aspects of the analysis. Results should be converted to the same year using an adjustor appropriate to the study.

Distributive implications

Cost-effectiveness analysis reports the cost per unit of effectiveness without regard to the incidence of the resource costs or the distribution of the benefits. As discussed in Chapter 1, distributive concerns may compete with or outweigh cost-effectiveness considerations in the context of particular decisions. In the discussion section, the researcher has the opportunity—and, many would argue, the responsibility—to describe the distributive implications of the interventions examined. The report may note, for example, the characteristics of the population experiencing the health benefits and risks associated with the intervention—young or old, wealthy or poor. It may also include a discussion of whether the health outcomes reported in the CEA reflect small improvements for a large number of people or a large impact for a few. It may note whether the beneficiaries are persons who are initially in good or poor health.

Some analyses will have unique distributive implications. For example, patterns of morbidity and mortality may influence the cost-effectiveness of an intervention, independently of the intervention itself. An HIV prevention program that averts an equal number of HIV transmissions among a group of intravenous drug users and a general, non-drug-using population might save fewer years of life in the former group because of the lower life expectancy of drug users. This issue arises more generally when interventions affecting the elderly are compared with those affecting younger populations or when interventions differentially affect gender or racial groups having different life expectancy.

As discussed in Chapter 6, income transfers related to an intervention entail an explicit redistribution of resources. For example, a statewide program to prevent teen pregnancy might have the effect of reducing expenditures for Medicaid and Aid to Families with Dependent Children (AFDC). This effect would not be captured by the cost-effectiveness analysis. However, the redistribution of resources from this program to another one with different beneficiaries—or to taxpayers—might well be of interest to the audience of the study.

Conclusions about cost-effectiveness

The cost-effectiveness of an intervention can only be established relative to other interventions or by an identified cost-effectiveness criterion. Unlike cost-benefit analysis, which determines whether the benefits of an activity outweigh its costs, cost-effectiveness analysis provides only a standardized "price" for an intervention. The choice of whether to implement the intervention depends on the resources available, alternative uses of resources, and other constraints considered by the decision maker.

Because cost-effectiveness is relative, it is difficult to make absolute statements regarding cost-effectiveness. (The exception is for interventions that result in a net economic savings as well as a savings in QALYs, but these are better described as "cost-saving" than as "cost-effective"; see Doubilet et al., 1986.) In some instances, the claim that an intervention is "cost-effective" implies that the author is making a comparison within a certain set of alternatives. Thus, if a type of surgery is described as "clearly cost-ineffective," the author may be suggesting that this intervention costs far more per QALY saved than other forms of medical treatment. Alternatively, the author may be implying that the intervention does not fall within society's assumed "willingness to pay" for the outcomes obtained.

However, these conclusions are vague and easily subject to misinterpretation. Interventions are better described as being more or less cost-effective than others. Specific examples of interventions society chooses to implement or not to implement are often useful benchmarks. For example, cost-effectiveness ratios for dialysis for end-stage renal disease and treatment for hypertension have been used often as benchmarks for cost-effectiveness (e.g. Mark et al., 1995.) The simple conclusion that an intervention is "cost-effective" or "not cost-effective" should be used with caution.

Some authors have argued for specific classifications for cost-effectiveness. Laupacis and colleagues, for example, have proposed that interventions be graded into categories costing less than $20,000 per QALY, $20,000–$100,000 per QALY, and more than $100,000 per QALY (Laupacis et al., 1992). However, classifications such as these—to the extent that they imply a judgment about cost-effectiveness—are highly dependent on the societal and the decision context. We cannot recommend a cost-effectiveness criterion for generalized use.[1]

Abstract for the journal report

Many journals publish an abstract with CEA reports. We offer a sample format, similar to that used in public health and medical journals, in Table 9.3.

Table 9.3 Format for Journal Abstract

Abstract
Problem. Purpose of the study. Description of the intervention, comparators, and target populations *Methods.* Description of the analytic approach, including type of model and software. Sources of data on effectiveness, costs, and outcome values, and units for expressing costs (currency and year) and outcomes (e.g., life years or QALYs) *Results.* Main cost-effectiveness results *Conclusion.* Brief summary of study findings and conclusions

The Technical Report

The technical report provides additional information on the CEA for reviewers, users of the CEA, and other researchers. It may include extensive detail on methods and data, model validation, sensitivity analysis, and disaggregated results, although the content and emphasis will depend on the characteristics of the study. In general, standardization of the technical report is not critical; its objective is comprehensiveness, with the obvious caveat that to be useful, it must be reasonably organized and readily understandable.

Much of the analysis that will be described in the technical report is currently customary practice for analysts undertaking good-quality CEAs. While this information is sometimes presented in detailed reports or book chapters, as a general rule, there is no repository for the additional information the analyst gathers in the course of the analysis. The goal of the technical report is to preserve this information and improve access to it.

Methods and Data

The technical report provides an opportunity to lay out fully the analytic methods. The analyst can diagram and explain all models and submodels used and describe and interpret transitions among model states. Tables are useful for presenting the parameters in the model along with their values in each analysis and sensitivity analysis. Tables and/or equations may also be needed to elaborate on transition probabilities that change with age or time. For example, in a CEA of breast cancer screening, the analysis would likely include age-dependent probabilities of developing breast cancer and time-dependent probabilities of stages of cancer. The technical report might include tables giving the probability of cancer by age and the probability of each stage of cancer by time since onset of cancer. The data used as a basis for these inputs should be described, and any survival analysis, regression, or other modeling to obtain the input probabilities should be clearly laid out.

Similarly, a detailed description of data on cost and outcomes should be provided. If costs were obtained from a hospital accounting system, for example, the author might describe the cost elements included and excluded and the assumptions used in much greater detail than is feasible in the journal report. Methods for allocating overhead costs, for adjusting professional charges for actual collection fractions, and other features of the cost accounting system could be described. Details of surveys used to obtain time costs, such as patient diaries, could be reviewed, including a presentation of the instruments used to collect information from patients.

It is often difficult to treat the valuation of outcomes adequately within the journal report, and more extensive information can be provided in the technical report. When the study has assessed health states directly or used experts to describe the health states within the context of a measurement system that has community weights associated with it, details of the process and results can be provided. The report should describe the relevance of the selected measurement instrument to the problem being studied. In addition, the report might describe the methods for surveying experts regarding the most applicable measure and how the study population was assigned by experts to component health states associated with the measurement system.

When the author has collected preference weights (e.g., within the context of a clinical study), the technical report should include a full account of the methods used. The author should describe the study population and discuss relevant characteristics (e.g., socioeconomic status, race, age) that might bear on differences in the distributions of the preferences. For example, a study might observe that older peoples' preferences for health states vary systematically from those of younger people with identical health states. If preference weights were obtained during the course of a clinical study, the author might discuss the timing of their collection in relation to the study design.

The questionnaire or other instrument used to assess preferences can be provided in the technical report. For example, if the time-tradeoff method was used, the report would indicate what length of life was used in the question, whether a single open-ended question was asked or a sequence of binary choices, whether the "Ping-Pong" method was used to bound the final answer or whether a monotonic progression was used from below or above, and how health states worse than death were dealt with. The report would describe the medium used to administer the survey—for example, telephone, mailed questionnaire, face-to-face interview, group panels with feedback, interactive computer software. It should also describe the information given to subjects about the health state being valued.

For preference weights obtained from the literature, the technical report could contain a description of the methods used in the source study. While the author could refer to published material containing much of the above information, a summary of important features of the source studies would provide useful documentation of the inputs to the CEA.

Model Validation

Extensive tests of a model's validity should be performed before it is used for cost-effectiveness analysis. (See Chapter 5.) Summary evidence of the model's validity is part of the results section in the journal report, as discussed earlier. However, it usually will not be feasible to include the details of these tests and their results; these belong in the technical report.

The type of validation appropriate for the model in question depends upon the analysis, as discussed in Chapter 5. The technical report should generally include the results of a variety of tests demonstrating that the model can predict existing data or can predict future data consistent with expectations. For example, for a model of a cholesterol-reducing intervention, the analyst may have assessed the extent to which, under the assumption that no intervention is in place, the model can predict a verifiable incidence of myocardial infarctions and cardiac deaths. While the basic results of this test will have been noted in the journal report, the technical report can present the annual incidence of events predicted by the model juxtaposed with the actual incidence figures used for comparison. In a model of the HIV epidemic, infection would be transmitted from an initially infected population to its contacts. Validation checks could include comparisons of the predicted effects on HIV incidence, HIV prevalence, new AIDS cases, and deaths occurring in the modeled population with existing data. The tests, the analyst's expectations, and the model's results can all be presented in the technical report.

As described in Chapter 5, additional validation tests may assess the model's response to predictable manipulations. For example, if the calculations of numbers of cases depend on test characteristics, disease transmission rates, or disease progression rates, the analyst should obtain predictable results and output patterns by setting these rates to 0 or 1. Again, these tests and their results can be described in the technical analysis.

An electronic copy of the model should be made available to peer reviewers along with the technical report. This step will allow reviewers to test the model and gain an understanding of the model's dynamics. Providing access to a computer model may raise proprietary concerns on the part of the researchers who have developed a model with the intention of using it for continuing research. We encourage researchers to allow use of their models for peer review under the assumption that the same code of conduct applies to use of a model as to data collected as part of a clinical trial or other study.

Sensitivity Analyses

As discussed earlier, the types of sensitivity analyses performed and reported will vary depending on the analysis, but the analyst should explore every important variable and its interactions with others, to the point that the analyst is confident of the model's response to all reasonable tests. Because of space limitations, only a few of the sensitivity analyses performed can be presented in the journal article; the technical report will provide a vehicle for presenting additional sensitivity analyses. For example, while the journal report may report that a result is not sensitive over a reasonable range of an important variable, the technical report might describe a larger range, as well as threshold values for the variable. Sensitivity analyses should be reported with respect to the sampling variation in measured variables such as utilization rates or efficacy rates. Multiway sensitivity analyses should be included. If the analysis has made use of Monte Carlo simulation, the technical report should include tests of the assumptions made concerning the distributions of variables and their statistical independence or interdependence.

Disaggregated Results

As described earlier, the analyst may find it informative to present selected disaggregated results in the journal report. However, this information by its nature will require significant amounts of space, and most disaggregated results will be more practically handled in the technical report. It may not be feasible to disaggregate results over all dimensions in the analysis, but the technical report should provide such results to elucidate important aspects of the analysis. These may include, for example, a breakdown of the number of years in each health state and QALYs accumulated per year (or other time period). It may be useful to disaggregate costs, presenting discounted and undiscounted costs incurred per year (or other time period) in each alternative scenario; disaggregated costs by major service categories, especially those accounting for more than 10% of incremental costs (e.g., hospital, physician services, drugs, procedures); and disaggregation between screening costs, induced costs, and follow-up costs. Finally, these results may expand the population subgroups considered. Total cost and total outcome might be reported, for example, for different risk groups, ages, or preference subgroups contained within the population examined.

Disclosure

The complexity of cost-effectiveness analyses and the discretion involved in determining their structure and content has given rise to concern about the potential for bias in these studies (Kassirer and Angell, 1994). This book addresses the problem of discretion and bias by seeking to improve standardization among studies. In addition, it is important that authors adhere to recommended guidelines for disclosure of relationships between researchers and financial sponsors. These guidelines include identification of the source of funding for a study and declaration of any financial connection between the researcher and a company producing or competing with a product under study (Task Force on Principles for Economic Analysis of Health Care Technology 1995, Kassirer and Angell, 1994).

Conclusion

The report of a CEA is designed to communicate all of the important features of an analysis to a consumer and to emphasize any aspects of the study that are unusual or unexpected. Journal reports provide a concise means of reaching the study's audience, while technical reports offer a repository for the additional information of concern to reviewers, researchers, and those having a particular interest a given study.

Our general recommendations concerning the reporting of cost-effectiveness analyses are summarized below. In addition, we provide a checklist (Table 9.4) for the use of authors composing cost-effectiveness reports.

Table 9.4 Reporting Checklist

1. Framework	
Background of the problem	
General framing and design of the analysis	
Target population for intervention	
Other program descriptors (e.g., care setting, model of delivery, timing of intervention)	
Description of comparator programs	
Boundaries of the analysis	
Time horizon	
Statement of the perspective of the analysis	
2. Data and methods	
Description of event pathway	
Identification of outcomes of interest in analysis	
Description of model used	
Modeling assumptions	
Diagram of event pathway/model	
Software used	
Complete information on the sources of effectiveness data, cost data, and preference weights	
Methods for obtaining estimates of effectiveness, costs, and preferences	
Critique of data quality	
Statement of year of costs	
Statement of method used to adjust costs for inflation	
Statement of type of currency	
Source and methods for obtaining expert judgment	
Statement of discount rates	

Table 9.4 Reporting Checklist (*Continued*)

3. Results	
Results of model validation	
Reference Case results (discounted and undiscounted): total costs and effectiveness, incremental costs and effectiveness, and incremental cost-effectiveness ratios	
Results of sensitivity analyses	
Other estimates of uncertainty, if available	
Graphical representation of C/E results	
Aggregate cost and effectiveness information	
Disaggregated results, as relevant	
Secondary analyses using 5% discount rate	
Other secondary analyses, as relevant	
4. Discussion	
Summary of Reference Case results	
Summary of sensitivity of results to assumptions and uncertainties in the analysis	
Discussion of analysis assumptions having important ethical implications	
Limitations of the study	
Relevance of study results for specific policy questions or decisions	
Results of related CEAs	
Distributive implications of an intervention	

Recommendations

1. We encourage analysts to document cost-effectiveness studies in two parts, a *journal report* and a more comprehensive *technical report,* making the latter available on request to readers requiring more detail concerning the analysis.

2. For the specific purpose of journal review, we recommend that editors request and authors submit a concise *technical addendum* with the journal report to assist reviewers assessing the study's methodology. This material may or may not be published along with the journal report.

3. If a cost-effectiveness analysis is intended to allow comparisons among the interventions studied and health care interventions broadly, the report should highlight the Reference Case results. Key sensitivity analyses should be conducted with respect to the Reference Case.

4. The perspective(s) of the analysis should be explicitly identified in a cost-effectiveness report.

5. The following information comprises a basic set of results in the journal report: total costs, total effectiveness, incremental costs, incremental effectiveness, and incremental cost-effectiveness ratios, both discounted (at the Reference Case rate of 3%) and undiscounted.

6. An appropriate number of significant figures should be used to report C/E results, generally two significant figures unless the precision of the data warrants a greater number.

7. In reporting incremental cost-effectiveness ratios, options ruled out because of dominance or extended dominance should be excluded. Among undominated options, incremental C/E ratios should be reported in increasing order of cost and effectiveness, starting with the lowest-cost option considered (generally the status quo or ''do nothing'' option).

8. C/E ratios should be compared to available C/E ratios for other interventions that compete for resources with the intervention under study. Such interventions may be drawn from health care broadly if the decision context is broad, or from restricted areas, such as particular disease or intervention modalities.

Notes

1. Specific thresholds may be relevant within a given CEA. For example, an analyst might summarize the results of a study of mammography by saying that the C/E ratio for mammography is less than $50,000 per QALY for women between the ages of 50 and 75 but greater than $50,000 per QALY for other age groups. This usage does not presuppose a cost-effectiveness criterion.

References

Cantor, S.B. 1994. Cost-effectiveness analysis, extended dominance, and ethics: A quantitative assessment. *Med Decis Making* 14:259–65.

Doubilet, P., M.C. Weinstein, and B.J. McNeil. 1986. Use and misuse of the term ''cost-effective'' in medicine. *N Engl J Med* 314:253–256.

Drummond, M.F., G.L. Stoddart, and G.W. Torrance. 1987. *Methods for the economic evaluation of health care programmes.* New York: Oxford University Press.

Drummond, M., G. Torrance, and J. Mason. 1993. Cost-effectiveness league tables: More harm than good? *Soc Sci Med* 37:33–40.

Kassirer, J.P., and M. Angell. 1994. The Journal's policy on cost-effectiveness analysis. *N Engl J Med* 331:669–70.

Laupacis, A., D. Feeny, A.S. Detsky, and P.X. Tugwell. 1992. How attractive does a new technology have to be to warrant adoption and utilization? Tentative guidelines for using clinical and economic evaluations. *Can Med Assoc J* 146:473–81.

Mark D.B., M. A. Hlatky, R.A. Califf, C.D. Naylor, K.L. Lee, P.W. Armstrong, G. Barbash, H. White, M.L. Simoons, C.L. Nelson, N. Clapp-Channing, D. Knight, F.E. Harrell Jr, J. Simes, and E.J. Topol. 1995. Cost-effectiveness of thrombolytic therapy with tissue plasminogen activator as compared with streptokinase for acute myocardial infarction. *N Engl J Med* 332:1418–1424.

Task Force on Principles for Economic Analysis of Health Care Technology, 1995. Economic analysis of health care technology: A report on principles. *Ann Intern Med* 122:60–69.

Torrance, G.W., W.H. Thomas, and D.L. Sackett. 1972. A utility maximization model for evaluation of health care programmes. *Health Serv Res* 7:118–33.

Udvarhelyi, S., G.A. Colditz, A. Rai, and A.M. Epstein. 1992. Cost-effectiveness and cost-benefit analyses in the medical literature: Are the methods being used correctly? *Ann Intern Med* 116:238-44.

Weinstein, M.C. 1990. Principles of cost-effective resource allocation in health care organizations. *Int J Technol Assess Health Care* 6:93–103.

Appendix A: Summary Recommendations

The following framing propositions and recommendations are compiled from the report of the Panel on Cost-Effectiveness in Health and Medicine. These recommendations, along with others that provide more detailed methodologic guidance, can be found within the body of the report. The number of the chapter from which either a recommendation or its supporting arguments arise is listed in *italics* following each statement.

Framing propositions indicate the nature and limits of CEA and serve as basic starting points in defining CEA. They are indicated by **F**. Although many of the listed recommendations will be useful in improving the conduct of all CEAs, those that are denoted by an **R** are intended for use in a Reference Case analysis, which seeks to improve comparability for analyses that will be done to inform resource allocation. Guidance recommendations, which are intended to improve the conduct of analyses, but which are not explicitly required for a Reference Case analysis, are denoted by **G**. An **s** notes instances when a sensitivity analysis would be of particular importance.

Both **R** and **G** and recommendations are followed by letters that indicate the rationales underlying the recommendations, which are discussed in detail within the chapters. Our purpose in distinguishing the types of rationales for the recommendations is to provide a basis for reevaluation and improvement as the field progresses. The six categories are:

Theoretical (T): These recommendations stem from theoretical considerations that are drawn from neoclassical welfare economics and expected utility theory.

Ethical (E): These recommendations are based on ethical considerations that the panel found might, under some circumstances, justify practices that deviate from a strict interpretation of welfare economic theory.

Accounting consistency (A): These recommendations are based on a need for logical consistency and the avoidance of double counting of health effects or resources in CEAs.

Pragmatic (P): These recommendations are based on best empirical evidence, a combination of empirical evidence and applied microeconomic theory, and/or consideration of the practical limitations of current techniques.

Conventional (C): These recommendations either conform to or establish a convention that produces standard procedures.

User considerations (U): These recommendations stem from an effort to ensure that CEA responds to the particular needs of its users, including health care decision makers.

I. The Nature and Limits of CEA and of the Reference Case

1. Cost-effectiveness analysis (CEA) is a methodology for evaluating the outcomes and costs of interventions designed to improve health. **F** *Chapter 1*
2. CEA evaluates a given health intervention through the use of a "cost-effectiveness ratio." In this ratio, all health effects of the intervention (relative to a stated alternative) are captured in the denominator, and changes in resource use (relative to the alternative) are captured in the numerator and valued in monetary terms. **F** *Chapter 1*
3. CEA is an aid to decision making, not a complete procedure for making resource allocation decisions in health and medicine, because it cannot incorporate all the values relevant to such decisions. **F** *Chapter 1*
4. CEA, cost-consequence analysis, and cost-benefit analysis are complementary, rather than mutually exclusive, forms of analysis. The use of one does not preclude the use of any of the others in a given study. **F** *Chapter 3*
5. When a CEA is intended to contribute to decisions on the broad allocation of health resources, a Reference Case analysis should be done to enhance comparability across studies. The Reference Case includes not only the associated baseline computation but also a meaningful set of sensitivity analyses. **F** *Introduction*
6. The Reference Case is based on the societal perspective. This perspective requires that an analysis consider all health effects and all changes in resource use. **R (T, E)** *Chapters 1, 2*
    - 6.1 Evaluation of effectiveness should incorporate both benefits and harms of alternative interventions. **R (T)** *Chapters 1, 5*
    - 6.2 The boundaries of a study should be defined broadly enough to encompass the range of groups of people affected by the intervention and all types of cost and health consequences. **R (T)** *Chapter 3*
    - 6.3 The time horizon adopted in a CEA should be long enough to capture all relevant future effects of a health care intervention. **R (T)** *Chapter 3*
    - 6.4 Decisions about costs and health effects to include in a CEA, such as the precision with which costs and effects are measured, the time horizon of the study, and the definition of the study boundaries, should strike a reasonable balance between expense and difficulty, and potential importance in the analysis. **R (P)** *Chapter 3*
7. The Reference Case analysis should compare the health intervention of interest to existing practice (the "status quo"). If existing practice appears not to be a cost-effective option itself, relative to other available options, the analyst should incorporate other relevant alternatives into the analysis, such as a best-available alternative, a viable low-cost alternative, or a "do-nothing" alternative. **R (C)** *Chapter 3*
    - 7.1 When varying levels of program intensity are relevant, alternative program options (e.g., as defined by variation in duration or frequency of the intervention)

should be included in the analysis and compared using the incremental cost-effectiveness algorithm. **R (C)** *Chapters 3, 9*

8. The estimates of resource consumption and effects of relevance for a CEA are those for the population or group that is actually affected by the health intervention. **R (T)** *Chapter 3*

II. Components Belonging to the Numerator and the Denominator

1. The major categories of resource use that should be reflected in the numerator of a C/E ratio include costs of health care services; costs of patient time expended for the intervention; costs associated with caregiving (paid or unpaid); other costs associated with illness such as childcare or travel expenses; and costs associated with nonhealth impacts of the intervention (e.g., on the education system or the environment). **R (T)** *Chapter 6*

2. Effects of a health intervention on length of life are incorporated in the denominator of the C/E ratio. A monetary value should not be imputed for lost life years and should not be included in the numerator of the C/E ratio. **R (A,C)** *Chapters 2, 6*

3. For a Reference Case analysis, health-related quality of life should be captured by an instrument that, at minimum, implicitly incorporates the effects of morbidity on productivity and leisure. Effects of a health intervention on subsequent morbidity, including the full value of morbidity time to patients, are incorporated in the denominator of the C/E ratio. **R (A,C)** *Chapters 2, 4, 6*

   3.1 Effects of lost productivity borne by others (e.g., employers, co-workers) including "friction costs," when significant, should be included in the numerator. **R (T,A,C)** *Chapters 2, 6*

4. Time spent seeking care or undergoing an intervention is a resource and a component of the intervention. It should be valued in monetary terms and incorporated in the numerator of a cost-effectiveness ratio. **R (T,A,C)** *Chapter 6*

   4.1 In some instances (e.g., when recuperating from surgery), time could be categorized either as morbidity time (valued in the denominator) or as input to the intervention itself (costed out in the numerator). As a general rule, in a Reference Case analysis, this time should be considered as morbidity time. **G (C)** *Chapter 6*

   4.2 In some instances, time may be a clear input to a health intervention, but the intervention will, in addition, produce a significant impact on health status. When relevant to a Reference Case analysis, the impact on health status should be captured in the denominator, leaving the time component (costed out) in the numerator. **G (C)** *Chapter 6*

III. Measuring Terms in the Numerator of the C/E Ratio

1. Changes in the use of resources caused by a health intervention should be valued at their opportunity cost. **R (T)** *Chapter 6*

   1.1 Costs should reflect the marginal or incremental resources consumed. **R (T)** *Chapter 6*

   1.2 Resource consumption should be assessed from a long-term perspective. **R (T)** *Chapter 6*

2. To the extent that prices reflect opportunity costs, they are an appropriate basis for valuing changes in resources. **R (T,P)** *Chapter 6*

   2.1 When prices do not adequately reflect opportunity costs because of market distortions, they should be adjusted appropriately. **R (T)** *Chapter 6*

   2.2 When substantial bias is present in prices, and adjustment is not feasible, more suitable proxies for opportunity costs should be considered. **G (T)** *Chapter 6*

3. In aggregating resource costs across time, CEAs should be conducted in constant dollars that remove general price inflation. If the prices of the goods in question change at a rate different from general price levels, this variation should be reflected in the adjustment used. **R (T)** *Chapter 6*

4. "Transfer payments" (e.g., cash transfers from tax payers to welfare recipients) associated with a health intervention redistribute resources from one individual to another. While administrative costs associated with suchtransfers are included in the numerator of a C/E ratio, the transfers themselves are not since, by definition, their impact on the transfer and the recipient cancel out. **R (T,A)** *Chapter 6*

5. For individuals in the labor force, wages are generally an acceptable measure of time costs. Wages corresponding to the target population should be used to approximate time costs. In general, age- and gender-specific wage estimates will provide adequately specific estimates. **R (T,P)** *Chapter 6*

   5.1 Use of group-specific wages may influence the conclusions of the analysis in ways that are ethically problematic. In these instances, sensitivity analysis should be conducted to explicitly indicate the nature of this influence. **R s (E)** *Chapter 6*

   5.2 The wage rate generally does not adequately reflect the value of time for persons engaged primarily in leisure or in activities for which they are not compensated. For individuals not engaged in compensated employment, wages, used as proxies, must be adjusted to reflect the full opportunity cost of time. **R (T)** *Chapter 6*

6. In theory, the numerator of a C/E ratio should include the net costs of health care and nonhealth consumption during years of life added by the intervention. However, because of problems in measuring these costs, and because of unresolved issues concerning the role of nonhealth costs in CEA, the Reference Case may either in-

clude or exclude health care costs associated with diseases other than those affected by the intervention, in added years of life. **R (T,P)** *Chapter 6*

  6.1 Whenever the inclusion or exclusion of health care costs of unrelated diseases makes a significant difference to the analysis, a sensitivity analysis should be performed to assess the effect on the C/E ratio. **R s (A,U)** *Chapter 6*

IV. Measuring Terms in the Denominator of a C/E Ratio

1. For a Reference Case analysis, incorporation of morbidity and mortality consequences into a single measure should be accomplished using QALYs. **R (P,C)** *Chapter 4*

  1.1 In general, since lives saved or extended by an intervention will not be in perfect health, a saved life year will count as less than 1 full QALY. **R (T)** *Chapter 4*

2. To satisfy the QALY concept, the quality weights must be preference-based, interval-scaled, and measured or transformed onto the interval scale where the reference point "death" has a score of 0.0 and the reference point "optimal health" has a score of 1.0. **R (T,A)** *Chapter 4*

3. A CEA should be based on a health-state classification scheme which reflects domains (attributes) that are important for the particular analysis. **R (A,P)** *Chapter 4*

  3.1 If the CEA is intended for Reference Case use, the preference measure used should be a generic one, or be capable of being compared to a generic system. **R (A,P)** *Chapter 4*

4. In general, community preferences for health states are the appropriate ones for use in the Reference Case analysis. **R (T,C)** *Chapter 4*

  4.1 When adequate information is unavailable regarding community preferences, patient preferences may be used as an approximation, but the manner in which they might differ from community preferences should be discussed and, where relevant, sensitivity analyses that reflect likely differences should be included. **R s (P)** *Chapter 4*

  4.2 If distinct subgroup preferences are identified that will markedly affect a C/E ratio, the study should provide this information and conduct sensitivity analyses that reflect this difference. **R s (E)** *Chapter 4*

5. The health-related quality of life of those whose lives have been saved or extended by a health intervention may be influenced by characteristics such as age, gender, or race. This may affect the Reference Case analysis in ways that are ethically problematic. In these instances, sensitivity analyses should be conducted to indicate explicitly how the results are affected by these characteristics. **R s (E)** *Chapter 4*

6. When designing primary data collection efforts, or deriving the necessary probability estimates from secondary data sources for estimation of effectiveness in a CEA, outcome probability values should be selected from the best designed (and least

biased) sources that are relevant to the question and population under study. **G (P)** *Chapter 4*

7. Evidence for estimation of effectiveness may be obtained from randomized controlled trials, observational data, uncontrolled experiments, descriptive series, and expert opinion. **G (U)** *Chapter 4*

   7.1 Good-quality meta-analysis and other synthesis methods can be used where any one study has insufficient power to detect effects, or where results conflict. **G (U)** *Chapter 4*

   7.2 Expert judgment should only be used to fill in values where no adequate data sources exist, or when the parameter is of secondary importance in the analysis. **G (U)** *Chapter 4*

8. Where direct primary or secondary empirical evaluation of effectiveness is not possible (e.g., in important subpopulations or in differing time frames), the use of modeling to estimate effectiveness is a valid mode of scientific inquiry for CEAs. **G (U)** *Chapter 4*

V. Discounting

1. Costs and health outcomes should be discounted to present value. **R (T)** *Chapter 7*
2. Costs should be discounted to present value at a rate consistent with the shadow-price-of-capital (SPC) approach to evaluating public investments. This rate (often termed the *social rate of time preference*) can be approximated by the real rate of return on long-term government bonds. **R (T)** *Chapter 7*
3. Costs and health outcomes should be discounted at the same rate. **R (T,P)** *Chapter 7*

   3.1 A real, riskless discount rate of 3% should be used. **R (T)** *Chapter 7*

   3.2 Because of the large number of CEAs that have adhered to a discount rate of 5%, analysts should perform sensitivity analyses using 5% as well as a reasonable range of rates (drawn from 0 to 7%). **R s (C)** *Chapter 7*

   3.3 The discount rate should be subject to review, and possible revision, over time in light of significant changes in the underlying economic data. However, to retain comparability with other analyses, both 3% and 5% should continue to be used in analyses for at least the next 10 years. **R s (C)** *Chapter 7*

VI. Uncertainty

1. At a minimum, univariate (one-way) sensitivity analyses should be conducted in order to determine where uncertainty or lack of agreement about some key para-

meter's value could have substantial impact on the CEA's conclusions. **R (U)** *Chapter 8*

2. Analysts should conduct multivariate (multiway) sensitivity analyses for important parameters. **R (U)** *Chapter 8*
3. Where possible, where parameter uncertainty is a major concern, a reasonable confidence interval or credible interval should be estimated based on either statistical methods or simulation. **G (U)** *Chapter 8*

VII. Reporting Guidelines: For a summary of detailed reporting guidelines, please refer to the *reporting checklist* in Table 9.4 in Chapter 9.

1. We encourage analysts to document cost-effectiveness studies in two parts, a *journal report* and a more comprehensive *technical report,* making the latter available on request to readers requiring more detail concerning the analysis. **G (U)** *Chapter 9*
2. For the specific purpose of journal review, we recommend that editors request and authors submit a concise *technical addendum* with the journal report to assist reviewers assessing the study's methodology. This material may or may not be published along with the journal report. **G (U)** *Chapter 9*
3. If a cost-effectiveness analysis is intended to allow comparisons among the interventions studied and health care interventions broadly, the report should highlight the Reference Case results. Key sensitivity analyses should be conducted with respect to the Reference Case. **R (U)** *Chapter 9*
4. The perspective(s) of the analysis should be explicitly identified in a cost-effectiveness report. **R (U)** *Chapter 9*
5. The following information comprises a basic set of results in the journal report: total costs, total effectiveness, incremental costs, incremental effectiveness, and incremental cost-effectiveness ratios, both discounted (at the Reference Case rate of 3%) and undiscounted. **G (U)** *Chapter 9*
6. An appropriate number of significant figures should be used to report C/E results, generally two significant figures unless the precision of the data warrants a greater number. **G (U)** *Chapter 9*
7. In reporting incremental cost-effectiveness ratios, options ruled out because of dominance or extended dominance should be excluded. Among undominated options, incremental C/E ratios should be reported in increasing order of cost and effectiveness, starting with the lowest-cost option considered (generally the status quo or "do nothing" option). **R (T,C)** *Chapter 9*
8. C/E ratios should be compared to available C/E ratios for other interventions that compete for resources with the intervention under study. Such interventions may be drawn from health care broadly if the decision context is broad, or from restricted areas, such as particular diseases or intervention modalities. **G (U)** *Chapter 9*

VIII. Research Recommendations

1. The use of CEA in decision making should be studied in a collaborative effort by decision makers and analysts to improve its usefulness. *Chapter 1*

2. When an intervention is deemed of sufficient importance because it addresses a condition with a high burden of illness or high cost, and where good-quality data do not exist, RCTs or large-scale observational studies should be conducted. *Chapter 5*

3. The use of CEA designs with the highest internal validity is hampered by the cost of these studies and by the shortage of data on intervention costs and effectiveness. Greater priority should be given to funding and conducting the studies needed to provide data for cost-effectiveness analysis. *Chapter 8*

4. The nature of the usual distribution of costs is such that larger studies will be needed for adequate samples for cost analysis than for effectiveness and efficacy. Individual trials intended to provide data on both costs and health effects should be large enough to provide adequate power for both. *Chapter 8*

5. Community weights for a standard set of health conditions and health states should be developed for use across studies intended to inform resource allocation. *Chapter 4*

6. Research is needed on the relationship of community preferences to patient preferences for different health states and conditions. *Chapter 4*

7. Research is needed to clarify the performance of different preference measures in different socioeconomic groups. *Chapter 4*

8. Preference results obtained from methods that employ simpler techniques, such as rating scales and paired comparisons, should be compared to those obtained using more traditional laboratory-tested methods (such as the standard gamble and time–tradeoff). Results obtained from self-administered interactive computer approaches should be compared to more traditional interview techniques. *Chapter 4*

9. Research to establish standard cost estimates for CEA will facilitate individual analyses and improve comparability among analyses. *Chapter 4*

10. Research to obtain reasonable values for the opportunity costs of time for population groups for whom traditional labor market methods do not apply—that is, children, the retired elderly, and persons unable to work—is encouraged. *Chapter 4*

11. In order to minimize variation in models, research is needed to understand the contribution to variation in CEA estimates of the modeling process itself. *Chapter 4*

Worked Examples

Appendices B and C contain two examples of cost-effectiveness analyses. The first assesses interventions to prevent neural tube defects and compares population-based with individual approaches; the second addresses cholesterol screening and treatment.

These two examples illustrate the application of the Reference Case recommendations contained in this book to specific cost-effectiveness analyses. The "worked examples" are not presented as "ideal" or prototype analyses. Instead, they are intended to demonstrate the types of concrete questions and methodologic choices that arise in cost-effectiveness research. Within the constraints of the resources allotted for these analyses, the studies demonstrate the authors' strategies for confronting data and analytic issues in the context of conducting a Reference Case analysis.

The authors have implemented Reference Case recommendations on the handling of outcomes, evidence of effectiveness, costs, time preference, and uncertainty. The elements of study framework and design outlined in Chapter 3 are discussed within the examples. Most of the components of the journal report can also be found in these examples, including the recommended format for presentation of results and discussion. However, because their emphasis is to a large extent didactic, the examples do not take the form of a cost-effectiveness journal report. (They are in fact considerably more discursive than a journal article would allow.) The information ordinarily found in a technical report of the CEA is, for the most part, additional to what is presented here.

These examples are primarily intended to illustrate methodology and do not address specific policy questions as fully as a CEA created for that purpose. For example, the study of cholesterol screening was limited to three illustrative risk-factor groups so that its presentation as a worked example would be manageable; for policy purposes, the authors would have included a more diverse population in the analysis. Similarly, in the neural tube defect example, the authors would have prefered to address in greater depth ethical issues concerning the valuation of outcomes associated with averted births of affected children.

312

Appendix B
Cost-Effectiveness of Strategies to Prevent Neural Tube Defects

Alison E. Kelly, Anne C. Haddix, Kelley S. Scanlon, Charles G. Helmick, and Joseph Mulinare

Background

Neural tube defects (NTDs) affect approximately 4,000 pregnancies in the United States annually (Cragan et al., 1995). Spina bifida and anencephaly are the two most common types of NTDs. Anencephaly is invariably fatal, and a substantial proportion of infants surviving with spina bifida have serious lifelong disabilities. Based on accumulated evidence from randomized clinical trials and other epidemiologic studies, the United States Public Health Service (PHS) recommends that all women who are capable of becoming pregnant consume at least 0.4 mg of folic acid daily to reduce their risk for these serious birth defects (CDC, 1992). However, the PHS cautions that care should be taken to keep total folate consumption at less than 1.0 mg per day, because the effects of higher intakes are not well known.[1]

One possible adverse effect of consuming doses of total folate greater than 1.0 mg is the potential for vitamin B_{12} deficiency to go undiagnosed. Vitamin B_{12} deficiency occurs in all age groups, but the most common form (also referred to as pernicious anemia) occurs primarily among the elderly. Although folate-related adverse effects have not been shown in controlled studies, some experts have expressed concern because the anemia associated with untreated vitamin B_{12} deficiency is responsive to folate, as well as to vitamin B_{12} (Butterworth and Tamura, 1989; Herbert, 1988); however, the neurologic manifestations of vitamin B_{12} deficiency can only be treated with vitamin B_{12}. This phenomenon is sometimes referred to as "masking." Because the presence of anemia is sometimes a diagnostic indicator of vitamin B_{12} deficiency, increased folate consumption could interfere with the prompt diagnosis of vitamin B_{12} deficiency, delaying the initiation of treatment with vitamin B_{12} and allowing the neurological manifestations to progress. The neurologic manifestations can be mild or severe; the most common are paresthesias ("pins and needles") of the hands and feet, but central nervous system impairments and a few deaths have been reported in severe cases.

Objectives of the Analysis

The PHS recommendation includes three possible strategies for increasing folic acid consumption in women of reproductive age: (1) improvement of dietary habits, (2) fortification of the U.S. food supply, and (3) use of dietary supplements. This analysis was conducted to evaluate the cost-effectiveness of food fortification and supplementation. This information filled a timely need; the U.S. Food and Drug Administration (FDA) has promulgated a rule that will require manufacturers to fortify cereal grain products with folic acid.

Audience for the Study

The primary audience for this study is policy makers examining the issue of folic acid food fortification and supplementation. This includes individuals throughout the Public Health Service and other agencies involved in nutritional programs. Secondary audiences include clinicians involved in providing care to populations affected by the decisions; members of these groups themselves (women of reproductive age, those at risk for vitamin B_{12} deficiency, individuals and families affected by neural tube defects); epidemiologists and public health program managers at the federal, state, and local levels; and advocacy groups concerned with problems affecting children and the elderly.

Perspective of the Analysis

A decision to pursue a program to reduce NTDs will be made by policy makers in the interest of society as a whole. Thus, the analysis is conducted from a societal perspective.

Type of Analysis

This study is a cost-effectiveness analysis. The outcomes used are quality-adjusted life years (QALYs) gained and years of life gained. The measure of QALYs gained captures two important aspects of the prevention of NTD-affected pregnancies: premature mortality and morbidity. The mortality associated with NTDs is significant. Infants born with anencephaly, 24% of all NTDs, are stillborn or live only a few days. Life expectancy for those with spina bifida is also lower than for infants born without the condition, although it has improved with advances in medical care during the past two decades (Bamforth and Baird, 1989). In addition to effects on length of life, NTDs can have a dramatic impact on the quality of life of the survivors. More than half of surviving adults experience at least moderate disabilities including incontinence and impairments of mobility, vision, and cognitive function (McLaurin et al., 1986; Elwood et al., 1992). In many cases, the disability resulting from NTDs affects individuals' ability to work.

Time Horizon

This analysis assesses the lifetime costs and effects of 1 year of the preventive interventions. All costs and benefits which occur as a result of actions taken during this year are included, regardless of when they occur.

Time Preference

All costs and outcomes were discounted to present value using a 3% annual discount rate.

Target Population for the Intervention

All women in the United States capable of becoming pregnant are the target population for this intervention. As many as 35–50% of pregnancies are unplanned (Williams and Pratt, 1990; Grimes, 1986) and folic acid must be taken early in pregnancy in order to be effective in preventing NTDs; folic acid interventions will therefore be significantly less successful if targeted only to pregnant women or those planning a pregnancy.

An estimated 20–30% of reproductive-age women currently consume a vitamin supplement containing ≥ 0.4 mg folic acid (Moss et al., 1989). In addition, a small number of women (less than 2%) get the recommended daily dose of at least 0.4 mg of folic acid in their diet, primarily through consumption of super-fortified cereals. Because little is known about characteristics that differentiate these women from the 70–80% of reproductive-age women who are not consuming adequate amounts of folic acid, a more targeted strategy is not feasible.

There is some evidence that there may be distinct subpopulations that experience differential benefits from consumption of additional folic acid. For example, higher rates of NTDs have been reported in certain geographic areas, particularly in Appalachia and on the United States–Mexico border (Greenberg et al., 1983; Texas Department of Health, 1992). There are also reported differences in the rates of NTDs among various racial and ethnic groups, with the highest rates occurring in Hispanics and the lowest rate in blacks (Elwood et al., 1992). Finally, limited data suggest that folic acid supplementation may be less effective in college-educated or Hispanic women (Shaw et al., 1995). However, until these subpopulations are studied more rigorously, few data are available with which to estimate potential differential effects.

Defining the Program

This analysis considers two main strategies for the prevention of neural tube defects: voluntary supplementation and food fortification. The voluntary supplementation strategy is a national public education and health-care-provider education program to encourage women of reproductive age to consume vitamin supplements providing 0.4 mg folic acid daily. The food fortification strategy takes a regulatory approach, requiring the addition of folic acid to cereal grain products. To develop the model's "no program" option, which served as our baseline comparator, we analyzed current food consumption patterns in the U.S. and estimated current folic acid and total folate intake. The "no program" option reflects the current annual incidence of NTD-affected pregnancies. We modeled the impact of these options on all members of the U.S. population aged 15 years or greater.

The Food Fortification Strategy

The fortification strategy evaluated here was based on the FDA's proposed rule to fortify enriched cereal grain products (FDA, 1993). This rule, initially proposed in October 1993, was recently enacted. The grain products affected include enriched bread, rolls and buns; enriched flour; enriched corn grits and corn meal; enriched farina and rice; and enriched noodle products.

When developing its proposed rule, the FDA examined fortification at three levels, 0.07, 0.14, and 0.35 mg of folic acid per 100 g of cereal grain product, to determine the amount of folic acid individuals would consume based on their diets. The 0.07-mg level would restore folate lost in the milling of cereal-grain products. The higher levels were examined because they would deliver the effective dose to a larger number of people. We examined three fortification levels: 0.14 (the FDA proposal which has now been enacted), 0.35 (the level initially proposed by CDC), and a higher level than had previously been evaluated, 0.70 mg per 100 g of cereal grains.

The advantage of fortification is that it is a passive intervention not requiring a behavior change. However, it is not a targeted intervention. Most people in the United States would experience an increase in their folic acid consumption. As mentioned previously, increased consumption of folate sometimes masks the anemia of vitamin B_{12} deficiency. Therefore, some experts are concerned that people with undiagnosed vitamin B_{12} deficiency might experience neurological complications resulting from a delay in diagnosis. Because the most common cause of vitamin B_{12} deficiency is age-related, this increase in risk would primarily affect a group who would not directly benefit from the intervention as currently conceived. For this reason, an alternative strategy to specifically increase folic acid intake in women of reproductive age has been proposed—supplementation.

The Supplementation Strategy

This strategy is based on the generally accepted model of public-health behavior-change programs. Through national- and state-based public information and education programs, women would be given information on NTDs and folic acid's preventive potential and would be encouraged to consider increasing their consumption of folic acid by using vitamin supplements containing folic acid. This strategy also includes education of health care providers and other professionals who serve women of reproductive age through presentations at professional meetings, curriculum development efforts, and newsletters. One of the advantages of supplementation is that it is targeted to the population group with the most clearly defined benefits; although this strategy may lead to total folate consumption in excess of 1.0 mg in some women, these women are generally at very low risk for vitamin B_{12} deficiency.

Scope of the Study

NTDs and the interventions that prevent them affect many parties. The interventions are intergenerational (the intervention is delivered to the mother and the effect is experienced by the offspring) and broad-based (fortification affects all people who consume cereal grains). In this study, outcomes are measured for two groups: (1) NTD-affected births of at least 20 weeks gestation and (2) people with vitamin B_{12}–related neurological complications resulting from masking of vitamin B_{12}–related anemia that delayed diagnosis. For NTD-affected pregnancies electively terminated prior to 20 weeks of gestation, costs, but not QALYs lost, are included in the Reference Case analysis.

Health-related quality of life is not considered for persons other than those with NTDs or vitamin B_{12}–related neurological complications. We have not included the psychological and physical impacts on parents and families with NTD-affected pregnancies, whether these pregnancies were terminated, stillborn, died shortly after birth, or were

Table B.1. Probabilities Used in Cost-Effectiveness Analysis of Alternative Strategies to Prevent Neural Tube Defects

Probability[a]	Baseline Value	Range for Sens. Analysis	Source
pWomen15–45	0.3		U.S. Census
pWConsum0.4+	0.282		USDA, 1990
pOConsum1.0+	0.021		USDA, 1990
pNTD0.4+	0.000035	0.000021–0.000049	Bower & Stanley, 1992; Cragan et al., 1995; MRC, 1991; Czeizel & Dudas, 1992; Mills et al., 1989; Milunsky et al., 1989; Mulinare et al., 1988; Smithells et al., 1983
pNTD<0.4	0.000085		Same as above
pSuppmts	0.272		USDA, 1990; Moss et al., 1989
pDiet0.4+	0.014		USDA, 1990
pBegSupp	0.15	0.0–100	CDC expert opinion
pWPostFort0.4+	(See below for fortification-level-dependent probabilities)		
0.14 mg level	0.042		USDA, 1990 (adjusted)
0.35 mg level	0.257		USDA, 1990 (adjusted)
0.70 mg level	0.663		USDA, 1990 (adjusted)
pOPostFort1.0+	(See below for fortification-level-dependent probabilities)		
0.14 mg level	0.028		USDA, 1990 (adjusted)
0.35 mg level	0.163		USDA, 1990 (adjusted)
0.70 mg level	0.434		USDA, 1990 (adjusted)
pOAdveff	0.000023	0.000007–0.000047	Healton et al., 1991; Herbert, 1988; Herbert & Das, 1994; Savage & Lindenbaum, 1995; Schafer et al., 1985; Kurland & Zinsmeister, 1993; Borch & Liedberg, 1984; expert opinion

Description and Definition of the Probabilities in the Decision Tree:

pWomen15–45 The probability that a member of the U.S. adult population is a woman aged 15–45.

pWConsum0.4+ The probability that prior to the intervention a woman aged 15–45 consumes at least 0.4 mg of folic acid daily either from dietary sources or by supplementation.

pOConsum1.0+ The probability that prior to the intervention an adult member of the U.S. population who is not a woman aged 15–45 consumes greater than 1.0 mg of total folate daily either from dietary sources or by supplementation.

pNTD0.4+ The probability that a woman age 15–45 who is consuming at least 0.4 mg folic acid daily will have an NTD-affected pregnancy. This probability is the product of the probability of a woman aged 15–45 becoming pregnant during the year of the intervention (0.07) and the probability of an NTD-affected pregnancy in a woman consuming the protective dose of folic acid (0.0005).

pNTD<0.4 The probability that a woman aged 15–45 who is consuming less than 0.4 mg folic acid daily will have an NTD-affected pregnancy. This probability is the product of the probability of a woman aged 15–45 becoming pregnant during the year of the intervention (0.07) and the probability of an NTD-affected pregnancy in a woman consuming less than the protective dose of folic acid (0.0012).

pSuppmts The probability that a woman aged 15–45 is taking a vitamin supplement containing folic acid prior to the intervention.

pDiet0.4+ The probability that a woman aged 15–45 not taking vitamin supplements containing folic acid consumes at least 0.4 mg folic acid daily from dietary sources.

pBegSupp The probability that a woman aged 15–45 not taking vitamin supplements containing folic acid prior to the intervention will begin taking supplements as a result of the intervention.

pWPostFort0.4+ The probability that a woman aged 15–45 who is not consuming at least 0.4 mg folic acid daily prior to food fortification will consume at least 0.4 mg folic acid daily after cereal grains are fortified. This probability is dependent on the fortification level.

pOPostFort1.0+ The probability that an adult who is not a woman aged 15–45 who consumes less than 1.0 mg total folate daily prior to fortification will consume greater than 1.0 mg total folate daily after the fortification of cereal grains with folic acid. This probability is dependent on the fortification level.

pOAdveff The probability that an adult who is not a woman aged 15–45 who consumes more than 1.0 mg total folate daily will have neurologic complications from the delayed diagnosis of vitamin B_{12} deficiency because their anemia was masked. This probability is the product of the probability that a person in this population group will have vitamin B_{12} deficiency (0.00032), the probability the increase in folic acid consumption as a result of fortification will mask the vitamin B_{12}-related anemia (0.40), and the probability that the person will experience neurologic complications that are clinically significant (0.167).

spina bifida survivors; on caregivers of either children or adults with spina bifida; or on caregivers of people disabled by vitamin B_{12}–related neurological complications. Although quality-of-life impacts on these parties are clearly important, their inclusion is not recommended in a Reference Case analysis because the methods for capturing these impacts are in early stages of development. Also, data on these quality-of-life impacts are not available. Including these QALYs would increase the benefits of all interventions.

Although this analysis considered the two main interventions currently contemplated, dietary improvement was not included. Dietary improvement is a strategy recommended by the PHS; however, little is known about the type of improvement that would effectively prevent NTDs. Folate is readily available in many raw foods, but its metabolic availability varies with the method by which food is prepared and with certain factors in the food itself which may inhibit or enhance folate absorption (Herbert, 1988). Although there is limited evidence that dietary folate will reduce the risk for an NTD-affected pregnancy there is little information regarding the specific dietary changes that would be required. As a result, the public debate has focused on supplementation as the most viable alternative to a fortification strategy.

Methods

This analysis uses SMLTREE[2] and spreadsheet calculations. Because neither of the two interventions we considered has previously been implemented, we constructed a model to estimate the costs and effectiveness of each under a given set of assumptions. A decision tree was used to model folic acid and total folate consumption and to compare the strategies. In comparing the strategies, the critical variables were the change in the number of women consuming the protective dose of 0.4 mg of folic acid (thus reducing their risk for an NTD- affected pregnancy) and the change in the number of individuals whose total folate consumption exceeds 1.0 mg (potentially increasing their risk for neurological complications from vitamin B_{12} deficiency). The strategies were compared in terms of their ability to prevent NTD-affected pregnancies resulting in live-born infants with NTDs, stillbirths at 20 weeks or greater of gestation, and NTD-affected pregnancies terminated before 20 weeks of gestation. As noted earlier, QALYs gained were calculated for prevented NTD-affected pregnancies that would have resulted in either a live birth or a stillbirth of at least 20 weeks of gestation. Figures B.1–B.3 depict the three intervention options. A definition and description of each of the variables in the analysis is provided in Table B.1.

As shown in Figure B.1 (''no program''), the population is separated into women of reproductive age (age 15–45) and others (all adults older than 15, excluding women of reproductive age). Some women currently consume more than 0.4 mg of folic acid

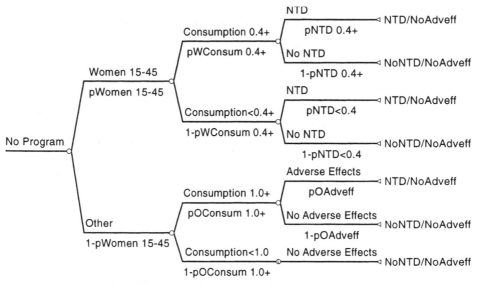

Figure B.1. Strategies for preventing NTDs—no program.

either from a supplement or from fortified cereals, thus reducing their risk for an NTD-affected pregnancy. A second group of women currently consume less than 0.4 mg of folic acid and are at increased risk of an NTD-affected pregnancy. At baseline, there are individuals in both population groups consuming more than 1.0 mg of total folate, potentially increasing their risk for neurological complications related to a delayed diagnosis of vitamin B_{12} deficiency.

Figure B.2, "fortification," is constructed similarly. However, as a result of fortification, consumption levels will be increased. Some women who were not consuming the protective dose at baseline will now be protected. In addition, some women will now be consuming greater than 1.0 mg of total folate. However, preliminary analyses indicated that because the risk for vitamin B_{12} deficiency for women aged 15–45 was very low and the number of women consuming greater than 1.0 mg of total folate was so small, there was less than one case of neurological complications in this population even at the highest level of fortification. Therefore, this branch was dropped from the model. This is not true in the population of others, which includes all people over the age of 45 in which the rates of vitamin B_{12} deficiency are higher.

The "supplementation" model is shown in Figure B.3. In this scenario, women are grouped by current supplement usage. It is assumed that women already taking supplements will not change their behavior as a result of the program, so their risk remains unchanged. Because their total folate consumption was already on the upper end of the

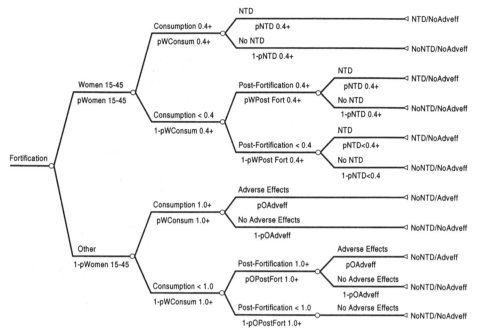

Figure B.2. Strategies for preventing NTDs—fortification.

distribution, these women were more likely to consume greater than 1.0 mg of total folate. However, because the risk of vitamin B_{12} deficiency is so low in this population, we did not observe an increase in neurological complications in this subgroup and this branch was removed from the tree. Of those women not taking supplements, some will begin to take them as a result of the program. Only these women will experience a change in risk.

Using this model, we computed two summary measures: (1) the incremental cost per additional quality-adjusted life year gained and (2) the incremental cost per additional life year gained. The model estimated the number of NTDs that would occur per year in the United States when each intervention is implemented and the number of new cases of vitamin B_{12}–related neurological complications resulting from delayed diagnosis of vitamin B_{12} deficiency because of increased folic acid consumption. We converted these intermediate health outcomes to the two final health outcome measures: QALYs and life years gained. The final measures are used because they allow comparison of the results of this study with the results of CEAs of other health-related interventions and conform to the Reference Case analysis recommended by the Panel on Cost-Effectiveness in Health and Medicine (PCEHM).

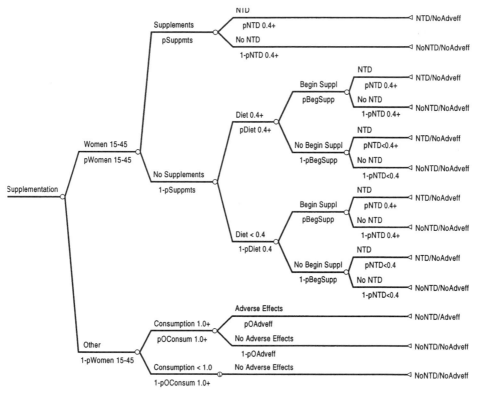

Figure B.3. Strategies for preventing NTDs—supplementation.

Data

Population estimates

Population estimates for the population over age 15 and the number of women age 15–45 were based on the 1990 census. Probabilities were assigned to the events detailed in the decision tree based on the assumptions outlined in Table B.1.

Current dietary patterns

Estimates of current dietary patterns were used to calculate consumption levels of the two population groups under the status quo "no program" strategy. In addition, patterns of consumption were used to predict the amount of folic acid and total folate that would be consumed by women of childbearing age and other adults under the fortification strategies.

Estimates of current total folate consumption were based on the Nationwide Food Consumption Survey (NFCS) (USDA, 1988). In the NFCS, 3 days of food intake data were collected on each participant by 24-hour recall (1 day) and self-administered food diaries (2 days). Individuals' daily consumption was the average of the amounts consumed during the 3-day study. The NFCS has been criticized for its low response rate (LSRO, 1984). However, at this time, it is the only national database that includes multiple days of folate intake information.

The NFCS also provides the total weight of cereal grains consumed by each individual. We estimated the consumption of cereal grain foods that would be fortified (e.g., the flour portion of bread) by multiplying the total weight of the grain products consumed by 0.275. This correction factor was used to approximate the fortifiable portion of cereal grain foods in previous analyses (FDA, 1993).

Because surveys that rely on an individual's recall or record of food intake generally underestimate intake, we multiplied reported total folate and grain intake by 1.25. This estimate is consistent with estimates of underreporting of energy intake in nutrition studies (Mertz et al., 1991).

Effectiveness of a supplementation program for delivering folic acid

Using data from the NFCS, we estimate that just over 27% of women of reproductive age currently consume at least 0.4 mg of folic acid in the form of vitamin supplements (USDA, 1988). The Reference Case analysis assumed that 15% of the 72% of women not currently taking supplements would begin to take them as a result of the supplementation program, bringing the total proportion of supplement users to 38%. The 15% compliance figure is an estimate developed through discussions with individuals working in the field of public health nutrition. There are few data available to validate this estimate of effectiveness. A small group of women (1.4%) currently consumes 0.4 mg of folic acid as a result of including fortified cereals in their diet. Although their risk for an NTD-affected pregnancy is already reduced, these women were assumed to be equally as likely to begin consuming supplements.

Effectiveness of food fortification for delivering folic acid

In examining the technical feasibility of folic acid food fortification, the FDA relied heavily on a 1974 Food and Nutrition Board report that identified cereal grains as appropriate vehicles for food fortification because they meet the criteria as carriers for most nutrients (NRC, 1974). The methodology used in the FDA analysis is described in the October 1993 proposed rule (FDA, 1993).

Estimation of potential adverse effects of folic acid

Because the anemia associated with vitamin B_{12} deficiency responds to folic acid, fortification of the food supply with folic acid has the potential for complicating the diagnosis of vitamin B_{12} deficiency, as described earlier.

Paresthesias (''pins and needles'') of the hands and feet occur in more than 70% of patients who experience neurologic symptoms (Healton et al., 1991). Gait ataxia and weaknesses of the legs and arms are also commonly reported, and central nervous system impairments such as memory loss and hallucinations are sometimes reported in severe cases. The majority of patients respond completely or partially to treatment with vitamin B_{12}; however, some are permanently disabled. In addition, some deaths attributed to neurologic manifestations of vitamin B_{12} deficiency have been reported (Healton et al., 1991).

The level of folate consumption at which the masking of anemia occurs is unclear (Herbert, 1988; Herbert and Das, 1994). Although much of the evidence of this type of masking is based on doses of around 5 mg of folic acid, there is some evidence that it may occur at lower levels of consumption (Savage and Lindenbaum, 1995). There is not, however, sufficient evidence to extrapolate a dose-response curve for the potential masking. Therefore, the FDA has based its proposal on an assumption of increased risk occurring at a threshold of 1 mg of total folate. This analysis has also used a safety threshold of 1 mg of total folate for the Reference Case.

There are no national population-based estimates for the incidence of vitamin B_{12} deficiency. There are, however, surveillance data for pernicious anemia (the most common form of vitamin B_{12} deficiency) from Olmsted County, Minnesota, which indicates an incidence of pernicious anemia of 20.9/100,000 in the population age 25 and over (Schafer et al., 1985; Kurland and Zinsmeister, personal communication, 1993). We adjusted the Olmsted County rates to the 1990 U.S. census population data to give a rate for pernicious anemia for adults over 15 years of age. Since pernicious anemia accounts for as much as 75% of vitamin B_{12} deficiency (Borch and Liedberg, 1984), we estimated the rate of vitamin B_{12} deficiency by dividing the age-adjusted pernicious anemia rates by 0.75.

Even in the absence of folic acid, an estimated 39.7% of individuals with pernicious anemia experience neurological signs and symptoms without hematologic evidence of disease (Schwartz et al., 1950). Because these people do not experience anemia, they may be at risk for delayed diagnosis. However, in these cases, the delay is not a result of the fortification intervention. We therefore adjusted our estimates to account for this group. Finally, we estimated that a delayed diagnosis would result in clinically important functional neurological deficits which would persist after appropriate treatment was initiated in 16.7% of those individuals whose anemia was masked (Healton et al., 1991).

Much of the literature on folate and vitamin B_{12} deficiency was written in the 1940s and 1950s and is based on significantly higher levels of folate intake. There are inadequate data on masking and neurological complications for daily intakes closer to values expected with a fortification program, and no data on these complications for daily intakes which are spread throughout the day (as in a fortification program) versus received all at once (as in a supplement or injection).

Current incidence of NTDs

Using rates calculated from the Metropolitan Atlanta Congenital Defects Program (MACDP) and several state-based surveillance systems, we estimated that NTDs occur in 1 per 1,000 pregnancies or 0.6 per 1,000 live births (Cragan et al., 1995). The MACDP is a population-based surveillance system of all births in the metropolitan Atlanta area. Although there are geographic and racial variations in NTD rates, the MACDP rates are very close to rates found in other surveillance systems. Of the approximately 4,000 NTD-affected pregnancies that occur in the United States each year, 32% are diagnosed and terminated before 20 weeks of gestation, 44% are infants born with spina bifida, and 24% are infants born with anencephaly.

Effectiveness of folic acid in preventing neural tube defects

The literature on the relationship between supplementation with folic acid and the risk for neural tube defects is extensive. It includes three randomized, controlled trials (Laurence et al., 1981; MRC, 1991; Czeizel and Dudas, 1992). Two of these trials focused on women with previous NTD-affected pregnancies. There are also two nonrandomized trials; both focused on women with previous NTD-affected pregnancies, one in the United Kingdom (Smithells et al., 1983) and the other in Cuba (Vergel et al., 1990). In addition, five case-control studies and one prospective cohort study were conducted among women without prior NTD-affected pregnancies (Mulinare et al., 1988; Mills et al., 1989; Bower and Stanley, 1992; Werler et al., 1993; Shaw et al., 1995; Milunsky et al., 1989). All of these studies except one (Mills et al., 1989) showed a protective effect of folic acid; the effect size ranged from approximately a 30% reduction in risk to 100% (CDC, 1992). In addition to the studies which evaluated the relationship between folic acid consumption and NTDs, two case-control studies have examined the relationship between dietary folate and neural tube defects, and also demonstrated a protective effect (Bower and Stanley, 1989; Watson-Duff and Cooper, 1994).

Based on this literature, we estimated that women consuming 0.4 mg of folic acid would experience a 50% reduction in their risk for an NTD-affected pregnancy (CDC, 1992). This population-based risk reduction was a reasonable estimate based on the published literature. A dose-response relationship may exist, but without adequate data to model the likely dose-response curve, 0.4 mg of folic acid was considered to be a threshold value, below which no prevention occurs.

Costs

This analysis includes the direct medical and nonmedical costs of the two interventions we evaluated and of changes in the major health outcomes resulting from these interventions: NTDs and vitamin B_{12}-related neurological complications. All costs are reported in 1993 U.S. dollars. Program costs are 1-year costs, and the costs of the health outcomes are lifetime costs. Costs were collected from a variety of published and unpublished sources and are summarized in Table B.2. Costs for years prior to 1993 were

Table B.2. Costs of Health Outcomes and Program Costs in 1993 Dollars and a 3% Annual Discount Rate

Health outcome: NTD	Cost, $	% NTDs[a]	Source
Elective termination			
15 weeks' prenatal care	1,500	32%	BC/BS[b]
Termination	650	32%	BC/BS
Anencephaly			
Neonatal ICU hospitalization	3,579	24%	Lipscomb, 1986; BC/BS
Spina bifida			
Medical, special education, and developmental services	156,033	44%	Waitzman et al., 1994 CDC, 1995
Caregiver	251,753	44%	Lipscomb, 1986 Haddix et al., 1996

Health outcome: vitamin B_{12}–related neurologic complications[c]	Cost, $	% cases[d]	Source
Diagnostic cost	856	100%	BC/BS
Hospitalization	11,510	10%	BC/BS
Outpatient therapy	260	90%	BC/BS
Six months' rehabilitative therapy	754	47%	BC/BS; Healton, 1991
Long-term rehabilitative therapy	21,700	6%	BC/BS; Healton, 1991

Program: fortification	Cost[e], $		Source
Label changes (annualized cost)	4.5m		FDA, 1993
Analytic testing	2.5m		FDA, 1993
0.07 mg folic acid/100 g grain	2.0m		FDA, 1993

Program: supplementation			
National education program	10m		—[f]
Vitamin supplements (1 year)	67m		—[g]

a. % of NTDs which incur cost (MACDP).

b. BC/BS indicates Blue Cross/Blue Shield, Center for Health Economics and Policy Research (Lapp, written communication).

c. Management profile for a case of masked B_{12} deficiency presenting with neurologic symptoms developed by consultation with experts.

d. % of persons with neurologic complications which incur cost.

e. m indicates millions of dollars.

f. Estimate was based on consultation with CDC Health Education and Promotion experts.

g. Estimate based on average retail price assuming 50% of women take multivitamin supplement and 50% of women take folic acid supplement.

adjusted to 1993 United States dollars using the Consumer Price Index (CPI) for all items.

Program Costs

Cost of fortification
We calculated the total cost of fortification of cereal grains in the United States for each fortification level analyzed based on FDA estimates (FDA, 1993). The total cost for each level of fortification ranges from $11 million for fortification with 0.14 mg per 100 g grain to $27 million for fortification with 0.70 mg per 100 g grain. The total annual cost of cereal grain fortification is comprised of three components: the cost of the folic acid ($2 million per additional 0.07 mg per 100 g of grain), the cost of analytic testing ($2.5 million annually), and an annualized cost for label changes ($4.5 million). The cost of analytic testing and the cost of label changes are fixed costs; only the cost of the folic acid changes with fortification level. Annual per capita costs calculated for the adult population over the age of 15 range from $0.06 to $0.15.

Cost of supplementation program
The cost of the supplementation program includes the cost of a public education campaign to promote the intake of folic acid supplements by women of childbearing years and the cost of the supplements consumed by women who begin taking supplements as a result of the educational campaign. Using estimates for similar physician-based and public education campaigns at CDC, we estimated that the cost is $10 million or $0.04 per U.S. adult 15 years of age or older. The estimated cost of the supplements was based on the average retail price for over-the-counter vitamin supplements, assuming that 50% of women would take a multivitamin supplement and 50% of women would take a folic acid supplement daily. The average annual cost of supplements for women who consume them is $11.

Costs Related to Health Outcomes

Cost of neural tube defects
The cost of a neural tube defect (NTD) used in this analysis encompasses the lifetime costs of spina bifida and anencephaly including medical costs, costs of special education and developmental services, cost of institutionalization, and the time costs for caregivers to children with spina bifida.

For the costs of children born with spina bifida, except for the cost of caregiver time, we used costs from two recently published studies on the economic costs of birth defects (Waitzman et al., 1994; CDC, 1995). These estimates reflect the direct medical costs and developmental and special education costs of a cohort of persons with spina bifida born in California in 1988. The authors subtracted the estimated costs of medical and other services used by children without spina bifida to obtain costs attributable to spina bifida. They estimated the number of new cases of spina bifida and excess mortality in the first year of life using data from the California Birth Defects Monitoring Program (CBDMP). Estimates of age-specific direct costs of spina bifida in these studies were obtained from several sources that reported charges and expenditures for children with the condition. Estimates of inpatient and outpatient medical costs, physician services, and long-term care were based on abstracts of all discharges from California nonfederal, acute care hospitals in 1988,[3] on claims for all MediCal beneficiaries in fiscal year 1988,[4] and on data from the California Department of Developmental Services. The authors adjusted charges to approximate actual costs using Medicare cost-to-charge ratios. The cost of developmental services, defined as nonmedical services provided to children outside the education system, was obtained from the California Department of Developmental Services master file, 1988–1989. Costs for special education services were obtained from the California Special Education Enrollment data, 1988–1989; the California Special Education Expenditure data, 1989; and the National Longitudinal Study of Special Education Services, 1985. The authors adjusted costs for differences between California and the nation. For the purposes of this analysis, the authors recalculated future costs using a 3% and a 0% discount rate (Waitzman, personal communication).

The aforementioned studies did not include the cost of caregiver time. We used unpublished data from Lipscomb (1986) to estimate the time spent providing care to a child with spina bifida compared to providing care for a child without the condition. These data were from survey responses of 104 parents of children with spina bifida. Lipscomb estimated an average weekly reduction in work of 5 hours for the father and 14 hours for the mother as a result of extra time rendered in the home to care for the affected child. We used $94 as the estimated value of a lost work day based on the weighted average annual mean earnings by age and sex for the proportion of the population in the labor force and the imputed value of nonwage housekeeping (based on labor force wage rates for similar tasks) by age and sex for the proportion of the population engaged as homemakers in 1990 (Haddix et al., 1996). The estimate was adjusted to 1993 dollars using the annual rate of increase in earnings (U.S. Bureau of Labor Statistics, 1995). Caregiver costs accrue until children with spina bifida reach age 20. By that age, most major surgeries and related therapies have been completed. We estimated the present value of the cost of caregiver time at $251,753.

The cost in this analysis of infants born with anencephaly includes only the direct medical costs of inpatient neonatal intensive care (ICU) for up to 28 days. Survival estimates for infants with anencephaly are based on Lipscomb's unpublished data. He used North Carolina mortality data from 1976 to 1980 to estimate that 25% are stillborn, 61% die within 24 hours of birth, 11% survive a week, and 3% survive as long as 28 days. Using an estimate of $1,600 for the 1993 cost per day for neonatal ICU from Blue Cross/Blue Shield (written communication, Lapp), we estimated the average cost for an infant with anencephaly at $3,579.

The cost of NTD-affected pregnancies that are diagnosed and terminated before 20 weeks of gestation includes the cost of prenatal care, diagnosis of the NTD, and elective termination. Costs were obtained from Blue Cross/Blue Shield. We estimated a cost of $2,150 per terminated pregnancy for the 32% of NTDs in this category.

Cost of neurological complications of undiagnosed vitamin B_{12} deficiency

Based on a review of the literature (Healton et al., 1991; Schwartz et al., 1950) and in consultation with three individual clinicians who routinely see patients with vitamin B_{12} deficiency, we developed patient management profiles reflecting current practice for diagnosis and treatment of the neurologic complications resulting from vitamin B_{12} deficiency including diagnosis, treatment of acute symptoms, and rehabilitation of persistent complications. Each of the three clinicians described the diagnosis and management of neurological conditions resulting from delayed diagnosis of vitamin B_{12} deficiency. Based on their experience, we estimated that 10% of patients presenting with neurological symptoms would require hospitalization, and 90% would receive outpatient treatment. After initial treatment, 47% of patients would experience complete resolution of symptoms, 47% would require 6 months of rehabilitation therapy for mild-to-moderate functional deficits, and 6% would require long-term therapy for severe permanent functional deficits. Two of the three experts estimated that approximately 3% of patients (50% of patients with severe permanent functional deficits) experience complications severe enough to cause death. The third expert did not attribute mortality as an outcome. We used a 3% mortality rate in our analysis.

Only the costs of cases of vitamin B_{12} deficiency that progressed to neurological complications because of misdiagnosis or delayed diagnosis due to the masking effect of total folate were included. These costs include diagnostic tests, outpatient and hospitalization costs for acute treatment, and rehabilitation costs. The costs of patient management were estimated from 1993 data on actual payments for medical services classified by diagnostic-related group (DRG) codes from Blue Cross/Blue Shield Center for Health Economics and Policy Research (written communication). To estimate the lifetime cost of rehabilitative therapy for patients with severe functional deficits resulting in permanent disability, we assumed the average age at onset of neurological complications was 60 years based on the panel of experts' clinical experience and that patients had a remaining life expectancy of 20 years. We estimated that the present value of the weighted average medical costs of neurological complications resulting from masked vitamin B_{12} deficiency is $3,897.

Other costs

In this worked example, we were not able to include estimates for the following costs: (1) time costs of people with spina bifida, (2) time costs for people with vitamin B_{12}–related neurological complications to seek and obtain treatment, (3) costs of caregiving for people disabled by vitamin B_{12}–related neurological complications, and (4) time costs for women receiving counseling on the benefits of folic acid supplementation during a routine physician visit. These costs should be included in the Reference Case analysis and are omitted here only because of constraints on the present analysis. We conducted sensitivity analyses using a wide range of costs of the health outcomes to estimate the impact of excluding these costs on the results of the evaluation.

Valuing Outcomes

The decision tree previously described was used to estimate the number of NTDs prevented by each strategy and the number of adverse effects from the delayed diagnosis of vitamin B_{12} deficiency. We then estimated the QALYs gained by preventing an NTD and the QALYs lost by causing an adverse effect. To calculate the net impact of each strategy, we multiplied the number of QALYs gained from preventing an NTD by the number of NTDs prevented with that strategy and then subtracted the QALYs lost as a result of adverse effects, calculated by multiplying the QALYs lost per adverse effect by the number of adverse effects that would occur with each strategy.

NTDs

The first step in estimating QALYs is to identify the relevant health outcomes. As discussed earlier, we considered three categories of NTDs in this analysis: spina bifida and anencephaly births of at least 20 weeks of gestation, and NTDs terminated prior to 20 weeks of gestation. The Reference Case includes QALYs only for the first two; the QALYs lost when a pregnancy is terminated—that is, the QALYs of the fetus—were not included in the Reference Case analysis. However, they were estimated and used for purposes of sensitivity analysis.

Children born with spina bifida generally survive for many years depending on the severity of the lesion and the sex of the child. Survivors experience a wide range of disabilities, which vary considerably in severity. Common disabilities include incontinence and impairments in mobility, vision, and cognitive function. Children with the most severe lesions must undergo numerous and painful surgeries (Bamforth and Baird, 1989; Elwood et al., 1992).

We classified lesions in three types for this analysis: thoracic/higher lumbar, lower lumbar, and sacral lesions. We used Lipscomb's estimates of the proportion of individuals with each lesion type and survival curves. Thoracic/higher lumbar lesions, 50% of spina bifida births, are the most severe, having the shortest survival and the greatest impact on the health of the individual. Most children do not survive adolescence. Thirty percent of spina bifida births are lower lumbar lesions, the second most severe lesion type. Although survival rates are much higher, individuals with lower lumbar lesions have lifelong, often serious, health problems. Sacral lesions, comprising 20% of spina bifida births, are the least severe. Persons with sacral lesions often survive a full life and carry on normal activities, including childbearing, despite some health problems (Bamforth and Baird, 1989; Elwood et al., 1992). As noted earlier, anencephaly, which occurs in 24% of all NTD-affected pregnancies of 20 weeks or greater, is invariably fatal—usually within the first few weeks of life.

Estimating Health-related Quality of Life and QALYs

In order to estimate QALYs lost as a result of an NTD-affected pregnancy or from adverse affects associated with consumption of total folate in excess of 1.0 mg, we first applied community values to the health states associated with the different outcomes. We estimated health-related quality of life for these health states using four different health state classification systems for which community values are available: the Health Utilities Index (HUI) (Drummond et al., 1987; Feeny et al., 1995; Torrance et al., 1995b; Torrance et al., 1992), the Quality of Well-Being Index (QWB) (Kaplan and Anderson, 1988), the EuroQol instrument (Essink-Bot et al., 1993; EuroQol Group, 1990; Williams 1995a,b), and the NCHS Years of Healthy Life (YHL) measure (Erickson et al., 1995; Torrance et al., 1995a) . We wished to explore how the use of different instruments, relying on differing levels of complexity in their description of health states, and different valuation tasks in obtaining preferences for the health states, would affect scores.

To apply community weights from the QWB, HUI II, and the EuroQol measures to the health states associated with different levels of spinal cord lesions, we first described those health states using the domains and levels within each domain of the different instruments. Because we did not have access to people who were directly experiencing spina-bifida-related health states, we asked experts to describe the ''average'' health state for persons with different levels of spinal cord lesions and stage of life. The experts were members of the Professional Advisory Council of the Spina Bifida Association of America or other clinicians with expertise in the care of persons with spina bifida. Using the domains and levels available within the QWB, the HUI II, and the EuroQol, six clinicians were asked to designate a ''typical'' health state for nine categories of persons; children, adolescents, and adults, with sacral, lower lumbar, and thoracic/higher lumbar lesions. Based on the selections of the clinicians, the average health state within each of the health-state classification systems (as described by its component domain and the levels within those domains) was calculated for the nine lesion-level and age subgroups. Community-gathered preference weights for the QWB, the HUI, and the EuroQol were then applied to these health states (personal communication, Ganiats, Torrance; Williams 1995a). The scores for the nine categories for each of the health status instruments are reported in Table B.3.

To estimate QALYs using the YHL we used secondary data collected in the National Health Interview Survey (NHIS) in which people born with spina bifida were asked to

Table B.3. Health-Related Quality of Life (HRQL) Scores for Spina Bifida by Age and Lesion Category Using Alternative Health Status Measures

	QWB[a]	HUI-II[a]	EuroQol[b]	YHL[a]
Sacral lesion				
Child[c]	0.601	0.83	0.731	0.94
Adolescent[d]	0.600	0.73	0.735	0.94
Adult[e]	0.564	0.79	0.736	0.88[f]
Lower lumbar lesion				
Child[c]	0.511	0.45	0.619	0.87
Adolescent[d]	0.529	0.42	0.621	0.87
Adult[e]	0.514	0.42	0.578	0.76[f]
Thoracic/higher lumbar lesion				
Child[c]	0.454	0.30	0.281	0.71
Adolescent[d]	0.462	0.18	0.268	0.70
Adult[e]	0.465	0.30	0.184	0.57[f]

a. HRQL scores range from 0 to 1; 0=death, 1=perfect health.

b. HRQL scores for EuroQol range from −0.594 to 1; 1=perfect health, 0=death, −0.402=unconscious. EuroQol allows for health states valued as worse than death.

c. Zero to 10 years of age.

d. Eleven to 21 years of age.

e. Twenty-two years of age and older.

f. Represents the mean of scores for age groups 18–24, 25–34, 35–44, 45–54, 55–64, 65–74.

classify their activity limitations and their general state of health. Condition-specific scores, based on the values for health states described by the two-domain YHL measure (Erickson et al., 1995), have been calculated (Gold et al., 1994). On the NHIS, individuals report conditions as well as self-perceived health (five levels ranging from "poor" to "excellent") and role function (six levels ranging from "not limited" to "limited in activities of daily living"). We used the population-weighted value of the average health state for all persons reporting spina bifida on the NHIS.

To integrate the values assigned to the health states with the quantity of life, we multiplied the scores for the different age-specific health outcomes by the probability of survival for each year of life for the three lesion categories. Lipscomb's estimates for life expectancy for infants born with and without spina bifida were used because they provide information on the basis of lesion level. More recent data on survival were not available. We summed over the life span, discounting future years at an annual rate of 3%. The final step was to multiply the total QALYs for a person with a lesion type by the probability of having that lesion type and summing for the three lesion types to obtain the average total QALYs for a person with spina bifida.

To determine the marginal QALYs gained by preventing spina bifida, we subtracted the total QALYs for a person with spina bifida from the total QALYs for the average person in the population with an average life expectancy. We used mean scores for each year of life of the general population for each of the four health classification

Table B.4. Comparison of Health Status Measures for Calculating QALYs Gained by Preventing an NTD or Lost Due to Vitamin B_{12}–Related Neurological Complications

Methodology	Spina Bifida[a]	Anencephaly & Terminations[a,b]	Neurological Complications[a]
QWB	15.44	24.20	0.31
HUI-II	18.91	26.43	0.29
YHL	13.05	26.70	0.17
EuroQol	15.73	24.06	0.29
Life years gained[c]	11.77	28.13	0

a. QALYs gained by preventing a condition are calculated by subtracting the total QALYs of a person with a condition from the total QALYs for the average person in the population. Incorporates both the yearly HRQL score and life expectancy. QALYs are discounted at a 3% annual rate.

b. Because terminations and anencephalic births are equivalent to the loss of a full life, the QALYs gained represent the lifetime discounted QALYs for the average person in the population with the average life expectancy.

c. No quality-of-life adjustments are included in years of life gained (or lost).

systems (Berthelot et al., 1995; personal communication, Franks; Williams 1995a; personal communication, Ganiats). For estimates of the QALYs gained by preventing an NTD that would have resulted in elective termination and by preventing anencephaly, we used the discounted sum of QALYs for an average person with an average life expectancy. The marginal QALYs gained by preventing spina bifida, anencephaly, and elective termination using the four different generic preference-based measures are shown in Table B.4.

We used a similar approach for the assignment of health states in people who experience neurological complications as a result of a delayed diagnosis of vitamin B_{12} deficiency. In this case we contacted a group of clinicians with experience in treating the neurological complications of vitamin B_{12} deficiency for information on health states, their duration, and mortality rates. We followed the methodology described above to assign scores to the health states, to integrate scores with life expectancy, and to estimate the marginal QALYs lost due to neurological complications for each of the four measures (Table B.4).

Although we calculated QALYs using four different measures, we used the QALYs estimated from QWB scores in the Reference Case analysis. We selected this measure for three reasons. First, it was the measure rated by the expert panel as the most sensitive to the health states of persons with spina bifida. Second, it produced a mid range score. Third, the community values used for the QWB were obtained from a population in the United States.

We also report results using years of life gained. To calculate the years of life gained by preventing an NTD and the years of life lost due to vitamin B_{12}–related neurological complications, we used the methods described above to estimate life expectancy but did not include a quality-of-life adjustment.

Results

Model Validation

Prior to analyzing the decision tree for the Reference Case, we tested the validity of the decision model to determine if the results produced by the "no program" option reflected the annual incidence of NTD-affected pregnancies in the United States. The "no program" option was structured to reflect the proportion of the U.S. adult population that are women age 15–45, the annual pregnancy rate in women in this group, and the risk of an NTD-affected pregnancy given the group's current folate intake pattern. The total number of cases of NTD- affected pregnancies produced by the "no program" option was 3,920. This is very close to the annual incidence of 1 per 1,000 pregnancies or approximately 4,000 NTD-affected pregnancies each year.

Reference Case

Table B.5 provides a breakdown of total costs (program costs and costs of health outcomes), the number of NTDs, and the number of vitamin-B_{12}-deficiency-related neurological complications that occur with each intervention in the Reference Case analysis. Annual program costs range from $11 to $27 million for fortification strategies and are $77 million for supplementation. The cost of all health outcomes is less under every intervention considered than it would be if no program were implemented, driven by the reduced number of NTD births in each scenario. The number of neurological

Table B.5. Total Program and Health Outcome Cost, NTDs, and Neurological Complications for Five Stategies to Increase Folic Acid Intake

Intervention[a]	Total Program Cost[b]	Total Cost of Health Outcomes[b,c]	Total NTDs in Birth Cohort	Total Neurological Complications[d]
Discounted results (3%)				
No program	0	$709m	3,920	0
Fort 0.14 mg	$11m	$694m	3,831	89
Supplement	$77m	$652m	3,602	0
Fort 0.35 mg	$17m	$611m	3,365	473
Fort 0.70 mg	$27m	$461m	2,517	1,388

a. Strategies ranked in order of effectiveness of preventing NTDs.

b. All costs are in 1993 dollars.

c. Total cost of health outcomes includes the cost of NTDs in the birth cohort and the cost of the vitamin B_{12}–related neurological complications caused by masking of anemia as a result of the intervention.

d. Includes only the cases of vitamin B_{12}–related neurological complications caused by masking of anemia as a result of the intervention.

complications ranges from 89 to 1388 in the fortification strategies, as compared to the absence of any program-related cases in either of the "no program" or the "supplementation" option.

In the Reference Case results, having "no program" results in total costs of about $709 million (1993 $) associated with the cases of NTD and neurological complications related to delayed diagnosis of vitamin B_{12} deficiency occurring during 1 year. Fortification, at all levels investigated, resulted in overall cost savings as well as gains in QALYs (Table B.6). Supplementation cost more than any other option (including the "no program" option) but gained QALYs relative to "no program" and "fortification" at 0.14 mg of folic acid. However, the "supplementation" program was dominated by "fortification" at the 0.35- and 0.70-mg levels, both of which gained more total QALYs at a lower total cost.

The three "fortification" options were increasingly cost saving. Fortification at the 0.70 level was the most effective and most cost saving, dominating the other "fortifi-

Table B.6. Reference Case Results—QALYs

Intervention	Total Cost (Millions)[a]	Total QALYs Lost[b]	Incr Cost (Millions)	Incr QALYs Gained	C/E, Incr $/ Incr QALYs
Discounted Results (3%)					
No program	$709	49,392	—	—	—
Fort 0.14 mg	$705	48,298	—	—	Cost saving, but dominated by 0.35 and 0.70
Supplement	$729	45,385	—	—	Dominated by 0.35 and 0.70
Fort 0.35 mg	$628	42,546	—	—	Cost saving, but dominated by 0.70
Fort 0.70 mg	$488	32,144	−$221.49	17,248	−$12,813
Undiscounted Results					
No program	$962	131,359	—	—	—
Fort 0.14 mg	$952	128,411	—	—	Cost saving, but dominated by 0.35 and 0.70
Supplement	$961	120,703	—	—	Dominated by 0.35 and 0.70
Fort 0.35 mg	$845	112,941	—	—	Cost saving, but dominated by 0.70
Fort 0.70 mg	$651	84,872	−$311.54	46,487	−$6,712
Discounted Results (5%)					
No program	$541	32,614	—	—	—
Fort 0.14 mg	$540	31,897	—	—	Cost saving, but dominated by 0.35 and 0.70
Supplement	$574	29,969	—	—	Dominated by 0.35 and 0.70
Fort 0.35 mg	$484	28,120	—	—	Cost saving, but dominated by 0.70
Fort 0.70 mg	$380	21,302	−$161.60	11,312	−$14,286

a. Total cost includes the total intervention cost for the U.S. adult population and the cost of the NTDs and the vitamin B_{12}–related neurological complications that occur when the intervention is implemented. All costs are in 1993 dollars.

b. Total QALYs lost are the QALYs lost in an annual U.S. birth cohort due to NTD-affected pregnancies that go to 20 weeks of gestation or greater and the QALYs lost from vitamin B_{12}–related neurological complications associated with total folate consumption in excess of 1.0 mg.

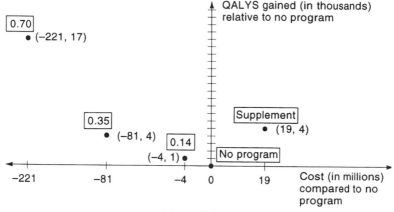

Figure B.4.

cation'' options. It resulted in cost savings of about $13,000 (1993 $) accompanying every QALY gained. These results are presented graphically in Figure B.4. The results of the analyses using life years as the measure of outcome were very similar (Table B.7) as were the results obtained using 0% and 5% discount rates (Tables B.6 and B.7).

Sensitivity Analyses

We performed both univariate and multivariate sensitivity analyses of critical probabilities in the model, and of the costs of the program and the health outcomes. These analyses were conducted in order to determine if varying the values of these parameters over a plausible range would change the results of the analysis. These analyses are discussed in detail below.

Univariate analyses

In evaluating the literature on the protective effect of folic acid, the reduction in the incidence of NTD-affected pregnancies varied considerably from no reduction to complete reduction. Our Reference Case estimate was a 50% reduction, but we also considered a 30% reduction and a 70% reduction, with no change in the conclusion that 0.70 mg was the most effective and overall most cost saving strategy.

Similarly, we evaluated a range of estimates for the likelihood of neurologic complications associated with a delay in diagnosis of vitamin B_{12} deficiency. Our Reference case estimate was based on Schwartz et al. (1950) and Healton et al. (1991), and to evaluate a wider range of estimates we adopted the values of the upper and lower confidence intervals as our parameters for sensitivity analysis. We also included in our sensitivity analysis of this variable the risk of neurologic complications for women age 15–45, and again, did not see a change in the preference order of the strategies.

Table B.7. Reference Case Results—Life Years

Intervention	Total Cost (Millions)[a]	Total Life Years Lost[b]	Incr Cost (Millions)	Incr Life Years Gained	C/E, Incr $/ Incr Life Years
Discounted results (3%)					
No program	$709	46,766	—	—	—
Fort 0.14 mg	$705	45,715	—	—	Cost saving, but dominated by 0.35 and 0.70
Supplement	$729	42,972	—	—	Dominated by 0.35 and 0.70
Fort 0.35 mg	$628	40,201	—	—	Cost saving, but dominated by 0.70
Fort 0.70 mg	$488	30,195	−$221.49	16,738	−$13,738
Undiscounted results					
No program	$962	125,440	—	—	—
Fort 0.14 mg	$952	122,619	—	—	Cost saving, but dominated by 0.35 and 0.70
Supplement	$961	115,264	—	—	Dominated by 0.35 and 0.70
Fort 0.35 mg	$845	107,822	—	—	Cost saving, but dominated by 0.70
Fort 0.70 mg	$651	80,960	−$312	44,480	−$7,014
Discounted results (5%)					
No program	$541	29,596	—	—	—
Fort 0.14 mg	$540	28,924	—	—	Cost saving, but dominated by 0.35 and 0.70
Supplement	$574	27,195	—	—	Dominated by 0.35 and 0.70
Fort 0.35 mg	$484	25,406	—	—	Cost saving, but dominated by 0.70
Fort 0.70 mg	$380	19,003	−$161.60	10,593	−$15,256

a. Total cost includes the total intervention cost for the U.S. adult population and the cost of the NTDs and the vitamin B_{12}-related neurological complications that occur when the intervention is implemented. All costs are in 1993 dollars.

b. Total life years lost are the life years lost in an annual U.S. birth cohort due to NTD-affected pregnancies that go to 20 weeks of gestation or greater and the life years lost from vitamin B_{12}-related neurological complications associated with total folate consumption in excess of 1.0 mg.

The third probability examined in a univariate analysis was the probability that women would begin taking supplements as the result of a supplementation program. There was considerable uncertainty regarding this variable. When compared with lower levels of fortification, the relative cost-effectiveness of supplementation is sensitive to women's compliance with supplemention intervention. However, at 0.70 mg per 100 g of grain, fortification would always dominate, even if compliance with supplementation was 100%.

Sensitivity analysis using the range of QALY estimates derived from alternative health status measurement instruments (Table B.4) showed that changes in the the number of QALYs gained per NTD prevented or lost per vitamin B_{12}-related neurologic complication had little impact on the results of the Reference Case analysis; fortification at 0.70 mg per 100 g folic acid remained the dominant strategy.

Finally, we performed a sensitivity analysis on the QALYs gained per NTD prevented by including QALYs lost per terminated NTD-affected pregnancy. For this scenario we assumed that the number of QALYs lost due to a termination were equivalent to the number of QALYs lost due to a stillborn NTD-affected pregnancy. The QALYs gained per NTD prevented increased from 12.6 to 20.34. Results of this sensitivity analysis showed that the assumption had no impact of the order of effectiveness of the alternative strategies. The cost-effectiveness of all strategies increased 64%.

Multivariate analyses

Multivariate sensitivity analyses were conducted by developing several scenarios under which a number of parameters were allowed to vary simultaneously. Unless otherwise noted, the parameters used in the multivariate analysis were the same as those used in the univariate analyses described above. Each scenario is described below.

In the best-case scenario, the parameter values were chosen to bias the analysis toward intervening to prevent NTDs by using the most optimistic value for the reduction in risk for women consuming 0.4 mg of folic acid and the lowest increase in risk for people consuming greater than 1.0 mg of total folate. The conclusion that fortification at 0.70 mg per 100 g of grain is the most effective and most cost-saving option remained unchanged. The worst-case scenario attempted to further bias the analysis away from choosing to intervene to prevent NTDs by adopting parameter values at the opposite extreme from the best-case scenario. Under this scenario, fortification at 0.14 mg no longer achieved cost savings, but the order of the programs remained the same.

Another multivariate sensitivity analysis was biased toward supplementation. The cost of fortification was doubled and the probability of adverse effects was set at its highest plausible value. In this scenario, fortification at 0.14 mg per 100 g of grain no longer achieves a cost saving. Fortification at the 0.70 mg per 100 g of grain level remains the most effective and most cost saving program for reducing the number of NTDs.

Finally, because we did not have estimates for several of the costs that should be included in the Reference Case analysis, we conducted sensitivity analyses using a scenario that approximated the inclusion of these costs. We doubled the cost of an NTD from $180,973 to $360,000 to approximate time costs of people with spina bifida and lifetime caregiver costs for people with spina bifida who have thoracic lesions. We increased the cost of a vitamin B_{12}-related neurological complication roughly ten-fold from $3,897 to $39,000 to reflect nursing home care for the 6% of people with severe irreversible complications and time costs to seek and obtain treatment including diagnosis, treatment, and physical therapy. We increased the cost of the supplementation program from $77 million to $85.5 million to include time costs of women receiving preconceptual counseling during a physician visit. Results from analysis of this scenario indicated that all strategies increased in their cost-effectiveness because the increase in the cost of an NTD far outweighed other cost increases; there was no change in the order of effectiveness of the alternative strategies.

Discussion

We conducted this cost-effectiveness analysis to examined the economic implications of two NTD prevention strategies, fortification and supplementation, in order to facilitate the public policy discussion regarding this issue. Fortification at 0.70 mg per 100 g of grain, the highest level examined in this analysis, proved to be the intervention of choice from a purely economic standpoint. This strategy gained the greatest number of QALYs and accompanied these health savings with the highest total savings in cost. The other fortification strategies, 0.14 and 0.35 mg folate, also produced cost savings associated with incremental gains in QALYs. The "supplementation" program resulted in new costs but gained QALYs relative to "no program" and to the low (0.14 mg)-level "fortification" program. However, it was dominated by the cost-saving and more effective higher-level "fortification" programs.

It should be noted that fortification at the highest level examined in this analysis prevents only 1,403 NTD-affected pregnancies, or about 70% of those judged to be preventable (CDC, 1992). Although higher levels of fortification are not considered in this analysis, it is possible that higher levels may be viable options.

This analysis supports the conclusions of a previously published cost-benefit analysis of fortification which reported a net benefit of $94 million for fortification at 0.14 mg, and $252 million at 0.35 mg (Romano et al., 1995). However, there are important differences in the assumptions used in each of the analyses. Based on limited data, Romano et al. assumed that 0.4 mg of total folate would be as effective as 0.4 mg of folic acid. Therefore, the number of NTDs prevented is significantly higher. The number of potential neurological complications is also greater, because they used a threshold of 0.85 mg of total folate for potential masking. The medical costs for neurological complications were assumed to be as costly as a case of subacute degeneration of the spinal cord, which is a fairly severe and costly outcome. In their comparison of fortification to supplementation, Romano et al. concluded that supplementation was more costly than fortification. However, compliance with a program of supplementation was not modeled, but was assumed to be 100%. Romano et al. also included $5 million in the cost of the fortification program to cover a surveillance system for potential adverse effects of increased folic acid consumption.

Finally, there were differences in the analyses that could be minimized as more analysts begin to include the Reference Case recommended by the PCEHM. For example, Romano et al.'s health outcome costs are significantly higher than in the current analysis, as they included indirect morbidity and mortality costs (productivity losses). They did not include time costs for caregiver services, and no health-related quality of life measures were used in this analysis.

Several limitations of the present analysis should be considered in interpreting its results. It is based on estimates of the national rates of NTD-affected pregnancies and vitamin B_{12} deficiency. There is no national surveillance program for vitamin B_{12} deficiency; thus, rates for Olmsted County, Minnesota, were applied to the entire population. Similarly, NTD rates from the metropolitan Atlanta area were used to estimate national rates. These rates may actually vary across racial and ethnic groups and geographic regions.

In this analysis we were dependent on very limited published data on the survival of persons born with spina bifida. The survival curves we used in this study are based on historical data that are unlikely to adequately reflect current medical practice. Recent developments in the treatment of spina bifida are likely to markedly improve survival rates of children born today. We have no information, however, on the long-term survival of these children.

Because neither the supplementation nor the fortification programs have been implemented, some uncertainties exist regarding the effectiveness of the programs. Many women of childbearing age, especially adolescents and low-income women, may be excluded from supplementation programs, because costs are borne largely by the women themselves. With limited data regarding likely compliance with supplementation, the estimates of effectiveness may be either overestimated or underestimated. However, sensitivity analyses indicate that fortification at higher levels always achieves a lower cost- effectiveness ratio than supplementation.

There are several reasons to believe that our Reference Case results may provide a lower bound estimate of the cost-effectiveness of these strategies. In the Reference Case, we limited our assessment of the impact on health-related quality of life to only three of the parties affected by an NTD-affected pregnancy: children born with spina bifida, children stillborn or dying in infancy due to anencephaly, and adults primarily over the age of 60 with neurological complications resulting from delayed diagnosis of vitamin B_{12} deficiency. The health-related quality of life of two other groups affected by NTD-affected pregnancies has not been included because of the lack of data and absence of methods to account for these impacts. First, the Reference Case does not include the lost QALYs of unborn children due to terminated pregnancies. An estimated 32% of NTD-affected pregnancies are prenatally diagnosed and electively terminated. We also did not account for the impact on the health-related quality of life of parents and families of NTD-affected children: neither the anguish associated with an NTD-affected pregnancy that ends in an elective termination, in stillbirth, or in early childhood death nor the anguish, stress, and caregiver burden imposed on families of a child who survives with spina bifida.

Limitations of the cost data

Important costs were excluded from the numerator of the C/E ratios that would have increased the cost-effectiveness of both fortification and supplementation. Because of lack of data and methodological guidance, we did not include the time costs for children with spina bifida seeking and receiving treatment. With adults, wages are used as a proxy for time spent in treatment. A suitable proxy for children's time is not available. We did include costs for caregivers to assist a person with spina bifida seeking and receiving treatment. This is, however, most likely an underestimate of the opportunity cost to the caregiver. Although the caregiver may not spend a 40-hour week assisting a person with spina bifida in seeking and receiving treatment, because of the frequent and often unpredictable demands, the caregiver, usually a parent, is often unable to hold either full-time or part-time employment.

We also did not include caregiver time for persons disabled by vitamin B_{12}–related neurological complications. Sensitivity analysis was conducted over a wide range in the cost of health outcomes. Including such costs would not have changed the results of the analysis; fortification at 0.70 remains cost saving and dominates all other strategies.

Difficulties in Assessing Health-Related Quality of Life

As discussed earlier, we used four different health-state classification systems to value the health-related quality of life associated with NTD-affected pregnancies. There was a 32% difference in the QALYs of persons born with spina bifida between the measure which produced the lowest estimate (YHL) and the measure which produced the highest estimate (HUI II) for health-related quality of life (Table B.4). For the Reference Case analysis, we used the QWB measure which produced a midrange score. The differences encountered here have been documented in previous studies and highlight the concern that comparability is somewhat compromised when differing health-state classification systems are used to estimate QALYs.

The use of a group of experts to describe prototypical health states associated with a particular condition provided us with a mechanism to gain information in a setting where primary data were unavailable. This limitation of data is the rule rather than the exception in cost-effectiveness evaluations of public health interventions which are almost exclusively done using secondary data sources. While the technique of relying on experts to ''describe'' rather than to ''value'' the health states allowed us to follow the PCEHM recommendations for use of community preferences, this technique had certain difficulties associated with it. First, on a questionnaire completed at the end of this exercise, some of the clinician experts reported discomfort with the task of characterizing a typical patient within lesion level. The different methods that each expert used in internally reconciling their subjective experiences of patients with different lesion levels raises the question of how accurate the average health state descriptions for the nine subgroups actually are. The mean health state reported within these classification systems by a representative sample of age-appropriate persons with the three levels of spinal cord lesion might provide a more accurate snapshot of the average patient. Further analyses looking at the variance in the scores between raters, and the test-retest reliability of the scores would be useful.

Second, spina bifida affects health status in a number of ways that some members of the advisory council felt were inadequately captured by these instruments. Unfortunately, even if primary data were available, asking persons with spinal cord lesions to holistically value their health state would preclude following the Reference Case recommendation that community, rather than patient weights be used.

Finally, our estimates of health-related quality of life of persons without spina bifida came from the published literature. In these studies health states have been gathered from representatives of the general population. The mean scores for health-related quality of life in these studies are less than 1 and decline with age. Although this is an appropriate selection of a baseline for use in a Reference Case analysis, it provided unlikely results in this analysis. It was not uncommon in this study for the mean score for an older adult with spina bifida to be *higher* than that of an adult without the condition. For example, the mean HUI-II score for a 75-year-old person without spina bifida was 0.78; the score for a 75-year-old person with the condition was 0.79. It is likely that expert assessments of the health state of persons with spina bifida accounted only for the impact of spina bifida and ignored the impact of other unrelated health conditions that emerge when population-based health states are used. The appropriate baseline score for calculating marginal impact of a health condition on the health-related quality of life needs further exploration and may depend on who is surveyed.

Although the use of preexisting YHL scores to estimate QALYs considerably lessened the difficulty of gathering data, this measure has only two domains and is therefore less likely than the other three to provide a nuanced description of the health states associated with spina bifida. This may not be a problem in broad-brushstroke resource-allocation studies; however, in comparing CEAs of competing therapies for a particular condition, this measure may fail to capture important differences in health outcomes. Finally, the sample size upon which the average is based is extremely small; only 17 persons in the NHIS sample were identified as having spina bifida, and this cannot be considered representative of the population of persons with spina bifida.

Public Policy Considerations

This analysis does not consider the extent to which fortification of the food supply would improve the folate nutritional status of the population. This benefit could be significant, as folate deficiency is one of the more common causes of nutritional anemia in the United States, particularly among pregnant and lactating women, the elderly, and adolescents of lower socioeconomic status (Bailey et al., 1980, 1982; Davis, 1986; Rosenberg et al., 1982). In addition, there is some evidence a folic acid food fortification program may decrease risk for other birth defects (Czeizel, 1995; Li et al., 1995; Shaw et al., 1995), myocardial infarction (Boushey et al., 1995; Stampher and Willet, 1993; Stampher et al., 1992), cervical dysplasia (Butterworth, 1993), and stroke (Brattsom et al., 1992). Although these associations are not well established, if they are borne out, they would have substantial impact in reducing the cost per QALY of fortification programs.

It has also been suggested that a fortification program could include both folic acid and vitamin B_{12}, in an effort to avert any potential negative consequences for people with undiagnosed vitamin B_{12} deficiency (Boushey et al., 1995). Further research is necessary before attempting to assess this option's effectiveness. While folate deficiency is most frequently caused by inadequate folate consumption, the most common cause of vitamin B_{12} deficiency is inadequate absorption rather than inadequate consumption (Herbert, 1988). Therefore, it is unclear whether enough vitamin B_{12} could be added to the food supply in order to overcome absorption problems.

The results of our analysis should be interpreted with regard for important differences in the distributive consequences associated with the intervention programs. The fortification programs impose costs and risks on populations other than those experiencing the benefits. The costs of a fortification program would be shared by all members of the population, not just those that are at risk for an NTD-affected pregnancy. The risk for masking vitamin B_{12} deficiency occurs among the older population, which, again, is not at risk for an NTD-affected pregnancy. A supplementation program does not have these distributive effects. The women consuming vitamin supplements are those experiencing the benefit of the program. In addition, the primary financial burden of a supplementation program is borne by those at risk for the preventable health outcome.

These distributive consequences are germane to decisions regarding the choice between supplementation and fortification interventions, but they also they bear on decisions among fortification programs. While higher levels of fortification programs save more QALYs and additional dollars, they also impose the risk of delayed or misdiagnosed vitamin B_{12} deficiency resulting in neurological complications on a greater number of people. However, if the potential benefits to other age groups described above are substantiated, the distributive consequences would shift.

Public policy regarding NTD prevention will be made not only on the basis of economics, but will also be made in order to maximize the prevention of NTDs while protecting the health of the general population, recognizing the legal, social, and ethical implications of each strategy. This analysis suggests that while fortification at 0.70 mg per 100 g of grain is the most cost-saving and most effective program, other fortification programs are also effective and save money. Supplementation is also effective, and may be a good use of resources if fortification—or higher levels of fortification—are ruled out on equity grounds. However, decision makers should be aware of the overall benefits to society that could be lost if some or all fortification options are excluded from consideration.

Notes

1. The terms "folic acid" and "folate" are sometimes used interchangeably in the literature. In this analysis, folic acid is used to describe the synthetic compound used in vitamin preparations and in fortification. Folate is the naturally occurring compound found in foods. Total folate is the sum of the two.

2. Version 2.9, Jim Hollenberg, Roslyn, NY.

3. Office of Statewide Health Planning and Development (OSHPD) hospital discharge abstract, 1988.

4. MediCal tape-to-tape claims file (MTTCF).

Acknowledgments

The authors would like to acknowledge the following individuals, without whom this analysis would not have been possible: Barbara Bowman, Glennis Elmore, J. David Erickson, Peter Franks, Ted Ganiats, Ralph Green, John Lindenbaum, Donald Lollar, Richard Olney, Steven M. Teutsch, and Alan Williams.

References

Bailey, L.B., Mahan C.S., and D. Dimperio. 1980. Folacin and iron status in low-income pregnancy adolescents and mature women. *Am J Clin Nutr* 33:1997–2001.

Bailey, L.B., P.A. Wagner, G.J. Christakis, C.G. Davis, H. Appledorf, P.E. Araujo, E. Dorsey, and J.S. Dinning. 1982. Folacin and iron status and hematological findings in Black and Spanish-American adolescents from urban low income households. *Am J Clin Nutr* 35:1023–32.

Bamforth, S.J., and P.A. Baird. 1989. Spina bifida and hydrocephalus: A population study over a 35-year period. *Am J Hum Genet* 44:225–32.

Berthelot, J.M., R. Roberge, and M.C. Wolfson. 1992. Calculation of health-adjusted life expectancy for a Canadian province using a multi-attribute utility function: A first attempt. In *Proceedings of the Sixth Meeting of the International Network on Health Expectancy (REVES-6)*, Montpellier, France, October 7–12, 1992.

Borch, K., and G. Liedberg. 1984. Prevalence and incidence of pernicious anemia. *Scand J Gastroenterol* 19:154–60.

Boushey, C.J., S.A.A. Beresford, G.S. Omenn, and A.G. Motulsky. 1995. A quantitative assessment of plasma homocysteine as a risk factor for vascular disease: Probable benefits of increasing folic acid intakes. *JAMA* 274:1049–57.

Bower, C., and F.J. Stanley. 1992. Periconceptional vitamin supplementation and neural tube defects: Evidence from a case-control study in Western Australia and a review of recent publications. *J Epidemiol Community Health* 40:157–61.

Bower, C., and F.J. Stanley. 1989. Dietary folate as a risk factor for neural-tube defects: Evidence from a case-control study in Western Australia. *Med J Aust* 150(5):613–19.

Brattsom, L., A. Lindgren, B. Israelsson, M.R. Malinow, B. Norrving, B. Upson, and A. Hamfelt. 1992. Hyperhomocysteinaemia in stroke: Prevalence, cause and relationship to type of stroke and stroke risk factors. *Eur J Clin Invest* 22:214–21.

Butterworth, C.E., and T. Tamura. 1989. Folic acid safety and toxicity: A brief review. *Am J Clin Nutr* 50:353–58.

Butterworth, C.E. 1993. Folate status, women's health, pregnancy outcome, and cancer. *J Am Coll Nutr* 12:438–41.

Centers for Disease Control and Prevention. (CDC). 1995. Economic costs of birth defects and cerebral palsy—United States, 1992. *MMWR* 44:695–99. Centers for Disease Control and

Prevention. (CDC). 1992. Recommendations for the use of folic acid to reduce the number of cases of spina bifida and other neural tube defects. *MMWR* 41(No. RR-14):1–7.

Cragan, J.D., H.E. Roberts, L.D. Edmonds, M.J. Khoury, R.S. Kirby, G.M. Shaw, E.M. Velie, R.D. Merz, M.B. Forrester, R.A. Williamson, D.S. Krishnamurti, R.E. Stevenson, and J.H. Dean. 1995. Surveillance for anencephaly and spina bifida and the impact of prenatal diagnosis—United States, 1985–1994. *CDC Surveillance Summaries* 44:SS-4.

Czeizel, A.E. 1995. Nutritional supplementation and prevention of congenital abnormalities. *Current Opin Obstet Gynecol* 7:88–94.

Czeizel, A.E., and I. Dudas. 1992. Prevention of the first occurrence of neural-tube defects by periconceptional vitamin supplementation. *N Engl J Med* 327:1832–35.

Davis, R.E. 1986. Clinical chemistry of folic acid. *Adv Clin* 25:233–94.

Drummond, M.F., G.L. Stoddart, and G.W. Torrance. 1987. *Methods for the economic evaluation of health care programmes*. New York: Oxford University Press.

Elwood, J.M., J. Little, and J.H. Elwood. 1992. *Epidemiology and control of neural tube defects*. Monographs in Epidemiology and Statistics, Vol. 20. Oxford: Oxford University Press.

Erickson, P., R.W. Wilson, and I. Shannon. 1995. *Years of healthy life*. Statistical Note No. 7. Hyattsville, MD: National Center for Health Statistics.

Essink-Bot, M.L., M.E. Stouthard, and G.J. Bonsel. 1993. Generalizability of valuations on health states collected with the EuroQol questionnaire. *Health Econ* 2:237–46.

EuroQol Group. 1990. EuroQol: A new facility for the measurement of health-related quality of life. *Health Policy* 16:199.

Feeny, D., W. Furlong, M. Boyle, and G.W. Torrance. 1995. Multi-attribute health status classification systems: Health utilities index. *Pharmacoeconomics* 7:490–502.

Food and Drug Administration. (FDA). 1993. Food Standards: Amendment to the Standards of Identity for Enriched Grain Products to Require Addition of Folic Acid (Docket No. 91N-100S). *Federal Register* (58 FR 53305-53312).

Food and Nutrition Board, National Research Council. (NRC). 1974. *Proposed fortification policy for cereal grain products*. Washington, D.C.: National Academy of Sciences Printing and Publishing Office.

Franks, P. 1995. *Personal communication*.

Ganiats, T. 1995. *Personal communication*.

Gold, M.R., P. Franks, and K. McCoy. 1994. Condition weight for chronic diseases from a nationally representative sample (abstract) *Med Decis Making* 14:431.

Greenberg, F., L.M. James, and G.P. Oakely, Jr. 1983. Estimates of the birth prevalence rates of spina bifida in the United States from computer-generated maps. *Am J Obstet Gynecol* 145(5):570–73.

Grimes, D.A. 1986. Unplanned pregnancies in the U.S. *Obstet Gynecol* 67:438–42.

Haddix, A., S. Teutsch, P. Shaffer, and D. Dunet. 1996. *Prevention Effectiveness: A guide to decision analysis and economic evaluation*. New York: Oxford University Press.

Healton, E.B., D.G. Savage, J.C.M. Brust, T.J. Garrett, and J. Lindenbaum. 1991. Neurologic aspects of cobalamin deficiency. *Medicine* 70(35):894–98.

Herbert, V. Anemias. 1988. In *Clinical nutrition, 2nd edition*, ed. D.M. Paige, 593–608. St. Louis: C.V. Mosby.

Herbert, V., and K.C. Das. 1994. Folic acid and vitamin B_{12}. In *Modern nutrition in health and disease, 8th edition*, ed. M.E. Shils, J.E. Olson, and M. Shike, 402–25. Philadelphia: Lea and Febinger.

Kaplan, R.M., and J.P. Anderson. 1988. A general health policy model: Update and applications. *Health Serv Res* Jun 23:203–35.

Kurland, L.T., and A.R. Zinsmeister. 1993. *Personal communication*.

Laurence, K.M., N. James, M.H. Miller, G.B. Tennant, and H. Campbell. 1981. Double-blind randomised controlled trial of folate treatment before conception to prevent recurrence of neural-tube defects. *Br Med J* 282:1509–11.

Li, D.K., J.R. Daling, B.A. Mueller, D.E. Hickok, A.G. Fanzel, and N.S. Weiss. 1995. Periconceptual multivitamin use in relation to the risk of congenital urinary tract anomalies. *Epidemiology* 6:212–18.

Life Science Research Office (LSRO). 1984. Assessment of the folate nutritional status of the U.S. population based on data collected in the second National Health and Nutrition Examination Survey, 1976–1980. Bethesda, MD: Federation of American Societies for Experimental Biology.

Lipscomb, J. 1986. Human capital, willingness-to-pay and cost-effectiveness analysis of screening for birth defects in North Carolina. Unpublished manuscript.

McLaurin, R.L., S. Oppenheimer, L. Dias, and W.E. Kaplan, Eds. 1986. *Spina bifida: A multidisciplinary approach.* New York: Praeger.

Medical Research Council (MRC) Vitamin Study Research Group. 1991. Prevention of neural tube defects: Results of the Medical Research Council study. *Lancet* 338:131–37.

Mertz, W., J.C. Tsui, J.T. Judd, S. Reiser, J. Hallfrisch, E.R. Morris, P.D. Steele, and E. Lashley. 1991. What are people really eating: The relation between energy intake derived from estimated diet records and intake determined to maintain body weight. *Am J Clin Nutr* 54:291–95.

Mills, J.L., G.G. Rhoads, J.L. Simpson, G.C. Cunningham, M.R. Conley, M.R. Lassman, M.E. Walden, D.R. Depp, and H.J. Hoffman. 1989. The absence of a relation between the periconceptional use of vitamins and neural-tube defects. *N Engl J Med* 321:430–35.

Milunsky, A., H. Jick, S.S. Jick, C.L. Bruell, D.E. MacLaughlin, K.J. Rothman, and W. Willett. 1989. Multivitamin/folic acid supplementation in early pregnancy reduced the prevalence of NTD. *JAMA* 262:2847–52.

Moss, A.J., A.S. Levy, I. Kim I, and Y.K. Park. 1989. Use of vitamin and mineral supplements in the United States: Current users, types of products, and nutrients. In *Advance data from vital and health statistics, No. 174,* Hyattsville, MD: National Center for Health Statistics.

Mulinare, J., J.F. Cordero, J.D. Erickson, and R.J. Berry. 1988. Periconceptional use of multivitamins and the occurence of neural tube defects. *JAMA* 260:3141–45.

Romano, P.S., N.J. Waitzman, R.M. Scheffler, and R.D. Pi. 1995. Folic acid fortification of grain: An economic analysis. *Am J Public Health* 85(5):667–76.

Rosenberg, I.H., B.B. Bowman, B.A. Cooper, C.H. Halsted, and J. Lindenbaum. 1982. Folate nutrition in the elderly. *Am J Clin Nutr* 36:1060–66.

Savage, D.G., and J. Lindenbaum. 1995. Folate-cobalamin interactions. In *Folate in health and disease,* ed. L.B. Bailey, 237. New York: Marcel Dekker.

Schafer, L.W., D.E. Larson, L.J. Melton, J.A Higgins, and A.R. Zinsmeister. 1985. Risk of development of gastric carcinoma in patients with pernicious anemia: A population-based study in Rochester, Minnesota. *Mayo Clinic Proc* 60:444–48.

Schwartz, S.O., S.R. Kaplan, and B.E. Armstrong. 1950. The long-term evaluation of folic acid in the treatment of pernicious anemia. *J Lab Clin Med* 35:894–98.

Shaw, G.M., E.J. Lammer, C.R. Wasserman, C.D. O'Malley, and M.M. Tolovara. 1995. Risks of orofacial clefts in children born to women using multivitamins containing folic acid periconceptually. *Lancet* 346:393–96.

Shaw, G.M., D. Schaffer, E.M. Velie, K. Morland, and J.A. Harris. 1995. Periconceptional vitamin use, dietary folate, and the occurence of neural tube defects. *Epidemiology* 6(3):219–26.

Smithells, R.W., M.J. Seller, R. Harris, D.W. Fielding, C.J. Schorah, N.C. Nevin, S. Sheppard,

A.P. Read, S. Walker, and J. Wild. 1983. Further experience of vitamin supplementation for prevention of neural tube defect recurrences. *Lancet* 1:1027–31.

Stampher, M.J., and W.C. Willet. 1993. Homocysteine and marginal vitamin deficiency: The importance of adequate vitamin intake (editorial). *JAMA* 270:2726–27.

Stampher, M.J., M.R. Malinow, W.C. Willett, L.M. Newcomer, B. Upson, D. Ullmann, P.V. Tishler, and C.H. Hennekens. 1992. A prospective study of plasma homocyst(e)ine and risk of myocardial infarction in US physicians. *JAMA* 268:877–81.

Texas Department of Health. 1992. An investigation of a cluster of neural tube defects.

Torrance, G.W., P. Erickson, D. Patrick, and J. Feldman. 1995a. Technical Notes. In *Years of healthy life*. Statistical Note No. 7, by P. Erickson, R.W. Wilson, and I. Shannon, 10–14. Hyattsville, MD.: National Center for Health Statistics.

Torrance, G.W., W. Furlong, D. Feeny, and M. Boyle. 1995b. Multi-attribute preference functions: Health utilities index. *Pharmacoeconomics* 9:503–20.

Torrance, G.W., Y. Zhang, D. Feeny, W.J. Furlong, and R. Barr. 1992. *Multi-attribute preference functions for a comprehensive health status classification system*. Working Paper No. 92-18. Hamilton, Ontario: McMaster University, Centre for Health Economics and Policy Analysis.

U.S. Bureau of Labor Statistics. 1995. *Employment and earnings*. Washington, D.C.: U.S. Department of Labor.

U.S. Department of Agriculture (USDA). 1990. *Nationwide food consumption survey/individual intake 1987–1988*. Springfield, VA: National Technical Information Service.

Vergel, R.G., L.R. Sánchez, B.L. Heredero, P.L. Rodríguez, and A.J. Martínez. 1990. Primary prevention of neural tube defects with folic acid supplementation: Cuban experience. *Prenat Diagn* 10:149–52.

Waitzman, N.J., P.S. Romano, and R.M. Scheffler. 1994. Estimates of the economic costs of birth defects. *Inquiry* 33:188–205.

Watson-Duff, E.M., and E.S. Cooper. 1994. Neural tube defects in Jamaica following Hurricane Gilbert. *Am J Public Health* 84:473–76.

Werler, M.M., S. Shapiro, and A.A. Mitchell. 1993. Periconceptional folic acid exposure and risk of occurrent neural tube defects. *JAMA* 269:1257–61.

Williams, A. 1995a. The measurement and valuation of health: A chronicle. Discussion Paper 136. York, Great Britain: Centre for Health Economics, University of York.

Williams, A. 1995b. The role of the EuroQol instrument in QALY calculations. Discussion Paper 130. York, Great Britain: Centre for Health Economics, University of York.

Williams, L.B., and W.F. Pratt. 1990. Wanted and unwanted childbearing in the United States: 1973–1988. Data from the National Survey of Family Growth. *Advance Data from the Vital and Health Statistics, No. 189*. Hyattsville, MD: U.S. Department of Health and Human Services, Public Health Service, Centers for Disease Control, National Center for Health Statistics.

Appendix C: The Cost-Effectiveness of Dietary and Pharmacologic Therapy for Cholesterol Reduction in Adults

AARON A. STINNETT, MURRAY A. MITTLEMAN,
MILTON C. WEINSTEIN, KAREN M. KUNTZ,
DAVID J. COHEN, LAWRENCE W. WILLIAMS,
PAULA A. GOLDMAN, DOUGLAS O. STAIGER,
MARIA G.M. HUNINK, JOEL TSEVAT,
ANNA N.A. TOSTESON, LEE GOLDMAN

Framing the Analysis

Background

In recent years, the medical and public health communities have increasingly focused on the role of lipids as risk factors for coronary heart disease (CHD). This heightened attention has resulted from a proliferation of clinical and epidemiological evidence demonstrating the effectiveness of cholesterol-lowering strategies for preventing CHD, the leading cause of mortality and morbidity in the United States.[1-7] High levels of serum total cholesterol (TC) and low-density lipoprotein (LDL) are now recognized as positive risk factors for CHD, while a high level of serum high-density lipoprotein (HDL) reduces the risk of CHD. In addition, while clinical trials of some cholesterol-lowering therapies have failed to demonstrate improvements in patients' survival,[8,9] a body of evidence from both clinical trials and observational studies indicates that cholesterol reduction may lower both CHD-related and all-cause mortality rates.[10-16]

Reflecting the important role of lipids as risk factors for CHD, expert panels of the National Cholesterol Education Program (NCEP) have recently issued recommendations on clinical and public health strategies for cholesterol reduction in adults.[17-19] In these reports, the NCEP has made it clear that cost-effectiveness is an important consideration in the evaluation of alternative strategies for cholesterol reduction. This recognition that both health effects and costs should be evaluated reflects the limited supply of resources available for investment in health and the large volume of resources at stake in decisions concerning the prevention and treatment of CHD.

Objective

The objective of the present study was to evaluate the cost-effectiveness of alternative diet- and drug-based clinical strategies for cholesterol reduction in U.S. adults according to patients' CHD risk factor characteristics. The results are intended to inform future efforts at clinical guideline development and, more generally, resource allocation decisions at the societal level. The diet considered here is the Step I Diet, and the medications considered are niacin and lovastatin.

In this study, we have attempted to improve on the methods of previous analyses in several ways. First, previous evaluations (with the exception of Hamilton et al.[20]) have measured lipid changes in terms of only TC; the present study considers the separate effects of changes in LDL and HDL. Second, this study considers both dietary therapy and alternative pharmacologic therapies, whereas most analyses to this point have focused on single interventions; we also explicitly consider the possibility that patients will discontinue or switch therapies due to drug intolerance. Third, the present study goes beyond effects on lipids, coronary events, and patient survival by making adjustments for quality of life. Fourth, this study estimates costs neglected in some prior studies, including the costs of patient time and downstream costs of non-CHD health care associated with prolonged survival. Finally, we consider in a sensitivity analysis the controversial possibility that cholesterol reduction directly causes an increase in non-CHD mortality beyond the change that would be expected due to the principle of competing risks.

Audience

The immediate audience for this analysis consists of readers of this book who wish to see an example of how the recommendations of the Panel on Cost-Effectiveness in Health and Medicine may be followed in practice, or at least of how one team of analysts has attempted to follow them. A later, more complete version of this analysis (including the consideration of more patient subgroups) will be targeted primarily to decision makers responsible for establishing recommendations for primary and secondary prevention of CHD through cholesterol reduction; such groups include, but are not limited to, the NCEP and the U.S. Preventive Services Task Force (USPSTF).

Type of Analysis

The present study is a cost-effectiveness analysis (CEA). The results are presented as incremental cost-effectiveness ratios, with health effects expressed in units of quality-adjusted life years (QALYs) and costs expressed in 1993 U.S. dollars.

Perspective

Because this analysis is intended to inform resource allocation decisions at the societal level, the societal perspective has been adopted. From this perspective, all costs and other consequences are taken into account, regardless of whom they affect.

Target Population

The present study focuses on strategies targeted to adults ages 35 and over in the United States. The results of prior cost-effectiveness analyses of cholesterol lowering strategies have consistently found that the cost-effectiveness of interventions depends heavily on the risk factor profiles of the target population.[21–29] A more complete analysis would consider a broad range of target populations defined by various combinations of risk factors for CHD, but for the purposes of this analysis we will consider three illustrative groups of patients who are at high, moderate, and low risk of CHD, with separate analyses for males and females in each group.

The high-risk population studied in this analysis consists of persons who have high LDL ($\geq$ 190 mg/dL) and low HDL ($<$ 35 mg/dL), and who also smoke cigarettes and have high diastolic blood pressure ($\geq$ 105 mmHg). The moderate-risk population includes patients who have high LDL and moderate HDL (35–49 mg/dL) and who do not smoke and have only mild hypertension (DBP 95–104 mmHg). The low-risk group consists of nonhypertensive (DBP $<$ 95 mmHg), nonsmoking patients with only moderately high LDL (160–189 mg/dL) and high HDL ($\geq$ 50 mg/dL).

Strategies

The prevention strategies considered in this analysis were combinations of primary and secondary prevention interventions; for example, one strategy is to use dietary therapy for primary prevention and 20 mg/day lovastatin for secondary prevention. *Primary prevention* refers here to interventions targeted to persons without prior CHD, while *secondary prevention* refers to interventions for people with a history of CHD.

The interventions considered here are: dietary therapy with the Step I Diet; pharmacologic therapy with niacin (3 g/day); pharmacologic therapy with lovastatin (20 or

40 mg/day); and stepped care, in which patients take niacin if they can tolerate it and otherwise take lovastatin. A ''do-nothing'' intervention, in which no cholesterol-lowering therapy is administered, was also evaluated. Throughout this analysis, we assumed that any antihyperlipidemic medication would be accompanied by dietary therapy and that any patient unable to tolerate a strategy's drug regimen would switch to dietary therapy alone.

Table C.1 summarizes the strategies evaluated in this study. For each of these primary–secondary prevention combinations (e.g., diet for primary prevention and niacin for secondary prevention), two strategies were considered: intervening in persons ages 35–84, and intervening only in those 55–84. For those strategies including a primary prevention intervention (other than ''do nothing''), we varied the target age groups only for primary prevention, assuming a backdrop of secondary prevention in all age groups. Thus, for men and women in each of the three risk factor groups considered here, we evaluated 47 strategies: (23 primary–secondary prevention combinations, enumerated

Table C.1 Strategies for Cholesterol Reduction Considered in this Evaluation[a]

Intervention for Primary Prevention	Intervention for Secondary Prevention
No primary prevention	No secondary prevention Step I Diet Niacin (3 g/day) Lovastatin (20 mg/day) Lovastatin (40 mg/day) Stepped care (with 20 mg/day lovastatin)[b] Stepped care (with 40 mg/day lovastatin)[b]
Step I Diet	Step I Diet Niacin (3 g/day) Lovastatin (20 mg/day) Lovastatin (40 mg/day) Stepped care (with 20 mg/day lovastatin)[b] Stepped care (with 40 mg/day lovastatin)[b]
Niacin (3 g/day)	Niacin (3 g/day) Lovastatin (20 mg/day) Lovastatin (40 mg/day) Stepped care (with 20 mg/day lovastatin)[b] Stepped care (with 40 mg/day lovastatin)[b]
Lovastatin (20 mg/day)	Lovastatin (20 mg/day) Lovastatin (40 mg/day)
Stepped care (with 20 mg/day lovastatin)[b]	Lovastatin (20 mg/day) Lovastatin (40 mg/day) Stepped care (with 20 mg/day lovastatin)[b] Stepped care (with 40 mg/day lovastatin)[b]

[a] Note that strategies are defined as combinations of primary prevention interventions (for patients without CHD) and secondary prevention interventions (for patients with a history of CHD).

[b] For stepped care, all patients begin taking niacin (3 g/day). Those unable to tolerate the niacin switch to lovastatin at the indicated dose.

in Table C.1) × (2 target age groups), plus the "do-nothing" strategy in which no prevention is undertaken.

Boundaries of the Study

This study addresses the impact of preventive interventions on the health and quality of life of patients in the target population. While family members and others are clearly affected by the patients' experiences, the Reference Case analysis does not include those effects due to a lack of data and prior research in this area. Another limitation of this study is that it does not evaluate alternative frequencies for population screening of lipids; a background of annual screening is assumed because methods have not yet been developed to model alternative screening schedules in the model used in this analysis (the CHD Policy Model, discussed later in this section).

In addition, not all possible pharmacologic agents for antihyperlipidemic therapy are evaluated, nor have we considered combinations of drugs for individual patients. However, two of the excluded classes of medications (fibric acid derivatives and hormones) have been linked with increased rates of non-CHD mortality in clinical trials,[30] and a third (bile acid sequestrants) has previously been found to be more costly and less effective than both niacin and lovastatin, the two medications evaluated here.[31] In addition, niacin and lovastatin offer interesting contrasts that make them appealing choices for comparators. Niacin is the least-expensive antihyperlipidemic medication (in terms of medication costs), while lovastatin is among the most costly. Furthermore, lovastatin, an HMG-CoA reductase inhibitor, is perhaps the best-tolerated antihyperlipidemic medication, while bothersome side effects (primarily flushing) are common among patients using niacin. Both medications have substantial effects on lipids and are among the most common cholesterol-lowering agents used in clinical practice.[32] Note that the results in this study for lovastatin do not necessarily extend to other drugs in the same class. A variety of HMG-CoA reductase inhibitors are available, with different costs and effects; we chose to consider lovastatin in this study because it is the most widely used and most studied cholesterol-lowering drug in its class. We also have not considered in this study all possible therapeutic doses for niacin and lovastatin.

Additional limitations of the present analysis (particularly with respect to data quality and availability) are discussed separately in the relevant sections of this report.

Time Horizon

Resource costs and effects on quality-adjusted life expectancy were estimated over a period of 50 years, beginning in 1995. This time horizon was chosen in order to capture the full life span of the youngest cohort present in the model in 1995. As discussed later, the CHD Policy Model includes detailed simulations for persons ages 35–84. For persons surviving to age 85, the model adds on a remaining sex-specific discounted life expectancy estimated from life tables; they are also assumed to have the same average quality of life and annual health care costs as persons 75–84. Thus, a simulation of 50 years is sufficient to model the full lifetime of persons who were age 35 (the youngest age included in the model) in the initial year of simulation.

Analytic Approach

Net costs and effects on quality-adjusted life expectancy were estimated using the Coronary Heart Disease Policy Model, a deterministic, population-based computer simulation model. Data used in the model were derived from a variety of sources, including clinical trials, observational studies, and public health statistics. The CHD Policy Model was developed prior to this study as a tool for use in performing forecasts and cost-effectiveness analyses of interventions to prevent or treat CHD. Previously published CEAs using the model include a comparison of antihypertensive therapies and a cost-effectiveness analysis of lovastatin for primary and secondary prevention.[33,34]

Using the model's estimates of net costs and quality-adjusted survival, we applied the methods of incremental CEA to calculate incremental cost-effectiveness (C/E) ratios for the 47 mutually exclusive prevention strategies described above for men and women in each of the three risk factor groups. To perform this analysis, we created a computer program that first identifies strongly dominated and extendedly dominated strategies and then calculates incremental C/E ratios for the remaining, undominated strategies. A strongly dominated strategy is both less effective and more costly than another strategy with which it is mutually exclusive; an extendedly (or weakly) dominated strategy is both less effective and more costly than a linear combination of two other strategies with which it is mutually exclusive. The methods of incremental CEA prescribe that dominated programs be eliminated from further consideration on efficiency grounds, so C/E ratios are meaningful only for undominated strategies.[35]

Estimates of health consequences and costs in the CHD Policy Model are population-based, rather than cohort-based. In other words, the present value of quality-adjusted survival and costs over the specificied time horizon are calculated with respect to the entire adult U.S. population cross-sectionally, and not with respect to a particular target cohort longitudinally. As long as the time horizon is sufficiently long, the resulting incremental cost-effectiveness ratios comparing intervention strategies are virtually identical.

Time Preference

All costs and quality-adjusted life years were discounted to present value at an annual rate of 3%.

Estimating and Valuing Outcomes

In this section, we discuss our estimation and valuation of health outcomes for the Reference Case analysis. This process consisted of the following steps: First, we estimated the rates at which patients would discontinue therapy or switch drugs for each prevention strategy being evaluated. Next, we estimated the effects of each strategy on patients' serum TC, LDL, and HDL. Finally, we used the CHD Policy Model to translate these lipid effects into estimates of survival, simultaneously weighing each person year in the model by a health-related quality-of-life measure based on values elicited from patients with similar health characteristics.

Drug Discontinuation and Switching Rates

A recent study by Andrade and colleagues reported discontinuation rates for various antihyperlipidemic medications according to the reason for discontinuation, based on data from two health maintenance organizations (HMOs) over the period 1988–1990.[36] In the present study, we assumed that patients switch drugs only if they are unable to tolerate the first-line medication. Andrade reported discontinuation rates due to adverse effects of 6.5% and 26.3% for lovastatin and niacin, respectively; these are the switching rates assumed in the present analysis. Discontinuations attributed by Andrade to drug ineffectiveness were not taken into account here for the following reasons: First, it is not clear how their study defined "ineffectiveness." A drug may have its expected effect on lipid levels yet be considered ineffective because the levels reached fail to achieve a physician-defined goal (such as TC < 240 mg/dL). If this is the case, then: (a) the discontinuations due to ineffectiveness may have been concentrated among patients with very high initial lipid levels, so applying this rate of ineffectiveness across risk factor groups would be inappropriate, and (b) if the expected effects of a medication are not adequate for some patient groups, this lack of therapeutic effectiveness should be reflected in the results of the present study rather than being built into the model's assumptions. Alternatively, ineffectiveness may indicate that a drug failed to have its expected effects on a particular patient's lipid levels. However, the present study's estimates of drugs' effects represent the average effects across a population of patients; some patients experience more-favorable effects and some experience less-favorable effects. Thus, if patients in whom the effect is below average were modeled as switching to other drugs, then the estimate of the first-line drug's effects would need to be adjusted upward to indicate above-average effects; however, sufficient data are not available to make such adjustments. In addition, some of the patients characterized by Andrade as discontinuing a particular therapy actually continued to take the initial medication but supplemented it with another drug; for example, about 7% of patients who began therapy with niacin later supplemented it with another cholesterol-lowering agent and were therefore classified as discontinuing niacin therapy (Dr. Susan Andrade, personal communication). The estimated discontinuation rates used in the present study are also consistent with the results of several long-term open-label trials reviewed by Andrade.

Because lovastatin is so well tolerated, we assumed that anybody unable to tolerate lovastatin would also be unable to tolerate niacin. Thus, we assumed in this study that 6.5% of those patients beginning on lovastatin would be unable to tolerate the drug (and also unable to tolerate niacin), and would therefore switch to the Step I Diet with no medication. For patients whose initial therapy was niacin, we assumed that 26.3% would be unable to tolerate the drug and would switch to lovastatin. Of the 26.3% switching to lovastatin, we assumed that 19.8% would tolerate lovastatin and the remaining 6.5% would be uanable to tolerate any cholesterol lowering drug and would switch to the Step I Diet with no medication.

Effects on Lipids

Dietary therapy

The NCEP recommends a low-fat diet such as the Step I Diet as a first step for cholesterol reduction in adults; a detailed decription of this diet can befound in the report of the NCEP Adult Treatment Panel II. We estimated the effects of dietary therapy on TC, LDL, and HDL by pooling the results of five studies in which a total of 178 outpatients were given dietary advice and follow-up counseling based on the Step I Diet. The findings of these studies are summarized in Table C.2. Results were aggregated by constructing a weighted average of percentage changes, with weights corre-

Table C.2 Estimated Effects of the Step I Diet, Pharmacologic Therapy with Niacin, and Pharmacologic Therapy with Lovastatin on Levels of Serum Total Cholesterol (TC), Low-Density Lipoprotein (LDL), and High-Density Lipoprotein (HDL)

Step I Diet	n	%Δ TC	%Δ LDL	%Δ HDL
Denke (1994)	41	−5.3	−6.2	−5.5
Denke and Grundy (1994)	50	−8.1	−7.8	0.0
Denke and Grundy (1995)	26	−8.5	−9.0	+2.9
Wood et al. (1991)	40	−7.8	−10.7	+1.8
Keenan et al. (1991)	21	+0.1	−2.8	−3.8
Pooled estimate		−6.5	−7.7	−0.9
Niacin (3 g/day)				
Illingworth et al. (1994)	68	−12.3	−16.3	+27.0
Knopp et al. (1985)	26	−12.9	−17.2	+27.8
Pooled estimate		−12.5	−16.6	+27.4
Lovastatin				
Bradford et al. (1991) 20 mg	1,642	−17	−24	+6.6
Bradford et al. (1991) 40 mg	1,646	−24	−34	+8.6

sponding to the number of patients in each study. To ensure that these estimates reflect as closely as possible the results that would be expected in clinical practice, studies in which patients received prepared meals or food items were excluded.

The estimated effect on TC is consistent with estimates reported by the NCEP Adult Treatment Panel II and is nearly identical to the mean 6.7% reduction observed in the Multiple Risk Factor Intervention Trial.[37] The finding that diet's favorable effect on LDL is partially offset by a reduction in HDL is consistent with several other studies noting reductions in both LDL and HDL among people on low-fat diets.[38–44]

Niacin

To estimate the lipid effects of niacin (3 g/day), we pooled the results of two randomized trials of crystalline niacin, weighing each study by the number of participants.[45,46] The results are shown in Table C.2. The pooled estimates are within the ranges reported by the NCEP Adult Treatment Panel II.

Similar effects (13% reduction in TC, 31% increase in HDL) were reported in a study by Alderman and colleagues of 101 patients receiving niacin therapy.[47] We did not include this study in our estimation because it had a lower target dose (2 g/day) and because some patients received sustained-release rather than immediate-release niacin. Sustained-release niacin has been reported to have smaller lipid effects and more serious side effects than standard (immediate-release) niacin.[48]

Lovastatin

We based our estimates of lovastatin's lipid effects on the results of the Expanded Clinical Evaluation of Lovastatin (EXCEL) Study, a multicenter, double-blind, diet- and placebo-controlled trial evaluating the safety and efficacy of lovastatin in patients with moderate hypercholesterolemia.[49,50] Results are summarized in Table C.2. These estimates are very similar to those reported in other studies[51–55] and are also consistent with estimates reported by the NCEP Adult Treatment Panel II.

Combined dietary and pharmacologic therapy

Throughout this analysis, we assumed that any antihyperlipidemic medication would be accompanied by dietary therapy. The effects of diet and drug therapy were assumed to be additive. This is supported by studies of diet and lovastatin,[56,57] while a study of diet and simvastatin found that the effect of diet modification was greater in patients not receiving drug therapy.[58]

Effects on CHD and Survival

Evidence from clinical trials

The results of clinical trials of cholesterol-lowering therapies have prompted considerable controversy. While these trials commonly report favorable effects on CHD event rates, not all have found favorable effects on CHD mortality, and some have reported increased rates of non-CHD mortality. Meta-analyses of these trials have reached conflicting conclusions.[59-61] Most recently, Gould and colleagues concluded from a meta-analysis of 35 long-term trials (including trials of diet, niacin, and lovastatin) that cholesterol reduction appears to reduce both CHD and all-cause mortality, with no effect on non-CHD mortality; adverse effects on non-CHD mortality observed in some trials appeared to result specifically from treatment with fibrates and hormones, rather than from cholesterol reduction per se.[62] Their study was distinguished from prior analyses in that it used trend analysis to relate the degree of cholesterol reduction to health outcomes and in that it allowed for the possibility that different types of interventions (e.g., diet versus estrogen therapy) may have different health effects.

Clinical trials of niacin and simvastatin (a member of the same drug class as lovastatin) for secondary prevention of CHD have reported statistically significant favorable effects on both CHD-related and all-cause mortality. In the Coronary Drug Project, patients in the niacin group (3 g/day) had mortality rates about 11% lower than the placebo control group after 15 years of follow-up.[63] In the Scandinavian Simvastatin Survival Study (4S), relative risks of 0.70 for all-cause mortality, 0.58 for coronary deaths, and 0.66 for major coronary events were reported after 6 years of follow-up for patients taking 10–40 mg/day simvastatin, compared with placebo.[64] In these trials, favorable effects on CHD events appeared to begin after about 1–2 years. Significant reductions in all-cause mortality began to appear after about 2 years in 4S and 6 years in the Coronary Drug Project; the reason for the longer delay in the Coronary Drug Project is not known. In the present study, we assume a 2-year delay between initiation of cholesterol-lowering therapy and the beginning of any health benefits.

Recent clinical trial data indicate that cholesterol reduction may also reduce all-cause mortality in persons with no history of CHD. In a study of primary prevention with pravastatin (40 mg/day) in 6,595 men with hypercholesterolemia but no history of CHD, the overall risk of death was 22% lower in the treatment group than in the placebo group after an average follow-up of 4.9 years ($p = 0.051$).[65] Differences in survival between the treatment and placebo groups appeared to begin within a year of initiating therapy. In their meta-analysis, which did not include the above study because it had not yet been published, Gould et al. estimated that the effects of primary prevention on CHD and all-cause mortality are similar in magnitude to the effects of secondary prevention, but the results for primary prevention were not statistically significant.

The CHD Policy Model
In the present study, the effects of cholesterol-lowering therapy on lipids were translated into effects on CHD and survival using the CHD Policy Model. This computer simulation model forecasts CHD incidence and prevalence, mortality, and resource costs under various assumptions regarding risk factor levels and treatment effects.[66-68] The model consists of three integrated submodels: the Demographic-Epidemiologic (DE) submodel, the Bridge submodel, and the Disease History (DH) submodel. The DE

submodel predicts CHD incidence and non-CHD mortality among subjects without prior CHD, stratified by sex, age (10-year age groups, 35–84), HDL level (<35, 35–49, ≥50 mg/dL), LDL level (<160, 160–189, ≥190 mg/dL), diastolic blood pressure (<95, 95–104, ≥105 mmHg), and smoking status (yes or no). Within the patient subgroups defined by these variables, patients are assumed to have the average value for each risk factor within that subgroup. Primary prevention interventions can be simulated by adjusting the mean risk factor levels within these subgroups of patients.

Patients who develop CHD move into the Bridge submodel. This portion of the model characterizes the initial CHD event (cardiac arrest, myocardial infarction, or angina pectoris) and estimates short-term mortality and treatment costs. Those who survive 30 days then move into the DH submodel, which predicts CHD events, revascularization procedures, CHD mortality, and non-CHD mortality among patients with a history of CHD. Two techniques for revascularization, coronary artery bypass grafting (CABG) and percutaneous transluminal coronary angioplasty (PTCA), are modeled.

The data sources used to develop the model have been described elsewhere.[69–71] The following discussion briefly summarizes some of the pertinent information. The U.S. population by age and sex for 1986 (the earliest year included in the model) and the estimated number of persons turning age 35 each year were obtained from the U.S. Bureau of the Census.[72] Mean levels of lipids, conditional on age and sex, were estimated from the Third National Health and Nutrition Examination Survey (NHANES III). Mean levels of diastolic blood pressure were obtained from the Second National Health and Nutrition Examination Survey (NHANES II), but because the survey was performed from 1976 to 1980, the values were updated to 1986 using observed trends in risk factors.[73,74] Smoking prevalence and the mean number of cigarettes smoked were estimated from the 1987 National Health Interview Survey.[75] The multivariate distribution of the five risk factors (TC, LDL, HDL, DBP, and smoking) was estimated by the method of iterative proportional fitting, based on the interactive structure of the data from NHANES II. Risk factor changes with age were estimated from cross-sectional analyses of the population in NHANES III (for lipids) and NHANES II (for blood pressure and smoking).

The age- and gender-specific prevalence of CHD at the beginning of 1986 was based on the 1986 National Health Interview Survey.[76] Based on 36-year follow-up data, multiple logistic risk functions were estimated for the CHD Policy Model by the Framingham Heart Study[77] to predict the annual probability of a CHD event or non-CHD death depending on risk factor levels, including interaction terms between risk factors and age. The CHD incidence risk function was calibrated so that age- and sex-specific CHD incidence in 1980 was equivalent to an estimate derived from a combination of data from Framingham, Massachusetts, and Olmsted County, Minnesota, adjusted for the racial composition of the U.S. population.[78–81] The frequencies of cardiac arrest, myocardial infarction (MI), and angina pectoris as the initial presenting evidence of CHD were also estimated using data from Framingham and Olmsted County. Thirty-day survival rates after cardiac arrest were estimated by pooling results from five papers.[82–86] Thirty-day survival rates after MI were obtained form the Worcester Heart Attack Study for the years 1986 and 1988 (Dr. Robert Goldberg, personal communication). Coronary attack rates (MI or arrest) conditional on a history of angina pectoris, and annual rates of recurrent MI, were estimated from Olmsted County data.[87]

The model was calibrated to data from 1980 and 1986 by comparing its predicted mortality with national data on the number of age- and gender-specific acute and chronic CHD and non-CHD deaths from U.S. *Vital Statistics*.[88,89] In addition, the predicted number of MIs in 1986 was compared with data from the U.S. Hospital Discharge Survey.[90] The calibration process involved the reestimation of several variables for which there were multiple estimates available and determining which combination of values from reliable sources led to the best agreement with *Vital Statistics* and hospital discharge data.

Delay in health effects

Based on studies noting a delay between the initiation of cholesterol-lowering therapy and changes in health outcomes,[91–93] we assumed that antihyperlipidemic therapy would not have any health effects until the third year of therapy. This is an imprecise estimate; effects on CHD events may actually begin sooner, but some studies (including the niacin portion of the Coronary Drug Project[94]) have noted even longer delays before a statistically significant effect on overall survival was observed.

Effects on Health-Related Quality of Life

We estimated health-related quality of life (HRQL) weights for people with a history of CHD based on whether or not they had angina or congestive heart failure (CHF). Primary data from the Framingham Heart Study were used to estimate the prevalence of angina and CHF as a function of age, gender, and history of MI. CHF and angina were assumed to be conditionally independent, because the sample included too few patients with both angina and CHF to produce reliable prevalence estimates for this combination of conditions. To estimate the prevalence of angina, CHF, and the combination of angina and CHF for each state in the DH submodel of the CHD Policy Model, we made two additional assumptions. First, due to a lack of data on cardiac arrest survivors, we assumed that survivors of cardiac arrest have symptom distributions identical to those of comparable CHD patients without cardiac arrest. Second, based on the results of the Coronary Artery Surgery Study (CASS), we assumed that revascularization reduces the long-term prevalence of angina by 50%.[95] Larger short-term effects have been reported, but these effects appear to wane with time.[96] Clinical trial results suggest that PTCA may have smaller short-term effects than CABG but that this difference diminishes with time.[97] In the absence of data, we assumed that revascularization has no effect on CHF.

HRQL weights were then estimated for each of four health states: the absence of angina and CHF ("asymptomatic"); angina without CHF; CHF without angina; and the combination of angina and CHF. We estimated these weights by pooling time-tradeoff (TTO) responses from patients involved in the Acute Myocardial Infarction (AMI) Patient Outcome Research Team (PORT) and the Beaver Dam Health Outcomes Study (BDHOS). The results are summarized in Table C.3.

Data from the AMI PORT included estimates for each of the four health states of interest (personal communication, Dr. Edward Guadagnoli and Dr. Paul Cleary, AMI PORT). However, the BDHOS did not stratify patients with angina according to whether or not they also had CHF (and vice versa);[98] therefore, we assumed that no patients in that study had both angina and CHF. To then estimate an HRQL weight for patients with both angina and CHF based on the BDHOS data, we assumed that CHF reduces patients' health-related quality of life by the same percentage whether or not they have angina. Thus, a BDHOS estimate for the health-related quality of life with angina and CHF was calculated as:

$$(\text{HRQL with angina}) \times (\text{HRQL with CHF/HRQL without symptoms})$$

We tested this estimation procedure using the AMI PORT data; the calculation yielded an estimate of 0.855 for the combination of angina andCHF, which is slightly higher than the estimate of 0.829 elicited directly from patients. This suggests that this estimation procedure is imperfect, but perhaps not entirely unreasonable in the absence of a direct estimate.

We pooled the TTO estimates from these two studies by taking an unweighted average of these estimates for each health state. The results are shown in Table C.3. We used the pooled estimate for health-related quality of life without angina or CHF both for asymptomatic persons with CHD and for all persons without CHD. We then com-

Table C.3 Estimated Health-Related Quality-of-Life Weights for Persons According to the Presence or Absence of Angina and Congestive Heart Failure (CHF)

| Health State | Time-Tradeoff Estimates | | |
	AMI PORT	Beaver Dam Health Outcomes Study	Pooled Estimate
Asymptomatic	0.935	0.869	0.902
	(n = 398)	(n= 1,225)	
Angina (no CHF)	0.896	0.786	0.841
	(n = 41)	(n = 65)	
CHF (no angina)	0.892	0.710	0.801
	(n = 316)	(n = 28)	
Angina and CHF	0.829	0.642	0.736
	(n = 290)	(calculated)	

bined these HRQL estimates with the estimates of CHF and angina prevalence discussed above to calculate average HRQL weights by age and sex for each state in the DH submodel of the CHD Policy Model.

While these weights were not estimated using a community-based preference weighting system, we judged them to be the best available proxies for community preferences. The BDHOS reported estimates using the Quality of Well-Being Scale (QWB), which relies on community weights, but the sample sizes for the BDHOS calculations for angina ($n = 68$) and CHF ($n = 30$) were quite small. By using the time-tradeoff results instead, we were able to pool studies so that data from more respondents could be incorporated. In addition, the BDHOS did not report HRQL weights for patients having both angina and CHF. Estimates from other community-based health-state classification systems were not available to estimate community preferences for the health states of interest.

Next, short-term HRQL adjustments were made to account for the disutility associated with events (MI, cardiac arrest, or revascularization) occurring in the Bridge and DH submodels of the CHD Policy Model. These adjustments assumed that patients have a utility of zero throughout periods of hospitalization for these events. Based on published reports, hospital lengths of stay were estimated to be 8 days for MI or cardiac arrest, 12 days for CABG, and 5 days for PTCA.[99–104] These short-term HRQL adjustments are not precise. The assumption of zero utility (which, by definition, corresponds to the utility of a health state considered preferentially equivalent to death) during hospitalization is not based on any empirical data. Some patients would assign a higher value to this state, while some other patients may value these periods of acute health problems as actually being ''worse than death.'' In addition, these length-of-stay estimates do not incorporate recovery time outside the hospital; health-related quality of life after leaving the hospital is assumed to be a function of angina and CHF prevalence (and any additional CHD events).

We assumed in this analysis that diet and medication do not directly affect patients' health-related quality of life. This assumption for dietary therapy is supported by a study that found no effects on quality of life in a randomized trial of a physician-directed diet treatment program ($n = 346$); in that study, quality of life was measured using scales measuring taste, cost, convenience, and ''perception that one is taking care of one's own health.''[105] The assumption for medication is supported by data from the BDHOS, which found that taking antihyperlipidemic medication ($n = 78$, out of 1356 participants) had no significant effect on either TTO or QWB scores.[106] This is also supported by an analysis of 1,100 patients participating in a randomized, double-blind, placebo-controlled trial of lovastatin for primary prevention, which found no effects on either general health perceptions or emotional well-being after 1 year of therapy.[107] In addition, as discussed above, the present study models patients experiencing adverse effects from pharmacologic therapy as switching to other therapies; thus, any lasting utility-lowering effects on these patients are unlikely.

Estimating Costs

Throughout this study, all costs were converted to 1993 U.S. dollars using the Medical Care Component of the Consumer Price Index (CPI).

Estimating Costs with Medicare Data

As discussed below, our estimates of costs for physician and hospital services in this study were based primarily on Medicare data. The extent to which these estimates differ from costs for people insured through sources other than Medicare is debatable. Miller et al. estimated that, on average, physician fees under Medicare were about 76% of the fees submitted to private insurers in 1990; Medicare fees were about 93%, 51%, and 46% of private fees for office visits, major procedures, and diagnostic tests, respectively.[108] Estimates reported by the Physician Payment Review Commission indicate that the gap between Medicare and private fees has been widening; they estimate that the ratio of Medicare to private fees (using the Medicare service mix) was 67% in 1989, 65% in 1990, and 61% in 1991.[109] However, due to well-documented market failures in the health care sector, the relationship between private fees and actual resource costs is not clear. Indeed, Medicare's fee schedule was designed in part to approximate the opportunity costs of resources more closely than do fees in the private sector.[110] It has also been noted that Medicare fees are about 67% higher than fees paid to physicians in Canada.[111]

Prevention costs

Office visits

The cost of an office visit was estimated as the value of a 15-minute visit for an established patient, based on Medicare's Resource-Based Relative Value Scale (RBRVS). Using 1994 RBRVS values, this procedure is valued at 0.97 relative value units (RVUs), with a primary care conversion factor of $33.718 per RVU.[112] Thus, each visit is estimated to cost $32.71 in 1994 U.S. dollars ($31.22 in 1993 dollars).

We assumed that all patients except those under the "do-nothing" (no prevention) strategy would require one office visit each year for lipid tests. Patients on dietary therapy were assumed to also require an annual midyear follow-up visit, as suggested by the NCEP Adult Treatment Panel II. We further assumed that patients taking medication would require an average of five visits in the first year of treatment and two visits per year in subsequent years (consistent with NCEP's guidelines). Patients switching from medication to diet alone were assumed to require one fewer visit in the first year than patients remaining on medication. Patients switching from niacin to lovastatin were assumed to require one extra office visit during the first year of therapy.

Patient time

The costs of patient travel, waiting, and treatment time associated with office visits were also estimated. We assumed that each visit would entail 15 minutes of medical care. This is consistent with four studies estimating median physician encounter times between 11 and 20 minutes for office visits by established patients; a fifth survey reported a median time of less than 10 minutes.[113] Estimates of patient travel time and waiting time were based on results from the 1987 National Medical Expenditure Survey.[114] Because there was very little variation in responses across gender or age groups, we used overall mean values for the survey population to estimate times for all patient subgroups. Survey results are presented in Table C.4. The average waiting time for patients in each interval was estimated as the midpoint of that interval; thus, times of 15 minutes and 45 minutes were assumed for patients reporting times of less than 30 minutes and 30–59 minutes, respectively. We assumed an average time of 75 minutes for patients reporting times greater than 60 minutes. This resulted in estimates of 41 minutes and 30 minutes for average round-trip travel time and average waiting time, respectively. This corresponds to a total of 86 minutes, or 1.43 hours, of patient time for each office visit.

To value patient time, we used the average hourly earnings of employed persons reporting earnings in the 1993 Current Population Survey as an estimate of the opportunity cost of time for all persons (employed or unemployed) in the corresponding age and gender group. Table C.5 reports the estimated average hourly earnings by age and sex. The total sample size for these calculations was nearly 100,000.

Laboratory costs

The costs of laboratory tests were estimated using the average Medicare payment for those tests in 1994. The estimated costs, in 1994 U.S. dollars, were $3.00 per specimen collection for phlebotomy; $6.23 per measurement of TC; $11.75 per measurement of HDL; and $15.50 per automated multichannel chemical profile.[115] The automated chemical profile was assumed to include measurement of both TC and triglycerides, as well as transaminases and other chemicals routinely monitored for patients on lovastatin and niacin; this chemical profile has almost the same cost as ordering separate tests of only TC ($6.23) and triglycerides ($8.20). These costs were deflated to 1993 dollars using the Medical Care Component of the CPI.

Table C.4 The Distribution of Patient Travel Time and Waiting Time for Usual Source of Medical Care[a]

	< 30 Minutes	30–59 Minutes	≥ 60 Minutes
Travel time (one-way)	84.2%	13.0%	2.5%
Waiting time	57.5%	22.8%	10.7%

a. Data taken from the results of the 1987 National Medical Expenditure Survey. Numbers do not add to 100% due to responses of "unknown."

Table C.5 Average Hourly Wages by Age Group and Sex, Based on 1993 Data
from the Current Population Survey

	Average Hourly Wages (1993 U.S. Dollars per Hour)	
Age Group	Male	Female
35–44	14.69	11.69
45–54	16.01	11.69
55–64	14.94	10.57
65–84	13.06	8.56

We assumed that annual visits for lipid testing would include a phlebotomy, chemical profile (including measurement of TC and triglycerides), and HDL measurement for each patient. Patients on dietary therapy were assumed to also have an additional phlebotomy and measurement of TC at a midyear follow-up visit. In addition to the annual lipid testing, patients on their first year of medication were modeled as receiving another four sample collections, chemical profiles, and HDL measurements. This was decreased to three extra visits for patients who discontinue medication in midyear and switch to diet, and was increased to five for patients who switch drugs (from niacin to lovastatin) during the year. In subsequent years, patients taking medication were assumed to receive a midyear phlebotomy, chemical profile, and HDL measurement in addition to their annual testing of lipids.

Medication costs

Based on compliance results reported by Knopp et al., we assumed that the average patient on niacin therapy takes 90% of the suggested dose.[116] Based on the results of a multicenter study of lovastatin, we assumed that the average patient on lovastatin therapy takes 95% of the suggested dose.[117]

We estimated medication costs using 1994 price levels.[118,119] For niacin, the cost was estimated using HCFA's Federal Upper Limit price, which determines Medicaid's reimbursement for multiple-source drugs. The estimated cost was $2.84 for 100 tablets (500 mg/tablet); this is lower than the average wholesale prices of the highest-cost manufacturers of niacin but higher than those reported by several lower-cost manufacturers. For lovastatin, costs were estimated using the 1994 average wholesale price, which was $1.997 per 20-mg tablet. Thus, incorporating the above estimates of noncompliance, annual medication costs (after deflating to 1993 dollars) were estimated to be $53.43, $660.95, and $1,321.90 for patients on daily doses of 3 g niacin, 20 mg lovastatin, and 40 mg lovastatin, respectively.

Patients who switch from medication to diet were assumed to incur half of the above annual medication costs for 1 year. For patients switching from niacin to lovastatin under a stepped-care approach, we assumed that the medication costs would be the average of the above costs for niacin and the appropriate dose of lovastatin during the first year and would be equal to the annual costs for lovastatin in subsequent years. We also assumed that patients taking niacin would require aspirin (one 325-mg tablet per day) to alleviate side effects during the first year of therapy.[120,121] Each dose of aspirin was assumed to cost $0.00629 (in 1993 dollars), which was calculated as the mean of the five lowest prices for 325-mg tablets in 1994.[122] Based on reports that problems with flushing abate with time,[123-126] we assumed that no aspirin would be required beyond the first year of therapy. Due to the limited time for which aspirin would be required, no effects of aspirin on CHD or survival were modeled in this study.

Costs of Treating CHD

The definitions and estimates of CHD-related cost variables in the CHD Policy Model are summarized in Table C.6.

Hospital costs
Hospital costs for cardiac procedures and MI, as well as annual hospital costs, were estimated from the Medicare Provider Analysis and Review (MEDPAR) files for Medicare beneficiaries admitted to a hospital in 1987 with a primary diagnosis of acute MI ($n = 218,427$), in conjunction with the AMI Patient Outcome Research Team (PORT). All costs were inflated to 1993 dollars using the Medical Care Component of the CPI. Total hospitalization costs were calculated by summing a number of component costs that reflect both accommodation and ancillary costs. The accommodation costs identify

Table C.6 Estimated Age-Specific CHD-Related Costs Used in the CHD Policy Model (in 1993 U.S. Dollars)

	Age-Specific Cost Estimates		
Description	35–64	65–74	75–84
Cost of AMI for survivors (first 30 days)	$12,600	$12,750	$13,160
Cost of AMI for those dying within 30 days	$9,050	$9,050	$9,050
Cost of cardiac catheterization (30-day)	$7,298	$7,868	$10,158
Cost of PTCA and catheterization (30-day)[a]	$18,343	$19,043	$22,733
Cost of CABG and catheterization (30-day)	$32,696	$33,116	$35,996
Cost of AMI and catheterization (30-day)	$16,698	$17,168	$19,008
Cost of AMI, PTCA, and catheterization (30-day)[a,b]	$26,213	$26,543	$28,253
Cost of AMI, CABG, and catheterization (30-day)	$40,372	$40,946	$44,446
Annual cost without prior revascularization (first year)	$2,352	$2,352	$2,352
Annual cost without prior revascularization (subsequent years)	$1,082	$1,082	$1,082
Annual cost following revascularization (first year)	$2,064	$2,064	$2,064
Annual cost following revascularization (subsequent years)	$949	$949	$949
Cost of hospitalization for CHF	$6,770	$6,770	$6,770
Cost of initial 30 days with angina	$2,762	$2,762	$2,762

a. PTCA costs are multiplied by 1.4 to reflect repeat procedures due to clinical restenosis (a rate of 30% is assumed); 7% of the marginal cost of CABG is added to PTCA costs to reflect emergency CABGs.

b. Proportion of hospital costs attributed to PTCA = 45%; 55% is attributed to MI.

routine, intensive care, and coronary care units and were obtained by applying a calculated per diem cost for each unit to the number of days in each unit given in the
Medicare Part A data. The ancillary costs identify the six largest departments and a
final "catch-all" category. For each ancillary component, a calculated ratio of cost to
charge (RCC) was applied to the Part A charges. Costs were available for patients ages
65 and over in 5-year age groups. The costs for patients under age 65 were assumed to
be equal to those for the 65–69-year age group, the closest age group for which we had
data.

Thirty-day costs with MI and no procedures. Patients who did not have a
cardiac catheterization, PTCA, or CABG in the first 30 days following their index MI
were stratified by whether or not they survived the first 30 days and by 5-year age
groups. An age trend was observed only for patients who survived the 30 days, ranging
from $10,281 for patients 65–69 to $10,841 for patients 75–84. Patients dying within
30 days had an average cost of $7,474.

Thirty-day costs with MI and cardiac procedure. Estimates of hospital costs
in the first 30 days after the index MI were stratified by age and by cardiac procedures
performed within the 30-day period. The resulting estimates (depending on age) were
$13,972–$16,282 for cardiac catheterization only, $17,019–$18,718 for cardiac catheterization and PTCA, and $35,221–$39,291 for cardiac catheterization and CABG.

Thirty-day costs without MI. Hospital costs for revascularization interventions
without MI were estimated from 30-day costs for procedures that were performed at
least 30 days after an index MI. Specifically, for the 1987 Medicare MI cohort, each
subsequent cardiac procedure (cardiac catheterization, PTCA, or CABG) through 1989
was identified and 30-day costs following that claim were obtained. Other cardiac admissions within the 30-day period defined the category for which the 30-day cost was
assigned (e.g., catheterization and CABG). If the 30-day window included an AMI,
then that 30-day cost was not included in the estimate. The resulting estimates (depending on age) were $6,891–$9,204 for cardiac catheterization only, $10,375–$13,493
for cardiac catheterization and PTCA, and $29,860–$33,160 for cardiac catheterization
and CABG.

Congestive heart failure. The total cost for hospitalization for CHF was obtained
from an ancillary study of the Survival and Ventricular Enlargement (SAVE) trial.[127]
The physician fee was calculated based on average length of stay estimated from SAVE
patients using the median reimbursement rate for the initial hospital day (Current Procedural Terminology [CPT] code = 99222), each subsequent day (CPT code = 99232),
and for the discharge day (CPT code = 99238).

Angina. We assumed that half of patients with new-onset angina are hospitalized, and the cost for those hospitalized was estimated using 1994 values from Medicare's Prospective Payment System for DRG 140 (angina pectoris). The resulting estimate for average hospital costs for the initial 30 days with angina was $1,262, in 1993 dollars. Having no data on physician fees in the initial 30 days of angina, we assumed a cost of $1,500 in 1993 dollars. Thus, the total cost was estimated to be $2,762 (in 1993 dollars). More accurate estimation of these costs is recommended as a topic for further research.

Annual costs. The annual hospitalization cost for the first year for patients who survive the first 30 days was estimated from the 1987 MI cohort for two patient groups: those who underwent revascularization in the first 30 days after MI ($897) and those who did not undergo revascularization during this 30-day period ($1,185). The relative cost relationship between the first and subsequent years reported by Hemenway et al.[128] (54% decrease in annual cost in subsequent years) was assumed to hold for both the revascularization and medical therapy groups. No age trend was observed in annual hospital costs. When a 30-day cost was used in a subsequent year for patients in the DH submodel of the CHD Policy Model, it was added to 11/12ths of the annual cost in that year.

Physician costs

The costs of physician services associated with cardiac catheterization, PTCA, and CABG were based on the Medicare Fee Schedule under RBRVS.[129] Estimated physician fees associated with MI include outpatient costs within the first 30 days after an MI.

Myocardial infarction. For patients who survive the first 30 days of an MI, the physician cost was estimated to be $2,319, after inflating to 1993 dollars. Physician costs for patients dying within 30 days of an AMI compared with survivors are assumed to be in the same proportion as the hospital costs (0.68), resulting in an estimate of $1,576.

Cardiac catheterization. We estimated the physician cost for cardiac catheterization as the sum of Medicare fees for left heart catheterization ($253.37), left ventricular injection ($52.65), and coronary injection ($101.02), for a total physician cost of $407.

Coronary angioplasty. We assumed that, on average, 50% of PTCAs are one-vessel (Medicare fee = $906.53) and 50% are two-vessel (Medicare fee $1,186.22), resulting in an estimated average physician cost for PTCA of $1,046.

Coronary artery bypass surgery. We assumed that all operations use an internal mammary graft (IMA) and that 50% of CABGs are two-vessel (1 IMA + 1 vein graft) and 50% are three-vessel (1 IMA + 2 vein grafts). Using Medicare physician fees of $2,126.36 for CABG with IMA, $201.46 for one vein graft, and $402.91 for two vein grafts, the resulting estimated average physician cost for CABG was $2,429.

Annual outpatient costs

The average annual cost of outpatient visits for patients with coronary artery disease (CAD) was calculated by multiplying the average number of outpatient visits per person with CAD by the average cost per outpatient visit. The average annual number of office visits to cardiovascular specialists over the period 1989–1990 was approximately 3,234,000.[130] For patients with angina pectoris, 35.3% of office visits were to a cardiovascular specialist. Assuming that this percentage applies across all CAD categories, the average annual number of office visits for persons with CAD is approximately 9,161,473 (= 3,234,000/0.35). The number of persons with CAD in 1989 was 6,948,000.[131] Thus, the average number of annual outpatient visits per person with CAD was 1.3186 (= 9,161,473/6,948,000). The average cost per outpatient visit was estimated from an analysis of Medicare beneficiaries at cardiovascular clinics in 1992; direct cost per visit was $131 and ancillary cost per visit was $122. Thus, we estimated the average annual cost of outpatient visits for a patient with coronary artery disease to be $333.61 (= $253 × 1.3186) in 1992 dollars and $353 in 1993 dollars.

Annual medication costs

Annual medication costs were estimated directly from the SAVE trial.[132] The costs of cardiac medications were estimated using 1991 wholesale prices[133] plus a dispensing fee of $4.24 per 1-month supply. In the SAVE trial, medication costs were determined for two groups of patients: those in the captopril group who received captopril ($631 per year) plus "other cardiac medications" ($338 per year) and those in the placebo group who received only "other cardiac medications" ($462 per year). For annual medication costs, an average of these two groups was used, yielding an estimate of $715.50 in 1991 dollars and $814 in 1993 dollars. Although resource consumption by patients participating in a clinical trial might not be representative of resource consumption by the average patient, no better estimates of average annual medication costs were available.

Non-CHD Health Care Costs

We included in our cost estimates age-specific average annual non-CHD health care costs. To do this, we first obtained estimates of per capita health care costs by age group based on data from the 1987 National Medical Expenditure Survey (NMES) (Agency for Health Care Policy and Research, personal communication). These estimates include expenses paid by individuals, private insurers, and public programs (Medicare, Medicaid, Civilian Health and Medical Program of the Uniformed Services and of the

Veteran's Administration [CHAMPUS/CHAMPVA], and the Indian Health Service) for hospital services, professional fees, prescribed drugs, home health care services, medical equipment, dental care, and vision care. Because these estimates include CHD-related costs, we then made adjustments to avoid double-counting these costs. To do so, we used the CHD Policy Model to estimate average CHD-related costs by age group for the year 1995. These costs were then subtracted from the NMES estimates of total health care costs per year to produce estimates of per capita non-CHD health care costs (with all costs expressed in 1993 U.S. dollars). The resulting estimates were $1,540 for persons 35–44, $2,930 for persons 45–64, and $6,020 for persons ages 65 and over.

These estimates do have shortcomings. First, they are not gender-specific; we had gender-specific estimates of CHD-related costs, but not of total health care costs. Second, any changes in real non-CHD health care costs per capita since 1987 are not reflected. These estimates also do not reflect any correlations between non-CHD costs and other risk factors in this model, such as smoking status. More precise estimation of these costs is recommended as a topic for further research. However, using these estimates more accurately reflects the true levels of non-CHD health care costs than omitting them altogether would.

Results of Reference Case Analysis

In this section, we focus our discussion on those strategies that were found not to be dominated. Full results, including dominated strategies, are attached as an Addendum.

High-Risk Patients

The results of the Reference Case analysis for high-risk males and females are shown in Table C.7. Note that the costs reported in this table represent sex-specific 50-year-discounted health care costs for persons 35 and over in the United States. Similarly, the reported values for quality-adjusted survival represent sex-specific 50-year discounted quality-adjusted survival for persons 35 and over in the United States. Costs and quality-adjusted survival reported in subsequent tables should be be interpreted in the same way.

Of the 47 strategies analyzed [(23 combinations of primary and secondary prevention interventions) × (2 target age groups) + the "no prevention" strategy], all but four for males and six for females are dominated. All undominated strategies for this risk factor group have incremental C/E ratios below $50,000/QALY.

Note that all of the undominated strategies in this group employ diet, niacin, or stepped care for primary prevention and either niacin or stepped care for secondary prevention. Strategies that employ no primary prevention and/or no secondary prevention are dominated—that is, they cost more and are less effective than strategies with primary and secondary prevention. Note also that lovastatin is dominated as a first-line

Table C.7 Results of Reference Case Analysis for High-Risk Males and Females[a]

Strategy		Results		
Primary Prevention	Secondary Prevention	Total Discounted Cost (1993 U.S. $)	Total Discounted QALYs	Incr. C/E Ratio
Males				
Niacin	Niacin	6,016,242,552,210	1,713,749,326	—
Niacin	Stepped care (20 mg)	6,016,246,980,274	1,713,752,677	1,321
Niacin	Stepped care (40 mg)	6,016,263,345,777	1,713,753,984	12,521
Stepped care (20 mg)	Stepped care (40 mg)	6,016,311,999,666	1,713,755,183	40,579
Females				
Diet (55–84)	Niacin	7,055,681,367,180	1,913,368,606	—
Niacin (55–84)	Niacin	7,055,706,336,711	1,913,387,197	1,343
Niacin	Niacin	7,055,715,274,581	1,913,392,198	1,787
Niacin	Stepped care (20 mg)	7,055,728,852,269	1,913,394,958	4,919
Niacin	Stepped care (40 mg)	7,055,745,113,996	1,913,396,039	15,043
Stepped care (20 mg)	Stepped care (40 mg)	7,055,865,850,533	1,913,398,580	47,515

a. The high-risk group considered here included patients with the following combination of characteristics: LDL $\geq$ 190 mg/dL; HDL $<$ 35 mg/dL; cigarette smokers; and DBP $\geq$ 105 mmHg. Due to their large number, results for dominated strategies are not presented here. All of the primary prevention interventions shown in this table entail intervening in persons ages 35–84 unless otherwise indicated. For stepped care, all patients begin therapy on niacin; those who cannot tolerate niacin switch to lovastatin at the indicated dose, and those who cannot tolerate lovastatin switch to the Step I Diet without medication. An incremental C/E ratio compares a strategy to the strategy listed directly above it in the table.

medication in this segment of the population; it may, however, be cost-effective as a fallback medication for patients who cannot tolerate niacin, as indicated by the results for strategies using stepped care. If the threshold C/E ratio is judged to be greater than $50,000/QALY, stepped care is cost-effective for both primary and secondary prevention in this population. Note also that all strategies employing no primary prevention and all but two strategies that limit primary prevention to patients 55 and over are dominated.

Moderate-Risk Patients

The results of the Reference Case analysis for males and females at moderate risk of CHD are shown in Table C.8. Overall, the results are similar to those for high-risk patients. All but seven strategies each for males and females are dominated. Of the undominated strategies, only the least cost-effective strategy for each sex employs lovastatin as a first-line medication, and even then only for secondary prevention. For a threshold C/E ratio of $150,000/QALY or less, lovastatin is not cost-effective as a first-line drug even for patients with CHD. Again, however, lovastatin may be judged to be relatively cost-effective as a fallback therapy for patients unable to tolerate niacin, for both primary and secondary prevention (incremental C/E ratios $<$ $50,000 QALY). As in the analysis for high-risk patients, strategies employing no primary prevention and/or no secondary prevention are dominated.

Table C.8 Results of Reference Case Cost-Effectiveness Analysis for Moderate-Risk Males and Females[a]

Strategy		Results		
Primary Prevention	Secondary Prevention	Total Discounted Cost (1993 U.S. $)	Total Discounted QALYs	Incr. C/E Ratio
Males				
Diet (55–84)	Niacin	6,016,423,989,106	1,713,968,290	—
Niacin (55–84)	Niacin	6,016,561,967,934	1,714,118,722	917
Niacin	Niacin	6,016,683,796,178	1,714,226,077	1,135
Niacin	Stepped care (20 mg)	6,016,829,652,915	1,714,268,613	3,429
Niacin	Stepped care (40 mg)	6,017,075,273,664	1,714,285,457	14,582
Stepped care (20 mg)	Stepped care (40 mg)	6,018,226,172,489	1,714,312,437	42,657
Stepped care (20 mg)	Lovastatin (40 mg)	6,020,443,944,769	1,714,313,179	2,988,912
Females				
Diet (55–84)	Diet	7,056,473,310,898	1,913,442,246	—
Diet (55–84)	Niacin	7,056,562,871,638	1,913,540,827	908
Niacin (55–84)	Niacin	7,057,003,416,773	1,913,702,700	2,722
Niacin	Stepped care (20 mg)	7,057,535,650,194	1,913,778,966	6,979
Niacin	Stepped care (40 mg)	7,057,717,221,940	1,913,790,183	16,187
Stepped care (20 mg)	Stepped care (40 mg)	7,058,911,623,693	1,913,817,225	44,168
Stepped care (20 mg)	Lovastatin (40 mg)	7,060,202,135,306	1,913,825,501	155,934

a. The moderate-risk group considered here included patients with the following combination of characteristics: LDL ≥ 190 mg/dL; HDL < 35–49 mg/dL; not cigarette smokers; and DBP 95–104 mmHg. Due to their large number, results for dominated strategies are not presented here. All of the primary prevention interventions shown in this table entail intervening in persons ages 35–84 unless otherwise indicated. For stepped care, all patients begin therapy on niacin; those who cannot tolerate niacin switch to lovastatin at the indicated dose, and those who cannot tolerate lovastatin switch to the Step I Diet without medication. An incremental C/E ratio compares a strategy to the strategy listed directly above it in the table.

Low-Risk Patients

The results of the Reference Case analysis for low-risk males and females are shown in Table C.9. As in the high-risk group, all strategies employing lovastatin as a first-line medication are dominated. All undominated strategies include primary and secondary prevention with diet, niacin, or stepped care. Strategies combining niacin for primary prevention with stepped care for secondary prevention have incremental C/E ratios below $50,000/QALY. However, in contrast to the results for high-risk and moderate-risk patients, moving from this combination to a more aggressive strategy (using stepped care rather than niacin for primary prevention) is relatively cost-ineffective (incremental C/E ratios > $120,000/QALY).

Comparison of Results Across Risk Factor Groups

Inspection of Tables C.7–9 shows several similarities between the results for high-, moderate-, and low-risk patient groups. All strategies involving no primary prevention

Table C.9 Results of Reference Case Cost-Effectiveness Analysis for Low-Risk Males and Females[a]

Strategy		Results		
Primary Prevention	Secondary Prevention	Total Discounted Cost (1993 U.S. $)	Total Discounted QALYs	Incr. C/E Ratio
Males				
Diet (55–84)	Niacin	6,018,823,121,865	1,714,099,806	—
Niacin (55–84)	Niacin	6,019,845,049,828	1,714,403,612	3,364
Niacin (55–84)	Stepped care (20 mg)	6,020,177,609,776	1,714,459,529	5,947
Niacin	Stepped care (20 mg)	6,022,248,669,703	1,714,590,593	15,802
Niacin	Stepped care (40 mg)	6,022,623,160,562	1,714,612,835	16,837
Stepped care (20 mg)	Stepped care (40 mg)	6,027,027,192,462	1,714,648,073	124,980
Females				
Diet (55–84)	Diet	7,065,181,947,508	1,913,675,984	—
Diet (55–84)	Niacin	7,066,594,009,032	1,914,200,169	2,694
Niacin (55–84)	Niacin	7,071,621,011,754	1,915,032,197	6,042
Niacin (55–84)	Stepped care (20 mg)	7,072,606,136,143	1,915,147,885	8,515
Niacin (55–84)	Stepped care (40 mg)	7,073,417,398,408	1,915,192,476	18,193
Niacin	Stepped care (40 mg)	7,082,078,789,393	1,915,383,486	45,345
Stepped care (20 mg)	Stepped care (40 mg)	7,098,141,445,351	1,915,477,481	170,888

a. The low-risk group considered here included patients with the following combination of characteristics: LDL 160–189 mg/dL; HDL ≥ 50 mg/dL; not cigarette smokers; and DBP < 95 mmHg. Due to their large number, results for dominated strategies are not presented here. All of the primary prevention interventions shown in this table entail intervening in persons ages 35–84 unless otherwise indicated. For stepped care, all patients begin therapy on niacin; those who cannot tolerate niacin switch to lovastatin at the indicated dose, and those who cannot tolerate lovastatin switch to the Step I Diet without medication. An incremental C/E ratio compares a strategy to the strategy listed directly above it in the table.

and/or no secondary prevention are dominated. Furthermore, all undominated strategies combining niacin for primary prevention with stepped care for secondary prevention have incremental C/E ratios below $50,000/QALY for men and women in each risk factor group.

Nearly all strategies employing lovastatin as a first-line medication are dominated. The only exceptions occur in the moderate-risk group, where the combination of stepped care for primary prevention and high-dose lovastatin for secondary prevention is not dominated for men or women. However, while not dominated, these strategies cannot be considered cost-effective unless the threshold C/E ratio is judged to be very high ($3,000,000/QALY for men; $160,000/QALY for women).

Sensitivity Analysis

We performed several sensitivity analyses to explore the implications of uncertainty in our parameter estimates and modeling. While many other sensitivity analyses would also be quite reasonable, we discuss here an illustrative set of analyses intended to reflect some of the key sources of uncertainty in this analysis.

Effects of Cholesterol Reduction on Non-CHD Mortality

The Reference Case analysis assumed that cholesterol reduction has no direct effect on non-CHD mortality. Because of the controversy surrounding the evidence from clinical trials of cholesterol-lowering therapy, we performed a set of sensitivity analyses to explore the effect of assuming that reducing serum TC directly causes an increase in non-CHD mortality. We assumed that the relative risk was constant for any percentage decrease in total cholesterol, and the logistic regression coefficient used to estimate this effect was derived from a meta-analysis of published data.

As would be expected, this had the result of making all prevention strategies lead to lower total quality-adjusted survival than in the Reference Case analysis. Furthermore, because of lovastatin's large effect on serum TC (see Table C.2), this modeling change had the effect of making lovastatin appear less attractive compared with niacin than in the Reference Case analysis. For example, lovastatin was dominated as a first-line medication for moderate-risk males in this sensitivity analysis; in the Reference Case analysis, although very cost-ineffective (see Table C.8), it was not dominated. Only in moderate-risk women was lovastatin not universally dominated as a first-line drug in this sensitivity analysis; even in this group, however, no strategy involving lovastatin as a first-line drug would be considered cost-effective unless the threshold C/E ratio were as high as $230,000/QALY.

It is important to note that the adverse effect of cholesterol reduction modeled here did not render all antihyperlipidemic therapy ineffective or cost-ineffective. In this sensitivity analysis, the combination of niacin for primary prevention and stepped care for secondary prevention for all ages remained relatively cost-effective, with incremental C/E ratios consistently less than $20,000/QALY in all risk factor groups except for low-risk women (C/E = $67,000/QALY, compared to using the same interventions but limiting primary prevention to the elderly). However, moving to a more aggressive primary prevention therapy (stepped care rather than niacin), while maintaining stepped care as the therapy for secondary prevention, was significantly less cost-effective than in the Reference Case analysis. This result is explained by lovastatin's large effects on serum TC. In the low-risk group, all strategies involving stepped care for primary prevention were dominated. In the high-risk group, no strategy employing stepped care for primary prevention could be considered cost-effective unless the threshold C/E ratio were as high as $94,000/QALY for women or $110,000/QALY for men (compared with < $50,000/QALY in the Reference Case analysis, as shown in Table C.7). This change was also seen, but less dramatically, in the moderate-risk patients. For this group, the incremental cost-effectiveness of moving from niacin to stepped care for primary prevention (with stepped care for secondary prevention) changed from $43,000/QALY for men and $44,000/QALY for women in the Reference Case analysis (as shown in Table C.8) to $66,000 for men and $58,000 for women in this sensitivity analysis.

An important insight from this sensitivity analysis is that some antihyperlipidemic therapies may be cost-effective even if cholesterol reduction has an adverse effect on non-CHD mortality. However, due to the large degree of uncertainty surrounding the issue of possible non-CHD effects of cholesterol reduction, we urge caution in interpreting the results discussed here. In particular, we note that the results of this sensitivity analysis are driven specifically by the different effects of niacin and lovastatin on serum TC. This raises an important question for future research: If there is a harmful effect of antihyperlipidemic therapy on non-CHD mortality, is the effect associated directly with a change in serum TC or with some other effect of the therapy, such as a change in a specific lipoprotein? The answer to this question, which has not yet been addressed in the literature, may have important implications for the relative attractiveness of different antihyperlipidemic therapies. Until more is known about the specific means by which antihyperlipidemic therapy may increase non-CHD mortality, we suggest that the specific results of this sensitivity analysis be interpreted with great caution.

Effects of Lipid Changes on CHD

To further explore the effects of uncertainty in our estimation of health effects, we performed a set of sensitivity analyses in which we varied the logistic regression coefficients in the CHD Policy Model corresponding to the effects of HDL and LDL on the development of CHD. Consistent with all estimates of these coefficients available from large studies, the Reference Case analysis used an estimate for the coefficient for HDL that was more than two times the magnitude of the coefficient for LDL (before adjustment for age and gender). For sensitivity analysis, we based our regressions simultaneously on the smallest available HDL coefficient estimate (based on results for men in the Framingham Heart Study) and the largest available LDL coefficient estimate (based on results for women in the Framingham Heart Study). Thus, this sensitivity analysis assigned a more important role to LDL and a less important role to HDL in the development of CHD, compared to the Reference Case analysis.

The principal result of this change was that interventions employing lovastatin appeared more cost-effective than in the Reference Case analysis. This result was expected, and is explained by the fact that lovastatin has larger effects on LDL and smaller effects on HDL than does niacin (see Table C.2), so this change in modeling of coefficients has a more favorable effect for lovastatin.

In the high-risk and low-risk groups, the results were not dramatic and were probably not policy-relevant. Among these groups, the biggest changes were observed in the high-risk women; the results for this group are shown in Table C.10. In this patient population, the strategy of using stepped care for primary prevention and high-dose lovastatin for secondary prevention was dominated in the Reference Case analysis (see Table C.7)

Table C.10 Results of Sensitivity Analyses Assuming a More Important Role of LDL and a Less Important Role of HDL in the Development of CHD; Results Are Shown for Females at High Risk of CHD[a]

Strategy		Incremental Cost-Effectiveness Ratio ($/QALY)	
Primary Prevention	*Secondary Prevention*	*Reference Case Analysis*	*Sensitivity Analysis*
Diet (55–84)	Niacin	—	—
Niacin (55–84)	Niacin	1,343	dominated
Niacin	Niacin	1,787	806
Niacin	Stepped care (20 mg)	4,919	3,719
Niacin	Stepped care (40 mg)	15,043	11,869
Stepped care (20 mg)	Stepped care (40 mg)	47,515	37,527
Stepped care (20 mg)	Lovastatin (40 mg)	dominated	122,746

a. All strategies not shown were dominated. Primary prevention interventions shown in this table entail intervening in persons ages 35–84 unless otherwise indicated. An incremental C/E ratio compares a strategy to the strategy listed directly above it in the table.

but was not dominated in the sensitivity analysis. However, even under the alternative set of assumptions for lipid effects, this strategy is estimated to cost more than $120,000 for each additional QALY gained. Therefore, it is not clear that this change is large enough to influence policy decisions.

In the moderate-risk group, however, where elevated LDL is the primary source of risk for CHD, this change in the model had a significant effect. In this group, strategies involving high-dose lovastatin as a first-line medication for secondary prevention became much more cost-effective than in the Reference Case analyis. To illustrate, the results for moderate-risk men areshown in Table C.11. Here, high-dose lovastatin for secondary prevention (coupled with either niacin or stepped care for primary prevention) can be considered cost-effective if the threshold C/E ratio is about $40,000/QALY–$50,000/QALY or higher. Similar results were obtained for women.

These results suggest that further research into the precise roles of HDL and LDL in the development of CHD would be valuable for future economic evaluations of cholesterol reduction. Furthermore, this study indicates that such an analysis would be particularly important for evaluating prevention strategies for people whose CHD risk is largely attributable to the level of one or the other of these lipoproteins. Moderate-risk patients considered here had little risk of CHD except that owing to their high levels of LDL; thus, a model that makes LDL reduction more effective for preventing CHD would be expected to have relatively large effects on the cost-effectiveness of using lovastatin (which acts principally through lowering LDL) in this group. In contrast, the high-risk patients considered in this analysis had low HDL as well as high LDL. Thus, the improved effectiveness of drugs through LDL reduction was largely offsetby the reduced effects of HDL elevations caused by the same drugs; for this reason, lovastatin remained relatively cost-ineffective in this group. In low-risk patients, who did not have very high LDL or very low HDL, this change had very little impact.

Table C.11 Results of Sensitivity Analyses Assuming a More Important Role of LDL and a Less Important Role of HDL in the Development of CHD; Results Are Shown for Males at Moderate Risk of CHD[a]

Strategy		Incremental Cost-Effectiveness Ratio ($/QALY)	
Primary Prevention	*Secondary Prevention*	*Reference Case Analysis*	*Sensitivity Analysis*
Diet (55–84)	Niacin	—	—
Niacin (55–84)	Niacin	917	dominated
Niacin	Niacin	1,135	188
Niacin	Stepped care (20 mg)	3,429	1,870
Niacin	Stepped care (40 mg)	14,582	10,428
Stepped care (20 mg)	Stepped care (40 mg)	42,657	35,101
Niacin	Lovastatin (40 mg)	dominated	42,651
Stepped care (20 mg)	Lovastatin (40 mg)	2,988,912	51,382

a. All strategies not shown were dominated. Primary prevention interventions shown in this table entail intervening in persons ages 35–84 unless otherwise indicated. An incremental C/E ratio compares a strategy to the strategy listed directly above it in the table.

Sensitivity to Health-Related Quality-of-Life Weights

Next, we performed several analyses to explore the sensitivity of the Reference Case results to our selection of HRQL weights.

First, we performed a set of analyses using QWB estimates from the BDHOS to estimate health-related quality of life. In contrast to the weights used in the Reference Case analysis, which were elicited directly from patients, the QWB scale uses community preference weights. The weights used in this sensitivity analysis were 0.66 for angina, 0.63 for CHF, and 0.73 for people without angina or CHF. Using the estimation procedure discussed earlier in this report, we calculated an approximate weight of 0.57 for the combination of angina and CHF. Note that these values are uniformly lower than the pooled TTO weights used in the Reference Case analysis. (See Table C.3.)

Next, we explored the effects of using age-specific estimates of health-related quality of life. For this analysis, we again used QWB weights from the BDHOS, but now used age-specific weights for persons without angina or CHF: 0.76 for asymptomatic people ages 45–54, 0.74 for asymptomatic people ages 55–64, and 0.70 for asymptomatic people ages 65 and over. We made the conservative assumption that people ages 35–44 have the same health-related quality of life as people ages 45–54. For people with CHF and/or angina, age-specific weights were not available; however, as in the Reference Case analysis, health-related quality of life for people with CHD varies by age to the extent that the prevalences of angina and CHF vary by age.

Finally, we performed an analysis in which health effects were measured in years of life gained rather than QALYs gained. Thus, no adjustments for health-related quality of life were made in this analysis.

The results of these sensitivity analyses indicate that the findings of the present study are fairly insensitive to changes in the weights used for health-related quality of life. To illustrate, the results for high-risk males are shown in Table C.12. The overall results

Table C.12 Results of Sensitivity Analyses Using Alternative Estimates of Health-Related Quality of Life; Results Are Shown for Males at High Risk of CHD[a]

Strategy		Incremental Cost-Effectiveness Ratios[b]			
Primary Prevention	Secondary Prevention	Reference Case Analysis[c]	Using QWB	Using Age-Specific QWB	Using Life Years
Niacin	Niacin	—	—	—	—
Niacin	Stepped care (20 mg)	1,321	1,667	1,686	1,127
Niacin	Stepped care (40 mg)	12,521	15,782	15,966	10,662
Stepped care (20 mg)	Stepped care (40 mg)	40,579	47,888	51,323	42,308

a. All strategies not shown were dominated. All primary and secondary prevention interventions shown in this table entail intervening in persons ages 35–84. An incremental C/E ratio compares a strategy to the strategy listed directly above it in the table.

b. Ratios are reported in units of $/QALY, except for the column corresponding to life years, in which ratios are reported in units of $/LY.

c. In the reference case analysis, health-related quality of life was estimated using time-tradeoff weights elicited from patients in the AMI PORT and BDHOS studies (see Table C.3).

did not change; strategies were ranked in the same order, and dominated strategies remained dominated. As would be expected, the use of the QWB weights, which are uniformly lower than the pooled TTO estimates, resulted in higher incremental C/E ratios. In addition, the use of age-specific QWB weights resulted in even higher ratios. This result is explained by the fact that many of the life years saved by preventing CHD are late in life (i.e., in relatively older people), and people at these ages tend to have lower health-related quality of life than they had at younger ages.

In addition, as shown by the results in the last column of Table C.12, the use of HRQL weights had little effect on the estimated incremental C/E ratios in this study. That is, the C/E ratios estimated in the Reference Case analysis (in units of $/QALY) are similar to the C/E ratios (in units of $/LY) that were estimated in the sensitivity analysis that used life years gained as the outcome measure. Improvements in *survival* resulting from CHD prevention appear larger when measured in life years gained than when measured in QALYs gained, because they are assigned a weight of 1 rather than the lower HRQL weights used to calculate QALYs. In contrast, improvements in *health-related quality of life* may play a large role when health gains are measured in QALYs, but they are not taken into account at all when outcomes are measured in years of life gained. The results in Table C.12 indicate that these two differences essentially offset each other. Similar results were seen in the other risk factor groups.

Sensitivity to Medication Costs

Niacin is recognized as an inexpensive agent for cholesterol reduction, and lovastatin is among the most expensive antihyperlipidemic medications. However, lovastatin's average wholesale price (which was used as the basis for the Reference Case cost estimate) may currently exceed its marginal cost because the drug is still under patent, and the manufacturer may charge prices above marginal cost to recoup R&D costs. Whether or not lovastatin's current price exceeds marginal cost, future competition may result in more efficient production and lower costs once the patent expires. In addition, although our estimate of niacin's cost is higher than the average wholesale prices charged by several niacin manufacturers, some other manufacturers charge higher prices.

To analyze the importance of this cost disparity and to investigate how sensitive the results of the present analysis are to changes in the estimated drug costs, we conducted a set of sensitivity analyses in which we assumed a higher cost for niacin and a lower cost for lovastatin than was used in the Reference Case analysis. We increased our estimate of niacin's cost by a factor of five and simultaneously reduced our estimate of lovastatin's cost by 50%. This analysis would clearly be expected to result in more-favorable results for strategies involving lovastatin and less-favorable results for strategies involving niacin than were found in the Reference Case analysis.

Simultaneously quintupling our estimate of niacin's cost and halving our estimate of lovastatin's cost led to few important changes in our results. The lone exception was observed in moderate-risk women. Here, the strategy of using stepped care for primary prevention and lovastatin for secondary prevention was estimated to cost an additional $48,000 for each additional QALY gained, compared with the strategy of using stepped care for both primary and secondary prevention; in the Reference Case analysis, this incremental C/E ratio was estimated to be $160,000/QALY. (See Table C.8.) Lovastatin as a first-line medication continued to be relatively cost-ineffective for moderate-risk men ($870,000/QALY versus the $3,000,000/QALY reported in Table C.8 for the Reference Case analysis) and was dominated for high-risk and low-risk men and women. Effects on other strategies were relatively small and unlikely to affect policy decisions.

Sensitivity to Changes in the Discount Rate

Varying the discount rate from the Reference Case rate of 3% to values of 0% (no discounting) and 5% had virtually no effect on the results of this analysis. While it is commonly observed that prevention programs tend to fare better when lower discount rates are used, this observation applies only when prevention programs are being compared with nonprevention programs. In this analysis, however, the strategies involving no primary prevention and/or no secondary prevention are dominated. Thus, the incremental C/E ratios of interest compare various strategies for CHD prevention with one another, rather than comparing preventive with nonpreventive strategies. Changing the discount rate had similar effects on the various strategies considered here, so the incremental comparisons between them changed very little.

Discussion

Several insights may be drawn from this analysis. First, our results indicate that cholesterol reduction for both primary and secondary prevention of CHD can be relatively cost-effective in a variety of risk-factor groups. However, some strategies for lowering cholesterol appear to be significantly more cost-effective than others. Strategies based on intervening with dietary therapy, niacin, and/or stepped care (with some exceptions) tend to be relatively cost-effective compared with many health care interventions currently in common use. In contrast, nearly all strategies that employ lovastatin as a first-line medication are dominated; in most cases, therapy with stepped care rather than lovastatin yields greater health gains at a lower cost. Thus, lovastatin appears to be much more cost-effective as a fallback therapy for patients unable to tolerate niacin (in the stepped-care interventions) than as a first-line agent for antihyperlipidemic therapy. This result is explained by the fact that, although lovastatin is very effective in reducing LDL, it has little effect on HDL; niacin, on the other hand, has large favorable effects on both LDL and HDL. Moreover, niacin is a very inexpensive medication, while lovastatin is among the most expensive antihyperlipidemic agents currently available.

Our results differ significantly from previous cost-effectiveness analyses of lovastatin therapy primarily because we compare it to other interventions for cholesterol reduction (diet, niacin, and stepped care), whereas most previous studies have compared it only to the alternative of providing no antihyperlipemic therapy. For example, Goldman and colleagues[134] estimated that—compared with no prevention—lovastatin (40 mg/day) extends lives at a cost of about $50,000/life-year-gained or less (after converting their results to 1993 U.S. dollars using the Medical Care Component of the CPI) when used for secondary prevention in men and women with pretreatment serum TC $\geq$ 250 mg/dL; the sole exception was in women ages 35–44 (C/E = $66,000/life-year-gained). For primary prevention, they found that low-dose lovastatin (20 mg/day) was relatively cost-effective for many patients with other risk factors for CHD but relatively cost-ineffective for patients without other risk factors and for some patients under age 44 or over age 75. The differences between their findings and the results presented here highlight the importance in CEA of choosing comparators carefully; choosing a comparator that is less effective or more costly than other alternatives that are available biases the analysis in favor of the new intervention being analyzed.

We wish to emphasize that the results of this analysis should be interpreted with some degree of caution. As we noted earlier, the clinical trial evidence regarding the effects of cholesterol reduction on survival is a source of great controversy. Few clinical trials of cholesterol-lowering therapy have shown statistically significant improvements in patient survival. The Reference Case analysis in this study assumed that cholesterol reduction prevents CHD and has no direct adverse health effects; this is supported by the Scandinavian Simvastatin Survival Study (4S) for secondary prevention,[135] the West of Scotland study for primary prevention,[136] a recent meta-analysis,[137] and several observational studies.[138–140] However, this issue remains controversial. It is important to note that we found several strategies for cholesterol reduction based on diet and medication to be relatively cost-effective even in a sensitivity analysis where we made the controversial assumption that reducing serum TC leads directly to an increase in non-CHD mortality.

Other limitations of this study, as discussed earlier, should also be borne in mind. We modeled health effects only for the patients being intervened on; effects on family members and others concerned with the patient's well-being were not included in the analysis. In addition, we have not considered all possible therapies for cholesterol reduction. In particular, future analysts may wish to consider HMG-CoA reductase inhibitors other than lovastatin (such as simvastatin and pravastatin), combinations of drugs (such as niacin and colestipol), and doses of niacin and lovastatin other than those considered here. However, despite the limitations of this study, the sensitivity analyses indicated that the results are fairly robust with respect to several of the key sources of uncertainty in the analysis.

Finally, we have not yet addressed the distributive implications of this analysis. Because CHD is a widespread health problem for persons of both sexes and all races, programs to prevent CHD would offer large potential health gains for virtually all segments of the population. However, we note that CHD is most prevalent among older persons; therefore, these programs would tend to offer more direct health benefits to older patients than to younger persons. Of course, younger persons may also experience important benefits associated with the survival of these older persons. The gain actually experienced within any population subgroup would depend on a number of factors, such as the prevalence of competing health risks and the extent to which individuals have health insurance and access to health care providers.

The results of this study suggest that strategies for cholesterol reduction through various combinations of diet, niacin, and stepped care for primary and secondary prevention are relatively cost-effective for many patients. Lovastatin is often relatively cost-effective as a fallback therapy for patients unable to tolerate niacin but not as a first line of medication. To improve future analyses and to help make more informed choices about the prevention of CHD, we recommend additional research into the epidemiology of CHD, the effectiveness of antihyperlipidemic therapy for preventing coronary events and prolonging survival, the nature of community preferences for health states related to CHD, and the costs associated with preventing and treating CHD.

Addendum

The body of this report focused on the results for strategies that were found not to be dominated. In this addendum, more complete results are presented, including results

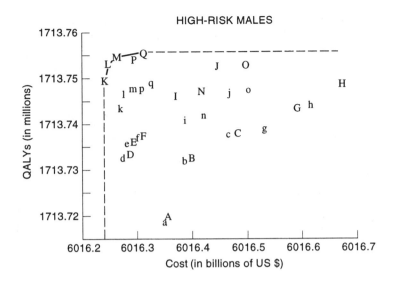

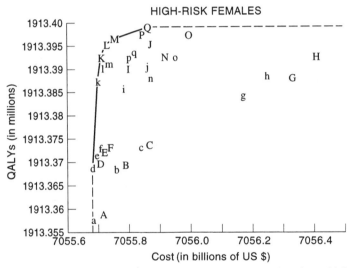

Figure C.A1. Results of Reference Case analysis for males and females at high risk of CHD. Costs are in 1993 U.S. dollars. The symbols in this graph are explained in the text of this addendum.

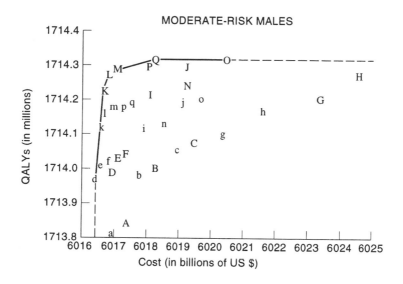

MODERATE-RISK MALES

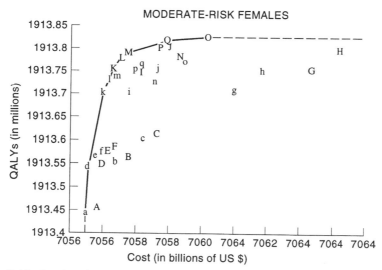

MODERATE-RISK FEMALES

Figure C.A2. Results of Reference Case analysis for males and females at moderate risk of CHD. Costs are in 1993 U.S. dollars. The symbols in this graph are explained in the text of this addendum.

for dominated strategies. Results from the Reference Case analyses for men and women are shown separately for the high-risk group in Figure C.A1, for the moderate-risk group in Figure C.A2, and for the low-risk group in Figure C.A3. In these figures, note that (as in Tables C.7–9 of this report) the costs reported are *sex-specific 50-year discounted costs* and that the QALY values represent *sex-specific 50-year discounted qual-*

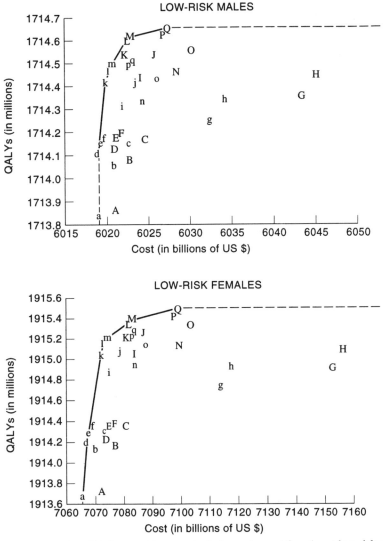

Figure C.A3. Results of Reference Cases analysis for males and females at low risk of CHD. Costs are in 1993 U.S. dollars. The symbols in this graph are explained in the text of this addendum.

ity-adjusted survival. These values include costs and quality-adjusted survival for all persons in the U.S. ages 35 and over during the 50-year time horizon of this analysis; note that these values are *not* just those for the group being intervened on.

In Figures C.A1–A3, we have used the following symbols to represent the various strategies analyzed:

	Primary Prevention	Secondary Prevention
A	Step I Diet	Step I Diet
B	Step I Diet	Lovastatin (20 mg)
C	Step I Diet	Lovastatin (40 mg)
D	Step I Diet	Niacin (3 g)
E	Step I Diet	Stepped care (20 mg)
F	Step I Diet	Stepped care (40 mg)
G	Lovastatin (20 mg)	Lovastatin (20 mg)
H	Lovastatin (20 mg)	Lovastatin (40 mg)
I	Niacin (3 g)	Lovastatin (20 mg)
J	Niacin (3 g)	Lovastatin (40 mg)
K	Niacin (3 g)	Niacin (3 g)
L	Niacin (3 g)	Stepped care (20 mg)
M	Niacin (3 g)	Stepped care (40 mg)
N	Stepped care (20 mg)	Lovastatin (20 mg)
O	Stepped care (20 mg)	Lovastatin (40 mg)
P	Stepped care (20 mg)	Stepped care (20 mg)
Q	Stepped care (20 mg)	Stepped care (40 mg)

In the figures, an uppercase letter corresponds to the strategy indicated above, with primary and secondary prevention in persons 35–84; a lowercase letter corresponds to the same strategy, except that primary prevention is delivered only to persons 55–84. Results are not shown for strategies involving no primary prevention because they were so much more costly than the other strategies that they did not fit well on the same figures as the others; all of these strategies were clearly dominated.

Note that the "efficient frontier" of undominated strategies can be easily identified from these plots by locating the points that define the outward-most convex set in each figure—that is, all other strategies (the dominated strategies) are to the "southeast" of the lines connecting the points on the efficient frontier.

References

1. Consensus Conference. 1985. Lowering blood cholesterol to prevent heart disease. *JAMA* 253:2080–86.

2. Lipid Research Clinics Program. 1984. The Lipid Research Clinics Coronary Primary Prevention Trial results: I. Reduction in the incidence of coronary heart disease. *JAMA* 251:365–74.

3. Lipid Research Clinics Program. 1984. The Lipid Research Clinics Coronary Primary Prevention Trial results: II. The relationship of reduction in incidence of coronary heart disease to cholesterol lowering. *JAMA* 251:365–74.

4. Keys A., A. Menotti, C. Aravanis, et al. 1984. The seven countries study: 2,289 deaths in 15 years. *Prev Med* 13:141–54.

5. Castelli W.P., R.J. Garrison, P.W.F. Wilson, et al. 1986. Incidence of coronary heart disease and lipoprotein cholesterol levels: The Framingham Study. *JAMA* 256:2835–38.

6. Martin M., S. Hulley, W. Browner, et al. 1986. Serum cholesterol, blood pressure, and mortality: Implications from a cohort of 361,662 men. *Lancet* 2:933–936.

7. Holme I. 1990. An analysis of randomized trials evaluating the effect of cholesterol reduction on total mortality and coronary heart disease incidence. *Circulation* 82:1916–24.

8. Davey Smith G. and J. Pekkanen. 1992. Should there be a moratorium on the use of cholesterol lowering drugs? *BMJ* 304:431–34.

9. Russell L.B. 1994. *Educated guesses: Making policy about medical screening tests.* Berkeley, CA: University of California Press.

10. Gould A.L., J.E. Roussouw, N.C. Santanello, et al. 1995. Cholesterol reduction yields clinical benefit: A new look at old data. *Circulation* 91:2274–82.

11. Scandinavian Simvastatin Survival Study Group. 1994. Randomised trial of cholesterol lowering in 4444 patients with coronary heart disease: the Scandinavian Simvastatin Survival Study (4S). *Lancet* 344:1383–89.

12. Shepherd J., S.M. Cobbe, I. Ford, et al. 1995. Prevention of coronary heart disease with pravastatin in men with hypercholesterolemia. *N Engl J Med* 333:1301–1307.

13. Canner P.L., K.G. Berge, N.K. Wenger, et al. 1986. Fifteen Year Mortality in Coronary Drug Project patients: Long-term benefit with niacin. *J Am Coll Cardiol* 8:1245–55.

14. Keys A., A. Menotti, M.J. Karvonen, et al. 1986. The diet and 15-year death rate in the seven countries study. *Am J Epidemiol* 124:903–15.

15. Anderson K.M., W.P. Castelli, and D. Levy. 1987. Cholesterol and mortality: 30 years of follow-up from the Framingham Study. *JAMA* 257:2176–80.

16. Neaton J.D., H. Blackburn, D. Jacobs, et al. 1992. Serum cholesterol level and mortality findings for men screened in the Multiple Risk Factor Intervention Trial. *Arch Intern Med* 152:1490–1500.

17. National Cholesterol Education Program. 1988. Report of the National Cholesterol Education Program Expert Panel on Detection, Evaluation, and Treatment of High Blood Cholesterol in Adults. *Arch Intern Med* 148:36–69.

18. Expert Panel on Detection, Evaluation, and Treatment of High Blood Cholesterol in Adults. 1993. Summary of the Second Report of the National Cholesterol Education Program (NCEP) Expert Panel on Detection, Evaluation, and Treatment of High Blood Cholesterol in Adults (Adult Treatment Panel II). *JAMA* 269:3015–3023.

19. National Cholesterol Education Program. 1991. Report of the Expert Panel on Population Strategies for Blood Cholesterol Reduction. *Circulation* 83:2154–232.

20. Hamilton V.H., F-E. Racicot, H. Zowall, et al. 1995. The cost-effectiveness of HMG-CoA reductase inhibitors to prevent coronary heart disease: Estimating the benefits of increasing HDL-C. *JAMA* 273:1032–1038.

21. Garber A.M., B. Littenberg, H.C. Sox, et al. 1991. Costs and health consequences of cholesterol screening for asymptomatic older Americans. *Arch Intern Med* 151:1089–1095.

22. Goldman L., D.J. Gordon, B.M. Rifkind, et al. 1992. Cost and health implications of cholesterol lowering. *Circulation* 85:1960–68.

23. Taylor W.C., T.M. Pass, D.S. Shepard, et al. 1990. Cost-effectiveness of cholesterol reduction for the primary prevention of coronary heart disease in men. In *Preventing disease: Beyond the rhetoric*, ed. R.B. Goldbloom and R.S. Lawrence, 437–441. New York, NY: Springer-Verlag.

24. Oster G. and A.M. Epstein. 1987. Cost-effectiveness of antihyperlipidemic therapy in the prevention of coronary heart disease: The case of cholestyramine. *JAMA* 258:2381–2387.

25. Weinstein M.C., and W.B. Stason. 1985. Cost-effectiveness of interventions to prevent or treat coronary heart disease. *Annu Rev Public Health* 6:41–63.

26. Himmelstein D.U., and S. Woolhandler. 1985. Costs and effects: The lipid research trial and the RAND experiment. *N Engl J Med* 311:1512–13.

27. Kinosian B., and J.M. Eisenberg. 1988. Cutting into cholesterol: Cost-effective alternatives for treating hypercholesterolemia. *JAMA* 259:249–54.

28. Goldman, L., M.C. Weinstein, P.A. Goldman, et al. 1991. Cost-effectiveness of HMG-CoA reductase inhibition for primary and secondary prevention of coronary heart disease. *JAMA* 265:1145–51.

29. Hamilton V.H., F-E. Racicot, H. Zowall, et al., *supra* note 20.

30. Gould A.L., J.E. Roussouw, N.C. Santanello, et al., *supra* note 10.

31. Schulman K.A., B. Kinosian, T.A. Jacobsen, et al. 1990. Reducing high blood cholesterol level with drugs: Cost-effectiveness of pharmacologic management. *JAMA* 264:3025–33.

32. Wysowski D.K., D.L. Kennedy, and T.P. Gross. 1990. Prescribed use of cholesterol-lowering drugs in the United States, 1978 through 1988. *JAMA* 263:2185–88.

33. Edelson J.T., M.C. Weinstein, A.N.A. Tosteson, et al. 1990. Long-term efficacy and cost-effectiveness of various monotherapies for mild to moderate hypertension. *JAMA* 263:408–13.

34. Goldman L., M.C. Weinstein, P.A. Goldman, et al., *supra* note 28.

35. Johannesson M., and M.C. Weinstein. 1993. On the decision rules of cost-effectiveness analysis. *J Health Econ* 12:459–467.

36. Andrade S.E., A.M. Walker, L.K. Gottlieb, et al. 1995. Discontinuation of antihyperlipidemic drugs—Do rates reported in clinical trials reflect rates in primary care settings? *N Engl J Med* 332:1125–31.

37. Caggiula A.W., G. Christakis, M. Farrand, et al. 1981. The Multiple Risk Factor Intervention Trial (MRFIT), IV. Intervention on blood lipids. *Prev Med* 10:443–75.

38. Grundy S.M. and M.A. Denke. 1990. Dietary influences on serum lipids and lipoproteins. *J Lipid Res* 31:1149–72.

39. Willett W. and F.M. Sacks. 1991. Chewing the fat: How much and what kind. *N Engl J Med* 324:121–123.

40. Sacks F.M. and W.W. Willett. 1991. More on chewing the fat: The good fat and the good cholesterol. *N Engl J Med* 325:1740–42.

41. Sacks F.M., G.H. Handysides, G.E. Marais, et al. 1986. Effects of a low-fat diet on plasma lipoprotein levels. *Arch Intern Med* 146:1573–77.

42. Ginsberg H.N., S.L. Barr, A. Gilbert, et al. 1990. Reduction of plasma cholesterol levels in normal men on American Heart Association Step 1 Diet or a Step 1 Diet with added monounsaturated fat. *N Engl J Med* 322:574–79.

43. Hunninghake D.B., E.A. Stein, C.A. Dujovne, et al. 1993. The efficacy of intensive dietary therapy alone or combined with lovastatin in outpatients with hypercholesterolemia. *N Engl J Med* 328:1213–19.

44. Mori R.A., R. Vandongen, L.J. Beilin, et al. 1994. Effects of varying dietary fat, fish, and fish oils on blood lipids in a randomized controlled trial in men at risk of heart disease. *Am J Clin Nutr* 59:1060–1668.

45. Illingworth D.R., E.A. Stein, Y.B. Mitchel, et al. 1994. Comparative effects of lovastatin and niacin in primary hypercholesterolemia. *Arch Intern Med* 154:1586–95.

46. Knopp R.H., J. Ginsberg, J.J. Albers, et al. 1985. Contrasting effects of unmodified and time-release forms of niacin on lipoproteins in hyperlipidemic subjects: Clues to mechanism of action of niacin. *Metabolism* 34:642–50.

47. Alderman J.D., R.C. Pasternak, F.M. Sacks, et al. 1989. Effect of a modified, well-tolerated niacin regimen on serum total cholesterol, high density lipoprotein cholesterol and the cholesterol to high density lipoprotein ratio. *Am J Cardiol* 64:725–9.

48. Knopp R.H., J. Ginsberg, J.J. Albers, et al., *supra* note 46.

49. Bradford R.H., C.L. Shear, A.N. Chremos, et al. 1991. Expanded Clinical Evaluation of Lovastatin (EXCEL) Study results I. Efficacy in modifying plasma lipoproteins and adverse event profile in 8245 patients with moderate hypercholesterolemia. *Arch Intern Med* 151:43–49.

50. Bradford R.H., C.L. Schear, A.N. Chremos, et al. 1991. Expanded Clinical Evaluation of Lovastatin (EXCEL) Study results III. Efficacy in modifying plasma lipoproteins and implications for managing patients with moderate hypercholesterolemia. *Am J Med* 91(suppl B):18S–24S.

51. Denke, M.A. and S.M. Grundy. 1995. Efficacy of low-dose cholesterol-lowering drug therapy in men with moderate hypercholesterolemia. *Arch Intern Med* 1995:393–99.

52. Illingworth R.D., E.A. Stein, Y.B. Mitchel, et al., *supra* note 45.

53. Havel R.J., D.B. Hunninghake, D.R. Illingworth, et al. 1987. Lovastatin (Mevinolin) in the treatment of heterozygous familial hypercholesterolemia. *Ann Intern Med* 107:609–15.

54. Tikkanen M.J., E. Helve, A. Jaattela, et al. 1988. Comparison between lovastatin and gemfibrozil in the treatment of primary hypercholesterolemia: The Finnish multicenter study. *Am J Cardiol* 62:35J–43J.

55. Lovastatin Study Groups I Through IV. 1993. Lovastatin 5-year safety and efficacy study. *Arch Intern Med* 153:1079–87.

56. Hunninghake D.B., E.A. Stein, C.A. Dujovne, et al., *supra* note 43.

57. Cobb M.M., H.S. Teitelbaum, and J.L. Breslow 1991. Lovastatin efficacy in reducing low-density lipoprotein cholesterol levels on high- vs. low-fat diets. *JAMA* 265:997–1001.

58. Clifton P.M., M.B. Wright, and P.J. Nestel. Is fat restriction needed with HMGCoA re-ductase inhibitor treatment? *Atherosclerosis* 93:59–70.

59. Muldoon M.F., S.B. Manuck, and K.A. Matthews. 1990. Lowering cholesterol concentra-tion and mortality: a quantitative review of primary prevention trials. *BMJ* 301:309–314.

60. Davey Smith G., F. Song, and T.A. Sheldon. 1993. Cholesterol lowering and mortality: the importance of considering initial level of risk. *BMJ* 306:1367–1373.

61. Roussow J.E., B. Lewis, and B.M. Rifkind. 1990. The value of lowering cholesterol after myocardial infarction. *N Engl J Med* 323:1112–19.

62. Gould A.L., J.E. Roussouw, N.C. Santanello, et al., *supra* note 10.

63. Canner P.L., K.G. Berge, N.K. Wenger, et al., *supra* note 13.

64. Scandinavian Simvastatin Survival Study Group, *supra* note 11.

65. Shepherd J., S.M. Cobbe, I. Ford, et al. 1995. Prevention of coronary heart disease with pravastatin in men with hypercholesterolemia. *N Engl J Med* 333:1301–1307.

66. Weinstein M.C., P.G. Coxson, L.W. Williams, et al. 1987. Forecasting coronary heart disease incidence, mortality, and cost: The Coronary Heart Disease Policy Model. *Am J Public Health* 77:1417–1426.

67. Tosteson A., M.C. Weinstein, L.W. Williams, et al. 1990. Long-term impact of smoking cessation on the incidence of coronary heart disease: Projections of the Coronary Heart Disease Policy Model. *Am J Public Health* 80:1481–86.

68. Tsevat J., M.C. Weinstein, L.W. Williams, et al. 1991. Expected gains in life expectancy from various coronary heart disease risk factor modifications. *Circulation* 83:1194–1201.

69. Weinstein M.C., P.G. Coxson, L.W. Williams, et al., *supra* note 66.

70. Tosteson A., M.C. Weinstein, L.W. Williams, et al. 1990. Long-term impact of smoking cessation on the incidence of coronary heart disease: Projections of the Coronary Heart Disease Policy Model. *Am J Public Health* 80:1481–86.

71. Tsevat J., M.C. Weinstein, L.W. Williams, et al., *supra* note 68.

72. U.S. Bureau of the Census. 1990. US Population estimates by age, sex, race, and Hispanic origin: 1989. *Current population reports, population estimates and projections.* Series P-25, No. 1057. Washington, DC: U.S. Department of Commerce.

73. Burke G.L., J.M. Sprafka, A.R. Folsom, et al. 1989. Trends in mortality, morbidity and risk factor levels from 1960–1986: The Minnesota Heart Survey. *Intern J Epidemiol* 18 (suppl I):S73–S81.

74. McGovern P.G., G.L. Burke, J.M. Sprafka, et al. 1992. Trends in mortality, morbidity, and risk factor levels for stroke from 1960 through 1990. *JAMA* 268:753–9.

75. National Cancer for Health Statistics. 1989. Vital and Health Statistics. Smoking and other tobacco use: United States, 1987. *Data from the National Health Survey Series 10,* No. 169, PHS 89-1597, Hyattsville, MD: US Department of Health and Human Services.

76. National Center for Health Statistics. 1987. Current estimates from the National Health Interview Survey, United States, 1986. *Data from the National Health Survey Series 10,* No. 164, PHS 87-1592, Hyattsville, MD: US Department of Health and Human Services.

77. U.S. Department of Health and Human Services. 1987. *The Framingham Study: an epidemiological investigation of cardiovascular disease. Some risk factors related to the annual incidence of cardiovascular disease and death using pooled repeated biennial measurements: Framingham Heart Study, 30-year follow-up.* Section 34, NIH Publication 87-2703. Bethesda, MD: National Heart, Lung and Blood Institute.

78. Elveback L.R., D.C. Connolly, and L.J. Melton. 1986. Coronary heart disease in residents of Rochester, Minnesota. VII. Incidence, 1950 through 1982. *Mayo Clin Proc* 61:896–900.

79. Pell, S., and W.E. Fayerweather. 1985. Trends in the incidence of myocardial infarction and in associated mortality and morbidity in a large employed population, 1975–1983. *N Engl J Med* 312:1005–11.

80. Weinstein M.C., P.G. Coxson, L.W. Williams, et al., *supra* note 66.

81. U.S. Department of Health and Human Services, *supra* note 77.

82. Longstreth W.T., L.A. Cobb, C.E. Fahrenbruch, et al. 1990. Does age affect outcomes of out-of-hospital cardiopulmonary resuscitation? *JAMA* 264:2109–10.

83. Valenzuela T.D., D.W. Spaite, H.W. Meislin, et al. 1992. Case and survival definition in out-of-hospital cardiac arrest. *JAMA* 267:272–4.

84. Wilcox-Gok, V.L. 1991. Survival from out-of-hospital cardiac arrest. A multivariate analysis. *Medical Care* 29:104–14.

85. Eisenberg M.S., B.T. Horwood, R.O. Cummins, et al. 1990. Cardiac arrest and resuscitation: a tale of 29 cities. *Ann Emerg Medicine* 19:179–86.

86. Eisenberg M.S., R.O. Cummins, S. Damon, et al. 1990. Survival rates from out-of-hospital cardiac arrest: recommendations for uniform definitions and data to report. *Ann Emerg Medicine* 19:1249–59.

87. Elveback L.R. and D.C. Connolly 1985. Coronary heart disease in residents of Rochester, Minnesota. V. Prognosis of patients with coronary heart disease based on initial manifestation. *Mayo Clin Proc* 60:305–11.

88. National Center for Health Statistics. 1985. *Vital statistics of the United States 1980* Volume II—Mortality, Part A. Hyattsville, MD: US Department of Health and Human Services.

89. National Center for Health Statistics. 1989. *Vital statistics of the United States 1986* Volume II—Mortality, Part A. Hyattsville, MD: US Department of Health and Human Services.

90. Centers for Disease Control. 1988. Detailed diagnoses and procedures for patients discharged from short-stay hospitals, National Health Survey, 1986. *Vital and health statistics, series 13* No. 95. Hyattsville, MD: US Department of Health and Human Services.

91. Canner P.L., K.G. Berge, N.K. Wenger, et al., *supra* note 13.

92. Lipid Research Clinics Program, *supra* note 2.

93. Scandinavian Simvastatin Survival Study Group, *supra* note 11.

94. The Coronary Drug Project Research Group. 1975. Clofibrate and niacin in coronary heart disease. *JAMA* 231:360–81.

95. CASS Principal Investigators and their Associates. 1983. Coronary Artery Surgery Study (CASS): a randomized trial of coronary artery bypass surgery. Survival data. *Circulation* 68:939–50.

96. Buda A.J., I.L. Macdonald, M.J. Anderson, et al. 1981. Longterm results following coronary bypass operation. *J Thorac Cardiovasc Surg* 82:383–90.

97. RITA Trial Participants. 1993. Coronary angioplasty versus coronary artery bypass surgery: the Randomised Intervention Treatment of Angina (RITA) trial. *Lancet* 341:573–80.

98. Fryback D.G., E.J. Dashbach, R. Klein, et al. 1993. The Beaver Dam Health Outcomes Study: Initial catalog of health-state quality factors. *Med Decis Making* 13:89–102.

99. Cleary P.D., S. Greenfield, A.G. Mulley, et al. 1991. Variations in length of stay and outcomes for six medical and surgical conditions in Massachusetts and California. *JAMA* 266:73–79.

100. HCIA and Ernst & Young. 1994. *The DRG handbook: Comparative clinical and financial standards.*

101. Topol E.J., S.G. Ellis, D.M. Cosgrove, et al. 1993. Analysis of coronary angioplasty practice in the United States with an insurance-claims data base. *Circulation* 87:1489–97.

102. Hlatky M.A., J. Lipscomb, C. Nelson, et al. 1990. Resource use and cost of initial coronary revascularization: Coronary angioplasty versus coronary bypass surgery. *Circulation* 82(Supp. IV):208–213.

103. Pilote L., N. Racine, and M.A. Hlatky. 1994. Differences in the treatment of myocardial infarction in the United States and Canada. *Arch Intern Med* 154:1090–96.

104. National Center for Health Statistics. 1994. National Hospital Discharge Survey: Annual Summary, 1992. *Vital and health statistics, series 13* 119. Hyattsville, MD: DHHS Publication No. (PHS) 94-1779.

105. Ammerman A.S., R.F. DeVellis, T.C. Keyserling, et al. 1994. Quality of life is not adversely effected by a dietary intervention to reduce cholesterol (abstract). *Abstracts of the 33rd Annual Conference on Cardiovascular Disease Epidemiology and Prevention.*

106. Lawrence W.F., D.G. Fryback, P.A. Martin, et al. 1994. Cholesterol and health status in the Beaver Dam Health Outcomes Study (abstract). *Med Decis Making* 14:436.

107. Downs J.R., G. Oster, and N.C. Santanello. 1993. HMG CoA reductase inhibitors and quality of life (letter). *JAMA* 269:3107–8.

108. Miller M.E., S. Zuckerman, and M. Gates. 1993. How do Medicare physician fees compare with private payers? *Health Care Financing Review* 14(3):25–39.

109. Physician Payment Review Commission. 1994. *Annual Report to Congress.*

110. Hsiao W.C., P. Braun, D. Dunn, and E. Becker. 1988. Resource-based relative values: an overview. *JAMA* 260:2347–53.

111. Welch P.W., S.J. Katz, and S. Zuckerman. 1993. Physician fee levels: Medicare versus Canada. *Health Care Financing Review* 14(3):41–54.

112. Health Care Financing Administration. 1993. Medicare program: Revisions to payment policies and adjustments to the relative value units under the physician fee schedule for calendar year 1994. *Federal Register* 58:63626–855.

113. Physician Payment Review Commission. 1993. *Annual report to Congress,* p. 39.

114. Cornelius L., K. Beauregard, and J. Cohen. 1991. Usual sources of medical care and their characteristics, AHCPR Pub. No. 91-0042. *National medical expenditure survey research findings 11,* Rockville, MD: Agency for Health Care Policy and Research, Public Health Service.

115. Health Care Financing Administration. 1995. *HCFA Part B extract and summary system.*

116. Knopp R.H., J. Ginsberg, J.J. Albers, et al., *supra* note 46.

117. The Lovastatin Study Group IV. 1990. A multicenter comparison of lovastatin and probucol for treatment of severe primary hypercholesterolemia. *Am J Cardiol* 66:22B–30B.

118. *Drug topics red book.* 1994. Montvale, NJ: Medical Economics Company, Inc.

119. *Blue book.* 1994. Hearst Corporation, New York.

120. Wilkin J.K., O. Wilkin, R. Kapp, et al. 1982. Aspirin blocks nicotinic acid-induced flushing. *Clin Pharmacol Ther* 31:478–82.

121. Drood J.M., P.J. Zimetbaum, and W.H. Frishman. 1991. Nicotinic acid for the treatment of hyperlipoproteinemia. *J Clin Pharmacol* 31:641–50.

122. Drug Topics Red Book. 1994. Montvale, NJ: Medical Economics Company, Inc.

123. Illingworth D.R., B.E. Phillipson, J.H. Rapp, and W.E. Connor. 1981. Colestipol plus nicotinic acid in treatment of heterozygous familial hypercholesterolaemia. *Lancet* 1:296–298.

124. Yovos J.G., S.T. Patel, J.M. Falko, et al. 1982. Effects of nicotinic acid therapy on plasma lipoproteins and very low density lipoprotein apoprotein C subspecies in hyperlipoproteinemia. *J Clin Endocrinol Metab* 54:1210–1215.

125. Kane J.P., M.J. Malloy, Tun, et al. 1981. Normalization of low-density-lipoprotein levels in heterozygous familial hypercholesterolemia with a combined drug regimen. *N Engl J Med* 304:251–258.

126. Figge H.L., J. Figge, P.F. Souney, et al. 1988. Nicotinic acid: A review of its clinical use in the treatment of lipid disorders. *Pharmacotherapy* 8(5):287–294.

127. Tsevat J., D. Duke, L. Goldman, et al. 1995. Cost-effectiveness of captopril therapy after myocardial infarction. *J Am Coll Cardiol* 26:914–919.

128. Hemenway D., H. Sherman, G.H. Mudge, Jr., et al. 1985. Comparative costs versus symptomatic and employment benefits of medical and surgical treatment of stable angina pectoris. *Med Care* 23:133–41.

129. Health Care Financing Administration. 1993. Medicare program; Revisions to payment policies and adjustments to the relative value units under the physician fee schedule for calendar year 1994. *Federal Register* 58:63626–855.

130. National Center for Health Statistics. 1993. Office visits to cardiovascular disease specialists: United States, 1989–1990. *Vital and Health Statistics, Advance Data* 226:6.

131. *Ibid.*

132. Tsevat J., D. Duke, L. Goldman, et al., *supra* note 127.

133. *Drug topics red book.* 1991. Oradell, NJ: Medical Economics Company.

134. Goldman L., M.C. Weinstein, P.A. Goldman, et al., *supra* note 28.

135. Scandinavian Simvastatin Survival Study Group, *supra* note 11.

136. Shepherd J., S.M. Cobbe, I. Ford, et al., *supra* note 65.

137. Gould A.L., J.E. Roussouw, N.C. Santanello, et al., *supra* note 10.

138. Keys A., A. Menotti., M.J. Karvonen, et al., *supra* note 14.

139. Anderson K.M., W.P. Castelli, and D. Levy, *supra* note 15.

140. Neaton J.D., H. Blackburn, D. Jacobs, et al., *supra* note 16.

Glossary

Terms in italics are defined elsewhere in the glossary.

administrative costs   Costs incurred by an organization for its direction and operation. These costs include costs of management, accounting, and personnel functions.

administrative prices   Prices fixed by governments and agencies, rather than set by markets. An example is prices set by Medicare's *Prospective Payment System*.

appropriateness   A judgment that an intervention is warranted. This judgment is generally the result of some formal process of expert consultation that considers issues of acceptability, feasibility, and costs.

area wage index   An index of labor costs used by the Health Care Financing Administration in paying hospitals for services delivered under Medicare. The index captures geographic differences in inpatient input costs.

attribute(s)   Generic element(s) of health status, also called *health concepts, domains*, or *dimensions*.

Bayes' rule   The algebraic formula used to express the *probability* that a hypothesis is true given observation of relevant evidence concerning the hypothesis. For example, Bayes's rule can be used to compute the *probability* of each possible diagnosis in light of test results or clinical observations.

Bayesian method   A branch of statistics that uses prior information on beliefs for estimation and inference. See *Bayes's rule*.

bootstrapping   A *simulation* method for deriving nonparametric estimates of variables of interest (e.g., the variance in the C/E ratio) from a data set.

capacity utilization   The extent to which productive facilities are utilized. For example, the fraction of beds filled in a 200-bed hospital is a measure of capacity utilization.

case-control study   A study comparing a case group, or series, of patients who have a disease of interest, with a control, or comparison, group of individuals without the disease. The proportion with the exposure of interest in each group is compared to that in the other.

case series study   Accumulated case reports that describe characteristics of a number of patients with a given disease.

category rating scales   Scales that are comprised of distinct categories. The categories are often numerical, such as 0, 1, 2, ... 10; the phenomenon being rated must be assigned to one and only one category. Numerical categories often are treated as equal-interval in analyses. In psychology, sometimes referred to as the method of equal-appearing intervals.

certainty equivalent   A sure outcome (e.g., 10 years of life) that the decision maker deems equivalent in value to an uncertain proposition (e.g., 10% chance of death today and 90% chance of living 20 years).

clinical epidemiology   Epidemiologic techniques applied to clinical questions, often dealing with the *effectiveness* of treatments and patient management. This rubric is used to differentiate the typical focus of clinical epidemiology studies from the more traditional use of "epidemiology" to refer to etiologic or chronic disease epidemiology, or public health epidemiology.

cohort case-control design   A *case-control study* conducted within a cohort study. (Also *nested case-control design.*)

compensation test   In economics, a gauge of the desirability of a program. A program is considered to be welfare enhancing if those who gain from it are willing to pay enough for their gains to compensate the losers. (Also *potential Pareto improvement* or *Kaldor-Hicks criterion.*)

conditional independence   Two random variables are conditionally independent given a third variable if the joint *probability* of the two given the third is formed from the product of their separate *conditional probabilities:* X and Y are conditionally independent of Z if $P(X,Y|Z) = P(X|Z)P(Y|Z)$. Calculations using *Bayes's rule* to express diagnostic *probabilities* conditioned on the results of several tests are greatly simplified if this condition is satisfied.

conditional probability   The conditional probability of a random variable, X, given a second random variable, Z, denoted "$P(X|Z)$," expresses the *probabilities* for values of X where the value of Z is known—that is, "conditioned" on knowledge of Z. For example, the *probability* that a test is positive given that the patient has the illness.

conditions of the commons   A situation where common access to a resource provides individuals with incentives to overuse the resource.

confidence interval   A $1-\alpha$ confidence interval for an unknown parameter is an interval of possible values of the parameter, based on sample data. It has the property that, in repeated sampling, $100(1-\alpha)\%$ of the intervals obtained will contain the true value.

confidence profile method A *Bayesian method* of *meta-analysis* that works by applying *Bayes's rule* to revise prior (subjective) *probability distributions* for unknown parameters, using the *likelihood functions* associated with observed data from clinical studies.

confounding A circumstance where the unique effects of two or more independent variables on a dependent variable cannot be statistically estimated because of unobserved or uncontrolled covariation in the variables.

construct An underlying, not directly observable concept of which measurement is desired. For example, ''severity'' of illness, ''intelligence'' of individuals, and ''quality'' of life are constructs.

construct validity An instrument exhibits construct validity when it is seen to correlate with other trusted measures of the phenomenon being measured and it is able to discriminate between groups that have known differences.

consumer price index (CPI) A measure of the average change in price over time in a fixed ''market basket'' of goods and services purchased either by urban wage earners and clerical workers or by all urban consumers.

consumption rate of interest The (after-tax) rate at which an individual is able to trade present for future consumption via market transactions. For example, if the consumption rate is 4%, the individual will have adjusted her purchases so that she is indifferent to $1 worth of consumption today versus $1.04 worth of consumption 1 year from now.

contamination effects In *randomized clinical trials* this refers to some members of the control group obtaining the treatment or some element of the treatment under study without the knowledge of investigators. Opportunity for this exists particularly after a treatment has become relatively widely used in advance of being evaluated by trials.

contingent valuation A method of placing a monetary value on a good or service that is not available in the marketplace by determining, contingent on it being available in the marketplace, the maximum amount that people would be willing to pay for it (buying price) and/or the minimum amount that people would be willing to accept to part with it (selling price).

convergent validity An instrument exhibits convergent validity when it is shown to co-vary (in the fashion expected of a good measure for the *construct* or phenomenon of interest) with a number of other distinct measures, each of which is thought to be a direct or indirect correlate for some distinct aspect of the *construct* or phenomenon. The correlations between the instrument being evaluated and these other measures are conceived of as representing convergent lines of evidence for the *validity* of the instrument.

cost-benefit analysis (CBA)   An analytic tool for estimating the net social benefit of a program or intervention as the incremental benefit of the program less the *incremental cost*, with all benefits and costs measured in dollars.

cost-consequence analysis   An analytic tool in which the components of *incremental costs* and consequences of alternative programs are computed and listed, without any attempt to aggregate these results.

cost-effectiveness analysis (CEA)   An analytic tool in which costs and effects of a program and at least one alternative are calculated and presented in a ratio of *incremental cost* to incremental effect. Effects are health outcomes, such as cases of a disease prevented, years of life gained, or *quality-adjusted life years*, rather than monetary measures as in *cost-benefit analysis*.

cost-effectiveness ratio   The *incremental cost* of obtaining a unit of health effect (such as dollars per year, or per quality-adjusted year, of life expectancy) from a given health intervention, when compared with an alternative.

cost-minimization analysis (CMA)   An analytic tool used to compare the net costs of programs that achieve the same outcome.

cost-of-illness study   An analysis of the total costs incurred by a society due to a specific disease.

cost subgroup   A group of individuals within the population receiving an intervention that are expected to experience similar costs or savings.

Cox proportional hazards model   In survival analysis the *hazard function* is the instantaneous likelihood of dying at a particular time, from which *survival probabilities* and survival curves are derived. The proportional hazards model is one algebraic form of the *hazard function* that assumes the impact of risk factors and other covariates is to multiply the baseline *hazard function* by some factor; hence their effect can be expressed as being proportional to the baseline hazard. Alternative hazard models such as the additive hazard model (where risk factors add to or subtract from the baseline hazard) are also used in survival analyses.

cross-sectional study   A study in which the status of an individual with respect to the presence or absence of both exposure and disease is assessed at the same point in time. Since exposure and disease are assessed contemporaneously, cross-sectional studies cannot fully distinguish whether the exposure preceded the development of the disease or whether the presence of the disease affected the individual's level of exposure.

decision analysis   An explicit, quantitative, systematic approach to decision making under conditions of *uncertainty* in which *probabilities* of each possible event, along with the consequences of those events, are stated explicitly.

decision tree   A graphical representation of a decision, incorporating alternative choices, uncertain events (and their *probabilities*), and outcomes.

Delphi method   A systematic process for eliciting the subjective opinion of a group of experts concerning the best estimate for a numerical parameter. Although there have been numerous ad hoc modifications to the process, originally it specified that the experts each initially communicate their numerical estimate privately to a facilitator. The facilitator then feeds back the group's initial estimates as anonymous numbers to the experts, who may then revise their initial estimates as they see fit. The revised estimates are then averaged to arrive at a single value to represent the group's opinion.

delta method   A mathematical method to approximate the variance of a function of several random variables in terms of the means and variances of those variables. Often used to compute an approximate *confidence interval* for a complex function of random variables. (This approximation has some potentially serious limitations when applied to C/E ratios where the denominator can approach zero.)

descriptive theory   A coherent group of general propositions or principles of which the objective is to explain phenomena.

deterministic model   For a health process, a model that computes quantities of interest (e.g., treatment *effect size*, *survival probabilities*, numbers of persons ending in various *health states*) directly by algebraic formulas. In particular, such a model does not use event simulation techniques to model the process.

dimension(s)   Generic element(s) of health status, also called *health concepts*, *attributes*, or *domains*.

direct costs   The value of all goods, services, and other resources that are consumed in the provision of an intervention or in dealing with the side effects or other current and future consequences linked to it.

direct medical costs   The value of health care resources, (e.g., tests, drugs, supplies, health care personnel, and medical facilities) consumed in the provision of an intervention or in dealing with the side effects or other current and future consequences linked to it.

direct nonmedical costs   The value of nonmedical goods, services, and other resources, such as child care or transportation, consumed in the provision of an intervention or in dealing with the side effects or other current and future consequences linked to it.

disability-adjusted life years (DALYs)   An indicator developed to assess the global burden of disease. DALYs are computed by adjusting age-specific life expectancy for loss of healthy life due to disability. The value of a year of life at each age is weighted, as are decrements to health from disability from specified diseases and injuries.

disability days   Days in which activity is restricted due to either a short-term or long-term health problem or condition.

discounting   The process of converting future dollars and future health outcomes to their *present value*.

discount rate   The interest rate used to compute *present value*, or the interest rate used in *discounting* future sums.

discrete-time model   A model in which the outcomes or events of interest are portrayed as occurring at specific, usually equally spaced, points in time. For purposes of *discounting*, a discrete-time model is one that assumes, for example, that outcomes (costs and effects) occur at the beginning or the end of each year rather than continuously or at various points during the years under study.

discriminant validity   An instrument exhibits discriminant validity to the extent that it does not correlate with variables and measures thought to be unrelated to the *construct* being measured.

disease history submodel   A simulation of the time course of the untreated disease used within a larger *simulation model*.

domain(s)   Generic element(s) of health status, also called *health concepts, attributes,* or *dimensions*.

dominance   The state when an intervention under study is both more effective and less costly than the alternative.

economies of scale   The situation where cost of production per unit of output decreases as the total volume of output increases. This may come about because of more efficient use of labor or equipment, or ability to specialize productive processes.

effectiveness   The extent to which medical interventions achieve health improvements in real practice settings.

effectiveness subgroups   Groups of individuals within the population receiving an intervention that are expected to experience similar levels and types of effects.

effect modification   A change in the magnitude of an effect measure according to the value of some third variable.

effect size   A standardized measure of change in some variable measured using a ''before and after'' design in a group or a difference in such changes between two groups. It is the mean change divided by the standard deviation of changes across individuals.

efficacy   The extent to which medical interventions achieve health improvements under ideal circumstances.

ex ante   A situation viewed from beforehand—that is, before the event occurs, before an action is taken, or before an outcome is known.

expected utility   A quantity used to represent the relative desirability of a specified course of action(s) where the outcome of the action cannot be specified before the fact with certainty. Each potential outcome is assigned a *utility*, to represent its desirability, and a *probability*, to represent the likelihood of its occurring if the course of action were adopted. The expected utility is the probability-weighted average *utility* of the potential outcomes.

expected utility theory   A framework for analyzing decisions under *uncertainty* positing that alternative actions are characterized by a set of possible outcomes and a set of *probabilities* corresponding to each outcome. The sum of the products of the *probability* of each outcome and the *utility* of that outcome is the expected value of *utility* and reflects the preferences of the decision maker. First axiomatized by J. von Neumann and O. Morgenstern in their 1947 book, *Theory of Games and Economic Behavior*, the theory sets forth conditions under which there exists a numerical measure of subjective attractiveness of outcomes (called a *utility function*) with the following properties: (1) this function represents the *ordinal* preferences of the decision maker if outcomes were to be received with certainty, and (2) the order of the expected utilities associated with various uncertain decision strategies represents the rankings of these strategies according to the decision-maker's preferences.

extended dominance   The state when a strategy under study is both less effective and more costly than a linear combination of two other strategies with which it is mutually exclusive.

externalities   The positive (beneficial) or negative (harmful) effects that market exchanges have on people who do not participate directly in those exchanges. Also called ''spillover'' effects.

external validity   The extent to which one can generalize the study conclusions to populations and settings of interest outside the study.

face validity   A judgment of the *validity* or reasonableness of a measurement or model based on its examination by persons with expertise in the health problem and intervention being measured or modeled.

first-copy costs   Costs accrued in order to produce the first unit of a drug or other medical service, but independent of the number of units provided after that—for example, research and development costs.

fixed costs   Costs that are held at a constant or fixed level, independent of the level of production and the time frame of the analysis.

frictional costs   Costs incurred as a result of a transaction—for example, the *administrative costs* of providing unemployment insurance or inefficiencies associated with use of replacement labor.

functional status   An individual's effective performance of or ability to perform roles, tasks, or activities (e.g., to work, play, maintain the house). Often functional status is divided into physical, emotional, mental, and social *domains*, although finer distinctions are possible.

hazard function   The instantaneous *probability* of mortality at any point in time.

health concept(s)   Generic element(s) of health status, also called *domains, attributes* or *dimensions*. "Health concept" is sometimes used to connote the broadest conceptual level in hierarchical conceptualizations of health status.

health-related quality of life   As a *construct*, health-related quality of life (HRQOL) refers to the impact of the health aspects of an individual's life on that person's *quality of life*, or overall well-being. Also used to refer to the value of a *health state* to an individual.

health state   The health of an individual at any particular point in time. A health state may be modified by the impairments, functional states, perceptions, and social opportunities that are influenced by disease, injury, treatment, or health policy.

health status measures   Systems used to define and describe *health states* (e.g., a multi-attribute health status classification system).

health status profile   An instrument that describes the health status of a person on each of a comprehensive set of *domains*.

healthy-years equivalent (HYE)   The number of years of perfect health (followed by death) that has the same *utility* as (is seen as equivalent to) the lifetime path of *health states* under consideration. It can be measured by two *standard gamble* questions or by one *time tradeoff* question.

home production   Unpaid services offered by family members and volunteers.

incremental cost   The cost of one alternative less the cost of another.

incremental cost-effectiveness (ratio)   The ratio of the difference in costs between two alternatives to the difference in *effectiveness* between the same two alternatives.

indirect costs   A term used in economics to refer to productivity gains or losses related to illness or death; in accounting is it used to describe *overhead* or *fixed costs* of production.

indivisibility   A production factor that cannot be segregated further into smaller elements. The input variable is restricted in some way, such as by size.

inference statistics Statistical methods used to draw conclusions about some parameter for a population based on data obtained in a sample of that population.

influence diagrams An alternative (to the *decision tree*) graphical representation of a decision problem, particularly useful in defining the structure of complex decision problems under *uncertainty*.

interrater reliability A measure of consistency among multiple judges.

interval estimate A range within which the true value is expected to lie with some specified *probability*.

interval scale A scale on which equal intervals (e.g., 0.1–0.2, 0.8–0.9) have an equivalent interpretation. An interval scale may have two arbitrarily anchored points.

intrarater reliability A measure of the stability of the rating an individual judge gives to the same question presented more than once during the same or a subsequent administration.

Kaldor-Hicks criterion See *compensation test.*

Keeler-Cretin paradox A logical argument (with accompanying mathematical proof) that if one *discounts* health outcomes at a lower rate than costs in CEA, the resulting C/E ratio can be successively improved (lowered) by successively delaying the start of the candidate intervention. This infinite regress can be avoided by *discounting* health outcomes and costs at the same rate.

lead-time bias Attribution of increased survival among screen-detected cases simply because the diagnosis was made earlier in the course of disease.

league table A table in which interventions are ranked by their (incremental) *cost-effectiveness ratios.*

length bias An erroneous inflation of improved survival among screen-detected cases relative to non-screen-detected cases due to the tendency of slower-growing, less-virulent disease to be more readily detected by screening than more aggressive disease, due to the longer preclinical phase of more indolent illness.

life-table methodology A procedure by which the mortality (or morbidity) of a fixed population is evaluated within successive small time intervals so that the time dependence of mortality can be elucidated.

likelihood functions The *conditional probability* (or *probability density*) for random variable X given a parameter, θ.

logistic regression model A data analysis technique to derive an equation to predict the *probability* of an event given one or more predictor variables. This model assumes the natural logarithm of the odds for the event (the "logit") is a linear sum of weighted values of the predictor variables. The weights are derived from data using the method of maximum likelihood.

magnitude estimation   A technique from psychophysics wherein judges are asked to rate the magnitude of the sensation produced by one stimulus versus another as a ratio (e.g., "2.5 times as much").

margin   The vantage from which the cost or the value of the next unit of a commodity is assessed.

marginal benefit   The added benefit generated by the next unit consumed.

marginal cost   The added cost of producing one additional unit of output.

marginal cost-effectiveness (ratio)   The *incremental cost-effectiveness ratio* between two alternatives that differ by one unit along some quantitative scale of intensity, dose, or duration. (This term is often used incorrectly as a synonym for *incremental cost-effectiveness*.)

marginal rate of return   The percent gain per time period (e.g., per year) from diverting $1 of consumption to investment. For example, if the marginal rate of return is 6% annually, a dollar invested today will yield $1.06 one year hence.

Markov models   A type of mathematical model containing a finite number of mutually exclusive and exhaustive *health states*, having time periods of uniform length, and in which the *probability* of movement from one state to another depends on the current state and remains constant over time. (See also *semi-Markov models*.)

Markov nodes   Branching points within the *decision tree* that lead into a Markov process.

maximin rule   A rule which seeks to maximize the well-being of the worst off member of society.

meta-analysis   A method for combining and integrating the results of independent studies of the effect of a given intervention. The label is used broadly to mean the averaging of results across studies. In a strict sense it refers to a defined method for acquiring reports of *randomized clinical trials*, rating and culling these reports for quality of the research, and statistically combining the results of the remaining studies.

micro-costing   A valuation technique which starts with a detailed identification and measurement of all the inputs consumed in a health care intervention and all of its sequelae. Once the resources consumed have been identified and quantified, they are then converted into value terms to produce a cost estimate.

minimum practice   A "do-nothing" alternative, if this alternative is acceptable practice. Otherwise, the lowest-cost alternative among effective practices.

model uncertainty   *Uncertainty* related to the model and modeling process used in a study. This *uncertainty* may be either "model structure uncertainty" (*uncertainty* about the correct mathematical formulation for combining parameters in the model), "modeling process uncertainty" (variation inherent in the fact that the model is one particular instance of an analyst, or analyst-team, constructing a complex model for the problem being addressed and not the only possible construction), or both.

Monte Carlo simulation   A type of *simulation modeling* that uses random numbers to capture the effects of *uncertainty*. Multiple simulations are run, with the value of each uncertain variable in the analysis selected at random from a *probability distribution* for the value of that variable, for each simulation. The simulation results are compiled, providing a *probability distribution* for the overall result.

nested case-control design   See *cohort case-control design.*

nominal price   In the context of *cost-effectiveness analysis*, a price that is not corrected for inflation or cross-sectional differences in cost of living.

normal distribution   A particular family of two-parameter statistical distributions used to characterize many random variables because of its flexibility and mathematical convenience; the graph of the density function is the familiar "bell-shaped curve" of introductory statistics books.

normative theory   A coherent group of general propositions or principles of which the objective is to define a norm or standard of correctness.

normative theory of social choice   Any group of coherent propositions that lead to prescriptions about the choices society ought to make under well-defined circumstances.

objective function   The summary quantity, expressed as a mathematical function of independent variables, that an investigator wished to maximize or minimize—for example, total cost.

observational cohort study   See *prospective cohort study.*

observer bias   The tendency of the patient or investigator to report results based on a preconceived notion. Observer bias can be avoided when the subject and/or the rater is "blinded" to either risk status and/or outcome (i.e., single or double blinded).

odds ratio   The ratio of exposure odds among cases to exposure odds among controls.

operations research   A set of scientific methods for providing a decision maker with a quantitative basis for decisions regarding the operations under his or her control. Encompasses *optimization* models and *simulation models* and includes such techniques as inventory models, linear programming, queuing theory, Program Evaluation and Review Technique (PERT), and *Monte Carlo simulation.*

opportunity cost   The value of time or any other "input" in its highest value use. The benefits lost because the next-best alternative was not selected.

optimization techniques   Mathematical methods (e.g., linear programming, nonlinear programming) used to find the solution to a problem stated in mathematical terms which both satisfies the constraints of the problem and maximizes or minimizes the *objective function.*

ordinal scale properties   As used here, a scale assigning numbers to *health states* so that the numerical order of greater than or less than implies "preferred to" or "not preferred to," but for which numerical differences are not meaningful with respect to how much more or less preferred.

overhead   The total cost to produce goods, excluding direct material and direct labor.

paired comparisons   A technique in which judges compare *health states* in pairs, and report which is better. Results are converted to an *interval scale* through *Thurstone's law of comparative judgment.*

parameter uncertainty   *Uncertainty* about the true numerical values of the parameters used as inputs.

Pareto improvement   A reallocation that makes at least one person better off and no one worse off.

Pareto optimality   A distribution of resources such that any change in the distribution must make at least one person worse off.

patient subgroup   A group of individuals or patients who are relatively homogenous on some aspect relevant to the problem but who differ from the larger patient population. Also *population subgroup.*

perspective   The viewpoint from which a *cost-effectiveness analysis* is conducted.

Ping-Pong method   A method of eliciting preferences by converging to the final answer while alternating steps from both sides. For example, finding the indifference *probability* in a *standard gamble* question by alternatingly asking about *probabilities* that are too high and too low while converging inward.

point estimate   A single estimate of a parameter of interest.

Poisson regression   A data analysis technique in which event *probabilities* are assumed to be represented by the Poisson distribution with an event-rate parameter expressed as a mathematical function of predictor variables. This technique is most often used in parametric survival analyses.

population subgroup   See *patient subgroup.*

positivity criterion   A decision rule defining the value of a test result that is used as the boundary between "test positive" and "test negative."

posterior distribution   A *probability distribution* that describes the likelihoods of all possible values in light of both the *prior distribution* and the data.

potential Pareto improvement   See *compensation test.*

power   See *statistical power.*

predictive validity   The ability of a model to make verifiably accurate predictions of quantities of interest. A measurement instrument that has predictive validity is one that allows accurate predictions of future states of the *construct* being measured.

preference score   See *preference weight.*

preference subgroup   A group of individuals within a larger population whose preferences for particular *health states* are relatively homogeneous and differ systematically from the average preferences of the population.

preference function   A mathematical expression describing preferences or *utility* as function of specific variables. See also, *utility function.*

preference weight   A numerical judgment of the desirability of a particular outcome or situation. Also known as *preference score* or *value.*

present value   The value to the decision maker now of outcomes occurring in the future.

prevalence   The proportion of individuals in a population who have a disease or condition at a specific point in time.

primary data   From the perspective of the CEA analyst, primary data are those data on costs and/or *effectiveness* that are collected specifically for the purpose of use in a CEA. Primary data may be collected using a variety of study designs, such as randomized controlled trials, observational studies, or *cross-sectional studies.*

prior distribution   The *probability distribution* for a random variable or hypothesis that is (or could be) specified prior to data collection.

probabilistic sensitivity analysis   A method of *decision analysis* in which *probability distributions* are specified for each uncertain parameter (e.g., *probabilities, utilities, costs*); a simulation is performed whereby values of each parameter are randomly drawn from the corresponding distribution; and the resulting *probability distribution* of *expected utilities* (and costs) is displayed.

probability   An expression of the degree of certainty than an event will occur, on a scale from 0 (certainty that the event will not occur) to 1 (certainty that the event will occur).

probability distribution   A numerical or mathematical representation of the relative likelihood of each possible value that a variable may take on (technically, a "probability density function").

probability theory   The aggregate body of mathematical definitions and theorems dealing with expressions of *probability*. Probability theory is usually taken as a branch of mathematics.

production function   The technical relationship between labor, capital, and other inputs and the outcomes of the process (e.g., health outcomes.)

productivity costs   The costs associated with lost or impaired ability to work or engage in leisure activities due to morbidity or due to death.

prospective cohort study   A study of disease-free individuals who are classified on the basis of exposure to the factor of interest and then followed forward in time to determine the rates of the disease development (incidence), or of deaths from the disease (mortality). Also, *observational cohort study*.

Prospective Payment System (PPS)   A payment scheme which Medicare uses to pay hospitals for its beneficiaries. A set amount of money is paid per DRG (diagnosis related group) case.

psychophysical methods   Methods (or protocols) for asking judges to give numerical assessments representing the psychological perception or sensation produced by physical stimuli. These methods have been adapted to ask people to give numerical responses to represent preferences or degrees of preference for *health states*.

publication bias   Bias resulting from the fact that negative studies are less likely to be published than positive ones.

quality-adjusted life expectancy   Life expectancy computed using *quality-adjusted life years* rather than nominal life years.

quality-adjusted life years (QALYs)   "A measure of health outcome which assigns to each period of time a weight, ranging from 0 to 1, corresponding to the *health-related quality of life* during that period, where a weight of 1 corresponds to optimal health, and a weight of 0 corresponds to a *health state* judged equivalent to death; these are then aggregated across time periods.

quality of life   A broad *construct* reflecting subjective or objective judgment concerning all aspects of an individual's existence, including health, economic, political, cultural, environmental, aesthetic, and spiritual aspects.

randomized clinical trial (RCT)   A clinical trial in which the treatments are randomly assigned to the subjects. The random allocation eliminates bias in the assignment of treatments to patients and establishes the basis for statistical analysis.

random sample   A sample drawn at random from a population. In random sampling with replacement, any member can be drawn at each draw. In random sampling without replacement, a member previously selected cannot be reselected.

real value The dollar value of a good or service after correction for inflation.

recall bias Bias that arises when the study subjects are asked to report past events based on their memory. May arise because individuals with a particular exposure or adverse health outcome are likely to remember their experiences differently from those who are not similarly affected.

reflective equilibrium The extent to which the implications of people's preferences are in accord with their directly elicited preferences.

relative price A comparison of the price of one product or service to the price of another comparable product or service.

relative risk An estimate of the magnitude of an association between exposure and disease which also indicates the likelihood of developing the disease among persons who are exposed relative to those who are not. It is defined as the ratio of incidence of disease in the exposed group divided by the corresponding incidence of disease in the nonexposed group.

reliability Consistency in repeated measures of a phenomenon by the same individual or across different groups of observers. The higher the reliability, the higher the test–retest correlation between replications of the measurement. Technically, the fraction of the variance in a measure that is the true value rather than measurement error. See also *intrarater reliability*, *interrater reliability*, and *test–retest reliability*.

reservation wage The least salary an employee will accept to take a job.

retrospective cohort study A study in which a defined group of persons with an exposure and an appropriate comparison group who were not exposed are identified retrospectively and followed from the time of exposure to the present, and in which incidence (or mortality) rates for the exposed and unexposed are assessed.

returns to scale The relationship between the quantity of output of a product and the quantities of factor inputs used to produce it. Refers to how output changes when all inputs are increased by the same multiplier.

risk premium The additional return required by investors to compensate them for assuming a given level of risk. The higher the risk premium, the more risky the investment (and vice versa).

sampling variability The variability in an estimate that results from using a sample of limited size.

secondary data From the perspective of the CEA analyst, these are data that have been collected prior to the CEA for other purposes. The CEA analyst abstracts relevant data from these sources, transforms them into the form required for the analysis (e.g., 10-year survival into annual *survival probabilities*), and incorporates them into the analysis or model. As with *primary data*, the data may arise from any type of study design.

semi-Markov models   A type of *Markov model* that allows for systematic changes in transition *probabilities* as a function of simulated time rather than having constant transition *probabilities*. For example, annual all-cause mortality rates can increase as the patient's simulated age increases. Also *time-varying Markov models*.

sensitivity   The *probability* of a positive test result in patients who have the disease of interest.

sensitivity analyses   Mathematical calculations that isolate factors involved in a *decision analysis* or economic analysis to indicate the degree of influence each factor has on the outcome of the entire analysis. Specifically measures the *uncertainty* of the *probability distributions*.

shadow price   The social *opportunity cost* of an outcome.

shadow-price-of-capital (SPC) approach   An approach to *discounting* in cost-benefit analysis in which, in theory, one transforms the time stream of investment costs and benefits into consumption losses and gains, respectively, and then *discounts* the algebraic sum of these in each period to *present value* using the *social rate of time preference* (SRTP). In practice, the analyst must select a *discount rate* that approximates the SRTP, while assuming that measured benefits and costs in each period mirror changes in consumption benefits and costs. In CEA, the SPC approach likewise serves to frame the choice of a rate for *discounting* costs.

simulation model   A model of a (complex) system or process is used to determine how a change in one or more variables affects the rest of the system. Used widely in cases where the problem is difficult to solve by mathematical analysis.

social opportunity approach   An approach to *discounting* in cost-benefit and *cost-effectiveness analysis* in which the *discount rate* (used for all monetized outcomes) is constructed as the weighted average of the rates applicable to the various economic sectors contributing resources to the program(s) under evaluation.

social rate of time preference   The rate at which the social decision maker is willing to trade off present for future consumption. Frequently approximated by the real (inflation-adjusted) return on low-risk government investments.

social utility function   An aggregate of individual *utilities*. Economists view the maximization of the social utility function as the ultimate goal of a resource allocation scheme.

societal perspective   A viewpoint for conducting a *cost-effectiveness analysis* that incorporates all costs and all health effects regardless of who incurs the costs and who obtains the effects.

standard gamble   In *cost-effectiveness analysis*, an approach to determining the *utility* of a particular outcome from a particular *perspective*. Judges are asked to compare life in a particular given *health state* that is ''a sure thing'' to a gamble with a *probability* p that perfect health is the outcome and $1-p$ that immediate death is the outcome. The *probability p* is varied until the preference for the sure thing, the certainty of the particular *health state*, is equal to the preference for the gamble. The *probability p* for which the *expected utility* of the two choices is equal is then a measure of the preference for the *health state* and for all intents and purposes satisfies (by construction) the requirements for a *von Neumann-Morgenstern utility*.

state-transition models   Models which allocate, and subsequently reallocate, members of a population among several categories or *health states*. Transitions from one state to another occur at defined, recurring time intervals according to transition *probabilities*. Through simulation, or mathematical calculation, the number of members of the population passing through each state at each point in time can be estimated. State-transition models can be used to calculate life expectancy or *quality-adjusted life expectancy*.

statistical power   The *probability* of detecting (as ''statistically significant'') a postulated level of effect. Technically, the *probability* of (correctly) rejecting the null hypothesis—that is, the *probability* of rejecting the null hypothesis when in fact the alternative is true.

stochastic   Involving chance or *probability*, probabilistic.

stochastic model   Health care process models that use computer-generated random numbers to simulate the occurrence of events over time. The computer programs are often used to simulate events happening to a cohort over time by modeling the time course for each individual as a series of random events controlled by specified *probabilities* in the simulation.

study arm   A group of patients assigned to the same treatment (or control condition) in a controlled study.

study boundaries   Also known as study scope. The analytical boundaries of a *cost-effectiveness analysis*, specifying what is included in the study and what is not.

survival probabilities   The *probability* that a specified individual will be alive at the end of a given period of time.

test–retest reliability   The correlation between scores on the same measure administered on two separate occasions.

threshold analysis   A type of analysis in which the analyst varies the parameter over a range to determine the values of the parameter that would lead to major changes in conclusions.

Thurstone's Law of Comparative Judgment   One of the earliest methods for deriving psychological scales; it is based on *paired-comparison* judgments. Thurstone's Law holds that stimulus differences which are detected equally often are subjectively equal.

time costs   The time a patient spends seeking care or participating in or undergoing an intervention.

time horizon   The period of time for which costs and effects are measured in a *cost-effectiveness analysis.*

time preference   The rate at which the decision maker is just willing to trade present for future consumption of some commodity of interest. A positive rate of time preference means the decision maker is willing to forgo some current consumption of the commodity in return for a sufficiently large gain in future consumption.

time tradeoff   A method of measuring *health-state utilities* in which patients are asked to trade off life years in a state of less-than-perfect health for a shorter life span in a state of perfect health. The ratio of the number of years of perfect health that is equivalent to longer life span in less-than-perfect health provides a measure of the preference for that *health state.*

time-varying Markov model   See *semi-Markov model.*

transfer cost   Also known as transfer payment. A payment made to an individual (usually by a government body) that does not perform any service in return. Examples are social security payments and unemployment compensation.

uncertainty   A state in which the true value of a parameter or the structure of a process is unknown.

utility   A concept in economics, psychology, and *decision analysis* referring to the preference for, or desirability of, a particular outcome. In the context of *health-related quality-of-life* measurement, utility refers to the preference of the rater (usually a patient or a member of the general public) for a particular health outcome or *health state.* For technical use in *decision analysis,* see *von Neumann-Morgenstern (vNM) utility.*

utility function   An algebraic expression stating that a decision maker's satisfaction is dependent on the types and amounts of commodities she consumes. Symbolically, $U = U(x_1, x_2 \ldots)$, where $x_1, x_2 \ldots$ are valued outcome attributes. According to *expected utility theory*, individuals behave so as to maximize the expected value of *utility*, subject to constraints.

utilitarianism   A theory of social justice that holds the policies that produce the greatest good for the greatest number improve social welfare. This theory incorporates everyone's well-being into the social process by balancing the *utility* of persons who gain from a given policy with the *utility* of those who lose as a result of the same policy.

validity   The extent to which a technique measures what it is intended to measure. See also *construct validity, convergent validity, discriminant validity, external validity, face validity,* and *predictive validity.*

value   See *preference weight.*

veil of ignorance   A philosophical *construct* in which a rational public decides what is the best course of action when blind to its own self-interest.

visual analogue scales   Direct rating methods using a line on paper (or similar visual device) without internal markings; raters are asked to place a mark at some point between the two anchor states appearing at the ends of the line.

von Neumann-Morgenstern (vNM) utility   A number representing relative desirability that satisfies axioms set forth by von Neumann and Morgenstern (1947) and suitable for computation of *expected utilities* to represent preferences among alternatives with uncertain outcomes.

welfare costs   In economics, the cost added due to inefficient operations, scale, or level or activity.

welfare economics   Also known as welfare theory. A normative branch of economics concerned with the development of principles for maximizing social welfare and economic output. It is based on the assumptions (1) that individuals maximize a well-defined *preference function* and (2) that the overall welfare of society is a function of these individual preferences.

willingness to pay   A method of measuring the value an individual places on a good, service, or reduction in the risk of death and illness by estimating the maximum dollar amount an individual would pay in order to obtain the good, service, or risk reduction.

Years of Healthy Life (YHL)   The duration of an individual's life, as modified by the changes in health and well-being experienced over a lifetime. Also called *quality-adjusted life years*, health-adjusted life years.

The following sources were invaluable in the development of some of the definitions for the terms described: Brown, B.M. and M. Hollander. 1977. *Statistics: A Biomedical Introduction* New York: John Wiley & Sons; CDC. 1994. *A Practical Guide to Prevention Effectiveness: Decision and Economic Analyses*; Hennekens, C.H. and J.E. Buring. 1987. *Epidemiology in Medicine* Boston: Little, Brown, and Company; Judd C.M., E.R. Smith, and L.H. Kidder. 1991 *Research Methods in Social Relations*, San Francisco: Holt, Rinehart, and Winston, Inc.; Kelsey, Thompson, and Evans. 1986.

Methods in Observational Epidemiology, New York: Oxford University Press; Miller R.L. 1978. *Intermediate Microeconomics: Theory, Issues, and Applications*, McGraw-Hill; Patrick, D.L. and P. Erickson. 1993. *Health Status and Health Policy: Allocating Resources to Health Care*, New York: Oxford University Press; Rothman, K.J. 1986. *Modern Epidemiology* Boston: Little, Brown, and Company; Shim, J.K. and J.G Siegel. 1995. *Dictionary of Economic Terms*, New York: John Wiley and Sons, Inc.

Index